SCHOOL HEALTH:
POLICY AND PRACTICE
Fifth Edition

Author:
Committee on School Health
American Academy of Pediatrics

Philip R. Nader, MD, Editor

American Academy of Pediatrics
PO Box 927
141 Northwest Point Blvd
Elk Grove Village, IL 60009-0927

Library of Congress Catalog Card No. 92-83866

ISBN No. 0-910761-42-6

MA0031

Quantity prices on request. Address all inquiries to:
American Academy of Pediatrics
141 Northwest Point Blvd, PO Box 927
Elk Grove Village, IL 60009-0927

The recommendations in this publication do not indicate an exclusive course of treatment or serve as a standard of medical care. Variations, taking into account individual circumstances, may be appropriate.

COMMITTEE ON SCHOOL HEALTH
1990-1993

Philip R. Nader, MD, Chairperson, 1991-present
Martin C. Ushkow, MD, Chairperson, 1990-1991

John R. Asbury, MD
Bradley J. Bradford, MD
Paula Duncan, MD

Steven R. Poole, MD
Debra E. Seltzer, MD
Daniel C. Worthington, MD

Liaison Representatives

Penny Anderson, RN, MSN, CPNP, National Association
of Pediatric Nurse Associates and Practitioners
Arthur B. Elster, MD, American Medical Association
Maureen Glendon, MSN, RN-C, National Association of
Pediatric Nurse Associates & Practitioners
Vivian Haines, RN, MA, SNP, National Association of
School Nurses
Paul W. Jung, EdD, American Association of School
Administrators
Patricia Lachelt, National Association of Pediatric Nurse
Associates and Practitioners
R. Dee Legako, MD, American Academy of Family Physicians
Susan Lordi, RN, MS, CPNP, National Association of School
Nurses, Inc
Lani Majer, MD, American School Health Association
John Santelli, MD, American School Health Association
Joan Stipetic, PhD, American Association of School
Administrators
Mary Vernon, MD, MPH, Centers for Disease Control and
Prevention
James H. Williams, MEd, National Education Association

Staff

Crystal A. Milazzo

FOREWORD

The fifth edition of *School Health: Policy and Practice*, prepared by the AAP Committee on School Health, is intended to provide health professionals and others with a framework and guidelines for developing comprehensive health-related programs for school-age children in a broad range of community settings.

Since most health professional readers of this guide already will possess basic information on clinical problems and procedures, we have chosen to emphasize health and illness management issues as they relate to the school and to educational problems, educational potential, or educational institutions.

Educational professionals referring to this guide are cautioned about the somewhat abbreviated handling of specific health problems or conditions, and they are urged to consult with a pediatrician or their own local medical advisor for more definitive, complete, and recent information.

There is increasing recognition of the interdependence of health and educational services in attempting to optimize the potential and the development of all children in this country. For this reason, many play or could play an important role in school health activities: pediatricians and other physicians who see and treat children and adolescents, school nurses and other nursing and physician-assistant personnel, teachers, counselors, special educators, administrators, school board members, and other interested citizens. Thus, the Committee on School Health commends to all who consult this guide an attitude that recognizes the legitimate interest and contribution that many can make toward improving the current and future health and educational status of youth.

Philip R. Nader, MD
Chairperson
Committee on School Health
American Academy of Pediatrics

ACKNOWLEDGMENTS

The Committee gratefully acknowledges the assistance of the following individuals who contributed to writing and reviewing this manual.

Stephen Barnett, MD, University of Texas, Galveston
Jeffrey L. Black, MD, Texas Scottish Rite Hospital, Dallas
Bradley J. Bradford, MD, Mercy Hospital, Pittsburgh, PA
David A. Brent, MD, University of Pittsburgh, Pittsburgh, PA
Susan Brink, DrPH, University of Texas, Houston
Stu Cohen, Education Development Center, Inc, Newton, MA, in cooperation with the National Education Association Health Information Network, Washington, DC
George Comerci, MD, Tucson, AZ
Alan W. Cross, MD, University of North Carolina, Chapel Hill
Paul H. Dworkin, MD, University of Connecticut, Farmington
Paul G. Dyment, MD, Tulane University, New Orleans, LA
David Elkind, PhD, Tufts University, Medford, MA
Marianne E. Felice, MD, University of Maryland, Baltimore
John Fontanesi, PhD, Kaiser Permanente, San Diego, CA
Robert D. Gross, MD, Children's Eye Specialists, Fort Worth, TX
Debra N. Haffner, Sex Information and Education Council of the United States (SIECUS), New York, NY
Richard B. Heyman, MD, Cincinnati, OH
Richard D. Krugman, MD, University of Colorado, Denver
Patricia Lachelt, Pasadena Unified School District, Pasadena, CA
Chris Y. Lovato, PhD, San Diego State University, San Diego, CA
Edgar K. Marcuse, MD, MPH, Children's Hospital, Seattle, WA
Philip R. Nader, MD, University of California-San Diego
George A. Nankervis, PhD, MD, Children's Hospital, Akron, OH
Jerry Newton, MD, University of Texas Health Science Center, San Antonio
Judith S. Palfrey, MD, Children's Hospital, Boston, MA
James M. Perrin, MD, Massachusetts General Hospital, Boston
Steven R. Poole, MD, Children's Hospital, Denver, CO

John S. Santelli, MD, MPH, Centers for Disease Control and Prevention, Atlanta, GA
Barton Schmitt, MD, Children's Hospital, Denver, CO
Martin W. Sklaire, MD, Madison, CT
James F. Steiner, DDS, Children's Hospital Medical Center, Cincinnati, OH
Howard L. Taras, MD, University of California-San Diego
Martin C. Ushkow, MD, Syracuse, NY
Daniel C. Worthington, MD, St Lukes Hospital, Cleveland, OH

Appreciation to:

Yvonne J. Hasse, Word Processor, Division of Child and Adolescent Health, American Academy of Pediatrics

Rebecca Parker, Administrative Assistant, Department of Pediatrics, University of California-San Diego

TABLE OF CONTENTS

PART I

SCHOOLS AND SCHOOL HEALTH

CHAPTER 1

DEFINITIONS AND SCOPE OF SCHOOL HEALTH

The Educational System and Where Schools Are Headed

Schools are a microcosm of society. Whatever social, health, or political issues are present in society will manifest themselves in the school. School health has historically been under-emphasized and neglected as a potential way to reach and impact a large number of children. Many of these children otherwise might have difficulty accessing health education and health care.

There is an increasing national emphasis to improve both educational and health outcomes for children. Schools have been the first to come under public scrutiny, with numerous expert and political groups calling for educational reforms. While reminiscent of previous educational reforms that tackled the school institution alone, the current call for reform also includes many institutions in the community that exist to serve many of the same families and children, but often with conflicting and confusing programs and services. Many resources are spent on remedial programs, and little is appropriated for programs that are preventive in nature. Schools have long realized that support for the home environment is crucial to educational achievement. Schools are now realizing that the school alone cannot successfully field all of the resources that will be required to make a major impact on the educational and health outcomes that are desired. The time is ripe to strengthen the preventive and health care components of school health programs. The only viable and effective options are cooperative and collaborative ways to deliver needed health and educational services to children and families. These new collaborative approaches demand a new definition of school health be formulated.

School Health Defined in Terms of a Broad Scope of Health Promotion in a Community

Traditional definitions of school health deal with three areas: health services, health education, and a healthy school environment. While all of these are important, it is necessary to now view school health as a broad range of school-based and community-based activities, engaged in by many different persons. These activities will coordinate educational, social, and health care institutions, to assist families and children in preventing disease, promoting and protecting health, and minimizing the complications of health problems of school-age children. It is important to note that school age in many states now reaches from birth to attainment of majority, especially for children with health or educational handicaps (Table 1).

Comprehensive school health has the potential to maximize health and educational outcomes of children and youth by attempting to focus the efforts of families, community institutions, and systems that impact them. Figure 1 illustrates this conceptualization. Health status and educational achievement are at the apex of the triangle of family, school, and community systems that support these outcomes. Included in the community sphere are influences of the media, because of the potential and real roles of the media in promoting health behaviors. Note arrows flow in both directions, indicating reciprocal interactions and influences of each component. Arrows also represent real programmatic interactions, with actual services and programs connected in meaningful and practical ways. While this conceptualization is idealized, each school or school district, with a collaborative effort from leaders interested in children's health, could strive to implement parts or all of such programs. Each community will decide the configuration of their school health programs at least in part by assessing local needs and resources. However, there will be a need to focus community interest on school health.

Potential Role of a Community Child Health Council

In order to raise awareness of the need for coordinated approaches to improving health and educational outcomes for children, and in order to forge the links required to implement the goals of a comprehensive school health program, it probably will be necessary to form or modify existing groups to form a "child/youth health council." This group should include the top leadership from all groups who have or should have a stake in influencing the health and educational outcomes of children and

Table 1. — Ages for Compulsory School Attendance and Compulsory Provision of Services for Special Education Students, by State: 1989-1990*†

State	Compulsory Attendance (Age & yr) (Nov 1989)		Compulsory Provision of Services for Special Education (Age & yr) (1989-1990)
Alabama		7 – 16	5 – 20
Alaska	1/	7 – 16	3 – 21
Arizona		8 – 16	2/ 5 – 21
Arkansas		5 – 17	5 – 20
California		6 – 16	2/ 5 – 21
Colorado		7 – 16	2/ 5 – 20
Connecticut		7 – 16	3 – 21
Delaware		5 – 16	3 – 20
District of Columbia		7 – 17	3/ 3 – 21
Florida		6 – 16	5 – 18
Georgia		7 – 16	5 – 21
Hawaii		6 – 18	3 – 20
Idaho		7 – 16	3 – 20
Illinois		7 – 16	3 – 20
Indiana		7 – 16	5 – 17
Iowa		7 – 16	Birth – 20
Kansas		7 – 16	5 – 21
Kentucky	4/	6 – 16	3 – 20
Louisiana		7 – 17	3 – 21
Maine		7 – 17	5 – 19
Maryland		6 – 16	Birth – 20
Massachusetts		6 – 16	3 – 21
Michigan		6 – 16	Birth – 25
Minnesota	5/	7 – 18	Birth – 20
Mississippi		6 – 14	5 – 20
Missouri		7 – 16	5 – 20
Montana	6/	7 – 16	6 – 18
Nebraska		7 – 16	Birth – 20
Nevada		7 – 17	5 – 21
New Hampshire		6 – 16	3 – 20
New Jersey		6 – 16	3 – 21
New Mexico		6 – 18	3 – 21
New York	7/	6 – 16	3/ 3 – 21
North Carolina		7 – 16	5 – 20
North Dakota		7 – 16	3 – 20
Ohio		6 – 18	5 – 21
Oklahoma		7 – 18	4 – 21
Oregon		7 – 18	5 – 20
Pennsylvania		8 – 17	2/ 5 – 21
Rhode Island		6 – 16	3 – 20

Table 1. — Ages for Compulsory School Attendance and Compulsory Provision of Services for Special Education Students, by State: 1989-1990*† (continued)

State	Compulsory Attendance (Age & yr) (Nov 1989)		Compulsory Provision of Services for Special Education (Age & yr) (1989-1990)	
South Carolina	8/	5 – 17		5 – 20
South Dakota	6/	7 – 16		3 – 20
Tennessee		7 – 17		4 – 21
Texas	9/	7 – 17		3 – 21
Utah		6 – 18	3/	3 – 21
Vermont		7 – 16	2/	5 – 21
Virginia		5 – 17		2 – 21
Washington		8 – 18		3 – 21
West Virginia		6 – 16		5 – 22
Wisconsin		6 – 18		3 – 20
Wyoming		7 – 16		3 – 20

*From US Department of Education, Office of Special Education and Rehabilitative Services, the 12th Annual Report to Congress on the Implementation of the Education of the Handicapped Act, 1990; Education Commission of the States; "Compulsory School Age Requirements, March 1987," and unpublished revisions (this table was prepared March 1991); and US Department of Education, Office of Educational Research and Improvement. 800/424-1616, Fred Beamer, information specialist.

†The Education of the Handicapped Act (EHA) Amendments of 1986 make it mandatory for all States receiving EHA funds to serve all 5- to 18-year-old handicapped children at present and all 3- to 5-year-old handicapped children by 1991.

1 – Ages 7 – 16 yr or high school graduation.
2 – State or local discretion determines at what point in year children become eligible for services.
3 – State has established two points in the program year by which children must be 3 yrs of age to be eligible for services.
4 – Must have parental signature for leaving school between ages of 16 and 18 yr.
5 – Takes effect in the year 2000. Currently 7 – 16 yr.
6 – May leave after completion of eighth grade.
7 – The ages are 6 – 17 yr for New York City and Buffalo.
8 – Permits parental waiver of kindergarten at age 5 yr.
9 – Must complete academic year in which 16th birthday occurs.

youth. This will likely include individuals who perhaps have not had much experience in working together. In addition to the schools, both private and public health departments, social services departments, community colleges and universities, hospitals, and business and labor groups are likely to be included.

Legal Mandates and Requirements Impacting on School Health

Both legal mandates and traditional organizational patterns for human services have an impact on school health. Too often, school health is not "owned" by anyone. In a recently published

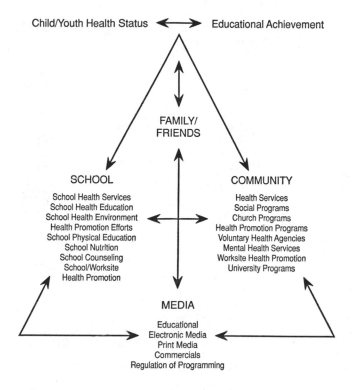

Child/Youth Health Status ◄——► Educational Achievement

Fig 1. From Nader PR. The Concept of "Comprehensiveness" in the Design and Implementation of School Health Programs. *J Sch Health.* 1990;60(4):134. Reprinted with permission.

survey, 44 of the 50 states had a state agency office responsible for school health, either in the education department or shared with the health department and education department. Nationally, many agencies have school-related activities in them. This lack of a single locus for responsibility for school health has been a distinct disadvantage in the past. This may become an advantage in the future in that innovative, cooperative structures will be required to implement comprehensive school health programs. The diffusion of responsibility may thereby aid in strengthening school health programs.

All states have legal requirements regulating age at school entry and specific medical requirements for entry. Table 2 lists such requirements as of 1989.

Table 2. — Number of States With Screening Requirements for Entry to Kindergarten*†

Requirements	Level of Policy		
	Mandated by Law N (%)	Recommended N (%)	No Policy N (%)
Screenings			
Hearing	33 (65)	12 (23)	6 (12)
Vision	32 (63)	13 (25)	6 (12)
Physical	18 (35)	21 (41)	12 (24)
Speech	13 (26)	19 (37)	19 (37)
Height and Weight	12 (23)	20 (39)	19 (37)
Dental	8 (16)	21 (41)	22 (43)
TB Test	12 (23)	2 (4)	26 (51)
Scoliosis	8 (16)	11 (22)	30 (59)
Immunizations			
DTP (diphtheria/ tetanus/pertussis)	50 (98)	1 (2)	—
Measles	50 (98)	1 (2)	—
Rubella	50 (98)	1 (2)	—
Polio	49 (96)	1 (2)	—
Mumps	38 (75)	11 (21)	2 (4)

*From American School Health Association. *School Health in America: An Assessment of State Policies to Protect and Improve the Health of Students*. 5th ed. Kent, OH: Library of Congress; 1989. ASHA Pub. No. G005-1990, LOC No. 90-82274. Reprinted with permission.
†Items not totaling 100% are due to missing data; items include data for District of Columbia.

Existence of specific requirements, such as those for immunizations, can form the backbone of support for developing a comprehensive school health program. However, requirements for specific screening activities of questionable scientific value can have deleterious effects, especially if they take resources away from more pressing issues or problems. Therefore, constant monitoring and active participation in the legislative process is vital to the development of rational school health programs.

Suggested Readings

American School Health Association. Proceedings of the national invitational conference on comprehensive school health programs. *J Sch Health*. 1990;60(4):133-138

American School Health Association. *School Health in America: An Assessment of State Policies to Protect and Improve the Health of Students*. 5th ed. Kent, OH: Library of Congress; 1989. ASHA Pub. No. G005-1990, LOC No. 90-82274

CHAPTER 2

GOALS AND OBJECTIVES OF A SCHOOL HEALTH PROGRAM

Goals and objectives are rarely explicitly stated in most school health programs. Because they seem to be self-evident, it is a vital but often overlooked step in program planning and evaluation. In fact, it is just because school health has not clarified its goals and objectives (except in the broadest terms: "to optimize a child's health in order to maximize learning") that convincing proof of the effectiveness of school health has been lacking. Program evaluation is essential if the practice of school health is to progress.

Goals and objectives for a given community will vary from one locale to the next. They must fit locally determined needs and resources. The goals listed below are suggested as a minimum set of goals that can be elaborated and modified as required. They will be expanded to include specific program objectives, which are *measurable*. This will assist in program evaluation (see chapter 10). The goals listed in Table 3, are discussed in general terms below. Each goal is further developed in chapters 6 through 10.

Goal 1: Assure Access to Primary Health Care

Historically, the reason that many school health programs have not been able to help each child overcome any health factors that might impede their success in school has been the lack of linkages between the school and a regular source of health care for the child. Some school health programs have always attempted to connect families with sources of ongoing primary health care. Attempting to link children with a regular source of health care should be an important goal for every school health program.

There has been recent interest in the role of the school health program in either providing direct health services in or near a school, or in more active brokering of health services with closer relationships and referral networks to existing sources of care in the community. Such efforts have utilized health aides and outreach workers, as well as expanding the roles of school nurses and nurse practitioners. Recent evaluations of school-based or school-linked direct primary care services have shown mixed

Table 3. — Goals of a School Health Program

Goal 1   Assure access to primary health care

Goal 2   Provide a system for dealing with crisis medical situations

Goal 3   Provide mandated screening and immunization monitoring

Goal 4   Provide systems for identification and solution of students' health and educational problems

Goal 5   Provide comprehensive and appropriate health education

Goal 6   Provide a healthful and safe school environment that facilitates learning

Goal 7   Provide a system of evaluation of the effectiveness of the school health program

results, with improvement in access but inconsistent effects on health outcomes. School-based clinics have had difficulty in securing ongoing funding and support for medical care delivered on the school site.

Schools are attractive as a relatively barrier-free system for contacting most children in a community when they need medical care, or for a crisis situation. Recent surveys in some underserved urban populations suggest that the school nurse, when available, is viewed by many families as a first-line source of advice concerning health and illness issues. It therefore makes sense to connect, through formal and informal means, with various systems of primary health care in that community. These linkages are mandatory since it is through the establishment of an ongoing medical home (source of regular medical care) that constant availability of health care will be accomplished.

Criticism of school-based primary health care services have included the fact that there is a danger that personnel and program may be isolated with little interaction with school staff. It is difficult, but crucial, to narrow the gap that exists between the health care systems and the schools, if truly comprehensive care is to be made available to all children.

Advantages and disadvantages can be listed for each of the two models that have been examined: the more prevalent model of referral for primary and secondary care and the less prevalent model of actual delivery of some primary health care services in the school setting. There is also a spectrum of services and programs that stretches between the two extremes. Many students will consult primary care services in the school setting when they otherwise might have difficulty getting to clinics or physicians' offices or if community health care facilities are too distant to be readily utilized. The Academy recommends that this care be provided by a physician and that attention be paid to not disrupting existing patterns of care. If care is given under direction or standing orders of a physician, there must be careful adherence to local standards of care and state regulations of medical practice as well as attention to medical liability issues. Access of patients to backup systems for secondary and tertiary care, as well as 24-hour coverage when school providers are not available, needs to be assured in any school-based delivery system. Traditional configurations of school health services (the referral model) often result in greater integration with educational programs and special education services. Difficulties may arise when there is incomplete or unclear communication between the child's regular physician and the school. The school nurse, who is often viewed as an integral part of the school team, should facilitate this needed communication. Regardless of the blend of models eventually used, assuring access to continuous high-quality primary health care services is a legitimate but often neglected goal of school health programs.

Goal 2: Provide a System for Dealing With Crisis Medical Situations

The school health service must provide for efficient and expert handling of emergency and life-threatening crisis medical situations (see chapter 7). First-aid policies and emergency management practices should be written out, and regular training of designated school staff carried out. Specific responsibilities and procedures, including accessing the 911 community telephone emergency system, should be known by school personnel. Students known to be subject to emergency medical crises should be identified to designated school personnel, who should also be taught what to do in the event of such a crisis. Systems of collection of student information and sources of medical care will facilitate handling of an emergency. Community disasters, suicides, and instances of violence can erupt on a school campus. Schools should plan for the ability to meet the immediate emotional needs of students and staff in such situations.

Goal 3: Provide Mandated Screening and Immunization Monitoring

Awareness of state and local requirements is a first step in designing programs and the resources that will be required to carry them out. Just as there is wide variation in the organization of school health programs, there is also wide variation in the extent and level of requirements for various procedures and activities.

Nearly all states have immunization requirements for entry into school. Schools may exclude children until proof of immunization is provided. The details of requirements, specification of immunizing agents, and timing of administration vary among states.

Screening is defined as a process by which to separate from a large group of apparently healthy individuals, those who have, or are at risk of having, a defined disorder. In relation to school screening programs, procedures that tend to yield a large number of false-positive results will only serve to overburden the community health system. False positives also will undermine confidence in the school health program by community health providers. On the other hand, a significant false-negative rate has major implications for missing the potentially serious nature of a disorder, especially if ready remediation is available. When considering the value of school screening, it is important to keep in mind the seriousness of the problem, the effectiveness of appropriate therapy, the relative efficiency of the screening procedure, the specificity and sensitivity and predictive ability of the procedure, and the availability of remediation to those children with positive screening results. If these criteria cannot be determined to have been met, actions should be undertaken to review and propose legislative repeal of mandates. Recent information on common school screening tests is reviewed in chapter 7.

Goal 4: Provide Systems for Identification and Solution of Students' Health and Educational Problems

School health staff interact daily with children and teachers, and are therefore in a strategic position to identify and take steps to remediate both health and educational problems. Some problems present themselves, others need to be detected. A child suddenly wheezing after strenuous exercise is not difficult to identify as a child who may have exercise-induced asthma. Immediate treatment, further evaluation, and prevention of future crisis episodes are indicated. On the other hand, a child presenting frequently to the nurse with stomach pains could be experiencing stress, related to school or other aspects of his or her life, or could be manifesting symptoms of peptic ulcer disease, sexual molestation, or regional ileitis (see chapter 13). In addition, the special needs of a child with a chronic condition or illness that actually or potentially affects schooling require attention.

The level of sophistication in the detection and management of identified problems will be directly proportional to the degree of experience and skill possessed by health personnel. The degree of successful resolution of identified problems can give an estimate of the effectiveness of the efforts of a school health program in this area.

Problems can be identified through analysis of students' reasons for visiting the school nurse, by regular conferences with teachers to identify students who are a concern, by regular classroom or schoolyard observation by health personnel, and by parental referral. Some schools have introduced child-initiated care; if reinforced by classroom and home discussion of decision making, this might begin to teach children appropriate use of health resources. Research on children exposed to such programs suggests that the children involved had increased confidence in their own ability to decide if they needed to see the nurse (see chapter 7).

To help solve an identified problem it is usually necessary to establish (if it does not already exist) a relationship with the child's home and those adults in parenting roles. Programs have utilized outreach workers, "home-school agents," to act as advocates for families and to help establish contacts with persons in the home. In a study, a target population identified to have difficulties completing referrals made from the school were shown to benefit from the services of outreach workers. Families became more knowledgeable about negotiating in the systems that provide needed services and assistance (see chapter 7).

Goal 5: Provide Comprehensive and Appropriate Health Education

One of the original and cardinal aims of education was to provide instruction that would enable students to avoid illness and maintain their health and that of their community. Comprehensive health education has long been an aim of many groups, yet health education is still not among the top priorities in a school. Steps to take to implement good health education programs in school are described in chapter 8.

If certain criteria are met, it is not unrealistic to expect an improvement in health habits or health behavioral outcomes as well as knowledge and attitudes from school-initiated health instruction. These criteria include: (1) instructional objectives and methods consistent with child development needs and skills in concert with major health objectives for a given age group; (2) instruction integrated into other curricula as well as the health curriculum; (3) some health education objectives integrated into services and environment, which include peers and teachers as partners in learning; and (4) some health education objectives implemented with parents/family as recipients of instruction to support the development of healthy habits among students.

Thus, newer instructional methods utilize home instruction, school nutrition, and school recreational programs, as well as classroom instruction to build children's skills in developing healthy dietary and physical activity habits. Further extension into community health programs and integration with school programs enhances both the scope and the effectiveness of school health education.

Goal 6: Provide a Healthful and Safe School Environment That Facilitates Learning

The environment of a school must be safe and clean. These objectives may require more elaborate and deliberate planning than they have in the past. Some construction materials used in old schools, such as asbestos, may represent a hazard, especially if disturbed. Community violence can and does spill into school campuses with alarming regularity. School nutrition programs are receiving attention, and modification, and more healthful food choices are increasingly available. School physical education programs are including more fitness activities and lifelong rec-

reational skills, as well as competitive sports. School environments should be smoke-free for students and teachers. Programs
are being developed to assist teachers and other school staff to
improve their own health status and ability to cope with stress.
In-service education on aspects of normal child development and
behavior should be a regular part of support available to teachers. The educational philosophy for all instruction will recognize
the necessity of tailoring instruction to the developmental level
of the student and will have a uniformly high expectation for the
achievement and quality of performance of students, teachers,
and administrators.

This manual addresses many of these issues in subsequent
chapters. Effective provision of programs and activities to accomplish the goal of a healthful and productive school environment
will depend on close collaboration with all divisions of a school
system, including the school board, and all aspects of administration and pupil services and instruction. Teachers' unions often
have a stake in many of these issues. Close working relationships
with agencies outside the school also will be mandatory to mount
effective programs in this area of school health.

Goal 7: Provide a System of Evaluation of the Effectiveness of the School Health Program

In times of scarce and diminishing resources, programs that
cannot demonstrate effectiveness are often subject to cutbacks
in financial allocations or elimination. The job of evaluation is
to provide data to those responsible for administering school
health programs and to those responsible for allocating resources. Beyond these needs, carefully executed program evaluation can provide data that can be used to improve efficiency and
effectiveness.

Many school health programs are so marginally supported that
few if any resources are devoted to evaluation. This places the
program further in jeopardy.

However, many routine school health activities lend themselves well to documentation, and school personnel are often
accustomed to recording information. Establishing ways to collate and codify these data may be an important initial step in
setting up an evaluation system. The availability of computer

systems to most schools is another advantage to data management and retrieval.

After evaluation is done, the results need to be made available to those who collected the data, those who evaluate the implications of the outcomes, and the general public, in order to increase awareness of the accomplishments of school health. Provision of case examples, along with statistical data, can add richness and meaning for decision makers who do not have extensive health backgrounds.

The goals enumerated in this chapter are proposed as a framework for development of more specific program activities. Ongoing decisions will need to be made with regard to priorities and identifying which needs are most crucial to children in a school district. Therefore, before initiating or modifying existing school health programs, it is advisable to carry out some form of a needs assessment and inventory of existing and potential community resources. Keeping in mind the broad definition of school health discussed in chapter 1 and the concept that the school cannot be expected to "do it all" will put the task of implementing a school health program in perspective; it will seem less formidable. The outcomes of even a partially implemented and effective school health program should have measurable impact on children.

CHAPTER 3

PERSONNEL INVOLVED IN SCHOOL HEALTH

In order to understand where school health can fit into the school bureaucracy, it is necessary to understand the governance of schools. Constitutionally, education is a function of each state. Policy and guidelines are set by the state board of education, along with the governor and the legislature. The state department of education, headed by a state chief school officer, has a staff that develops administrative regulations; provides training, certification, and technical assistance; and monitors pupil achievement and other program parameters. Curriculum is set in broad terms, but significant autonomy is delegated to the local school board, local superintendents, and other administrators. At the local school the building principal usually has broad leadership and administrative power. In addition, at the local school district and building level, there is usually a teachers' union, which has a keen interest in the education of children and teachers. Parent groups and parent-teacher organizations also can provide personnel and support for school health programming.

School Health Is Multidisciplinary

Many individuals in all walks of life can potentially be involved in school health programs. Three major systems influence the health and education of children: the home, the school, and the community (including health care systems).

Therefore, school health could be an extremely multidisciplinary field. Often, professionals involved with school health include school-related activities as only a part of their usual professional roles. Within the educational system it is not at all unusual to have key administrators in charge of school health programs without any background or training in health fields.

Table 4. — Non-Health School Personnel and Responsibilities to School Health*

Position or Title and Activities	Decision Making Relevant to School Health
School Superintendent Chief administrator of school system; directly responsible to school board. Budgets and public relations are generally priority concerns; almost always has experience in teaching and administration in various schools, moves to new community to become super-intendent.	Budgetary. Personnel hiring and firing. Represents "school" to parent. Controls deployment of local school and district resources. Controls teachers' time and distribution of effort.
Assistant Superintendent Similar to superintendent, but may be more directly involved with other admini-strators in schools, eg, monitors principal's meetings, works closely with curriculum directors, personnel director.	
Principal Chief administrator of individual school. School is considered his/her "house," therefore guests are expected to greet principal as they enter and leave. Principal is of crucial importance in deter-mining fate of change process in individual school.	Fosters implementation of school health program at local school site. Advocates/supplies expansion of services. Administrative supervision of health personnel assigned to school site. Has ultimate site responsibility for safety of staff and physical plant.
Classroom Teacher Works with children in regular educational program. Pupils receive most of their instruction from this team (many schools have "team teaching" at various grade levels so students may receive instruction from each teacher on the team).	Identification of students. Referral of students. Contacts parents. Willingness to implement special programs for specific children.

Position or Title and Activities	Decision Making Relevant to School Health

Special Educator, Resource Teacher

a. Self-contained, works with special education pupils on a full-day basis. Pupils receive all instruction from this teacher.

b. Resource room, teaches students who come from regular classroom to resource room as necessary for special instruction (small groups, sometimes individual tutoring).

Certification, individual investigation of need for services.
Carries out special or remedial instructional plan.
Willingness to coordinate effort with regular teacher.
Personal assessment and interaction with child.

Speech and Language Specialist

Often administers screening tests to students, provides individual and small group therapy.

Certification, individual assessment of need for services.
Carries out treatment programs for children with speech and/or language problems.

Counselor

Roles of counselors vary depending on need and other resource staff in school. Most are identified with certain responsibilities and areas, eg, vocational counselor monitors program and works with children in this track, academic counselor is concerned with individual academic programs of children, coordinates program and often serves as liaison between students and teachers, special education counselor provides pupil and parent counseling concerning problems arising out of child's handicapping condition.

Certification, individual assessment of need for services.
May coordinate special education for children.
May be liaison with parents, teachers in overall planning.

Table 4. — Non-Health School Personnel and Responsibilities to School Health* (continued)

Position or Title and Activities	Decision Making Relevant to School Health
School Psychologist May provide same services as educational diagnostician and associate psychologist, but is likely more involved in a consultation role to teachers, supportive professional personnel, parents, and community agencies.	Certification, individual assessment of need for services. May coordinate special education resources for children. May be liaison with parents, teachers in overall planning.
Associate Psychologist Role very similar to education diagnostician, however, can assess emotional and/or behavioral factors, may co-lead groups with social worker in school.	
Education Diagnostician Serves on support service team (appraisal team); is the psychometrist in the school, often is involved in developing individual educational plans and talking with parents.	
Social Worker Generally more of an outreach worker with children and families, consults with school personnel and community agencies and parents, may do individual and group counseling in school context.	May be part of certification of need. May coordinate liaison with parents and school staff. May carry out direct counseling with children, parents.
Outreach Worker May be paraprofessional from neighborhood of school, assist in obtaining services for families.	

Position or Title and Activities	Decision Making Relevant to School Health
Health Educator May have coordinating, classroom teaching, or combination role. Some districts and states combine health and physical education.	Coordinates, teaches health curriculum at all levels, K–12. Potentially could carry out educational programs integrated with school health services.
Health Office Aide, Teaching Aide Usually a high school graduate, aide may be utilized in classroom or clinic to assist professional with clerical duties and Individual supervision of children.	Provides direct services to children. May act as "gatekeeper" for children's complaints. Can facilitate record-keeping, parent contacts.

*From Nader.[1] Reprinted with permission.

Non-Health Personnel and School Health

Table 4 lists decision-making influences on school health made by non-health professionals in the school setting. Not included in this list are non-school-related personnel in health departments, governmental agencies, and regulatory bodies at state and local levels who may directly influence school health programs and policies.

Health Personnel and School Health

The school nurse represents the major provider of school health services in many schools in the country. The level of professional preparation and patterns of care by nursing personnel in schools has been challenged recently by economic considerations. Despite rigorous attempts by organizations such as the National Association of School Nurses, the American Nursing Association, and the American School Health Association to define roles and responsibilities of professional nurses, only 38 states require school nurses to be registered nurses, while 19 require the attainment of specific school nurse certification. School nurses perform or supervise most of the activities undertaken by school health programs, at least in the health services areas. Because of their strategic position in relationship to principals, teachers, students, and parents, involvement of the school nurse in all aspects of the school health program is vital. Various recommendations are made concerning the desired nurse-pupil ratio for a school, but in reality actual ratios are determined by available resources and the existence of special needs of the students in a given school. These aspects of staffing are considered in more detail in chapter 7.

There has been a recent interest in expanding the traditional role of the school nurse by equipping the nurse with more extensive examination and problem-solving skills. Various training programs (now most include master's degrees) result in preparation of (school/pediatric/family) nurse practitioners; 29 states require certification of the nurse practitioners; and all states have laws governing the nurse practitioner's scope of practice. In addition, other physician extenders and assistants have been utilized in school health programs. Since the latter generally must function under the immediate supervision of physicians, the application to an independent or separate professional site, such as a school, is not as feasible as for the nursing professionals. The presumed greater knowledge and problem-solving ability of the nurse practitioner is intended to facilitate management of more problems on site, to improve the information needed by parents and doctors to remediate a problem once it is referred, and to improve communication with sources of health care in the community. Nurse practitioners have been utilized in school-based primary care endeavors, as well as in carrying out of routine Early Periodic Screening, Detection, and Treatment (EPSDT) screening examinations and in performing physical examinations required for children in sports and special education programs. Utilization of nurse-practitioners almost always requires a formal backup relationship with a licensed physician in the community.

Health aides, clerks, and outreach workers have been employed by school health programs to carry out duties assigned and supervised by the school nurse. These often include carrying out triage or screening procedures (when permitted by law), recording health information, and record-keeping. About half of the states indicate that aides are utilized, but there is no indication of guidelines, supervision, or degree of autonomy permitted. Such individuals may play important first-line contact roles with students and parents, and therefore require careful consideration and training for the specific tasks they are assigned.

There are two major ways in which physicians interact with school health programs. The first is as a school district's medical advisor. While many state education departments recommend that schools retain school medical advisors, very few districts actually employ full- or part-time medical consultants. Some schools rely on informal relationships with physicians in the community, who may or may not have knowledge and expertise about children or school health issues. These informal relationships are frequently voluntary. Whether paid or volunteer, such consultation arrangements should be formalized and specified. How to develop such relationships is further considered in the following text.

The second, and most common, physician interaction with a school will be as a child's primary or specialist physician. Because of the nature of children's health problems and the care needed, specialist physicians often have more routine contact with school health personnel than primary physicians. Yet, many health maintenance concerns and commonly presenting health problems in a school-age child warrant useful dialogue and interaction with the school.

It is important to distinguish the two roles of a physician in relation to schools. Table 5 compares physician activities in relation to two common problems of school-age children: learning difficulties and asthma. The activities of a child's physician and a consultant to a school or school district are contrasted.

Guidelines for physician behavior in relation to schools can be helpful. The educational system is one in which the physician may not be expert or experienced. Physician opinion or suggestions may not be sought or welcomed. Tables 6 and 7 list guidelines that may be helpful in interacting with schools.

Physicians, of course, also routinely play many other important policy setting and advocacy roles that may relate to school health program objectives. Serving on an AAP committee or as a local school board member are just two ways physicians can advocate for school health. Active participation in the legislative

Table 5. — Physician's Role in Schools*

Clinical Issue/ Problem	Examples of Physician's Activities as Child's Primary Care Provider	Examples of Physician's Activities as Consultant to School or School System
Learning Disability	1. Requests teacher's perception of child's learning and behavior, results of individualized testing.	1. Serves on district committee to accomplish biannual review of handicapped children's progress.
	2. Shares results of medical evaluation of child with school.	2. Assists in setting up mechanism for providing follow-up behavioral and academic information to physicians who have placed students on psychoactive medication.
	3. Works cooperatively with school personnel and parent to develop educational and behavioral management plan for child (may include school visit).	3. Provides in-service session for classroom teachers on new concepts in attention deficit disorder.
	4. Sets up mechanism for follow-up on behavioral and educational progress of child.	4. Advises school board on need for movement training for children with learning disabilities.
Asthma (School-Age Children)	1. Requests school information on absenteeism, visits to school nurse, evidence of nonparticipation in physical education activities.	1. Reviews absenteeism data to identify groups of students with excessive absences that might be amenable to intervention.
	2. Sets up mechanism for regular administration of bronchodilator at school.	2. Assists curriculum director and nurse in developing educational program for children with asthma and their parents.
	3. Sets up follow-up mechanism for continued monitoring of school attendance, medication-taking compliance, and participation in appropriate physical activities.	3. Helps publicize program and communicates directly with students. Solicits primary care physicians' input and support for the educational program by reinforcing concepts in their patient visits.

*From Nader.[1] Reprinted with permission.

Table 6. — Guidelines for Physician Acting as Child's Care Provider

1. Approach all school personnel as co-professionals with skills and interests that complement your expertise and can provide information that you do not have. Recognize their interest in helping the children in their charge.

2. When contacting a school for the first time, contact the principal initially.

3. When calling a teacher, find when it is the best time for him/her to talk.

4. Always inform parents and obtain permission to communicate with the school. Keep them informed as to progress.

5. Encourage direct school-parent and parent-school communication.

6. Be willing to attend a school meeting if necessary to share information and/or make treatment plans.

7. Listen carefully to ascertain the school personnel's main concerns and questions, and attempt to respond to them.

process, as supporters of specific candidates or issues, is an option that can be exercised by interested physicians, as by any other citizen. Becoming an active member of boards of agencies related to education and health is another role that pediatricians can play.

Working With Schools: A Challenge Worth Meeting

Since most schools and school districts are not aware of what physician consultation can provide, it will be necessary to do some homework and preparation to establish a relationship with a school district. First, it is absolutely necessary to know both the educational system governance and the local needs and resources. It may be useful to talk over issues and concerns with your patients, friends, and contacts in the schools. You may wish to discuss with your colleagues and other physicians in the community your interests in establishing a relationship with the schools, to point out the potential benefits of better and closer communication with the schools.

Second, approach the top leadership in the system, either school board or superintendent, to present your ideas and to

Table 7. — Guidelines for Physician Acting as a School Health Consultant

1. Clearly distinguish roles of a primary health care provider and that of a school consultant.

2. Become aware of laws and regulations affecting schools, including those related to school finance, education for handicapped, bilingual education, and other education mandates.

3. Become knowledgeable about the formal and informal decision-making processes in schools related to "regular" and "special" education of children, including health education.

4. Act as a liaison to the rest of the medical community.

5. Establish a contract with the school defining mutually agreed on expectations and objectives.

6. Provide a regular report on consultation activities to the school district.

7. Attempt to set up relationships with all levels and departments of the school system in order to permit access from the board and superintendent level to the classroom teacher.

8. Become aware of group process dynamics and decision making in groups.

solicit their interest, reactions, and support. Describe what you have to offer and how, in your view, it would fit with district policies and procedures. Inquire about who in the system might be the best person to coordinate your activities. While the initial response may be to designate a building nurse coordinator, it may be wise to query other higher-level administrators, who can provide information about curriculum and other pupil service needs, such as special education. Whatever administrative arrangement is arrived at, keep communication lines open to the top level.

Third, it may be necessary to have a brief period of voluntary time commitment. During this time, some definite on-site and other activities will be carried out. This will give the physician a "feel" for the nature of the system, how it operates, and some of the problems facing children and staff. It also will give school staff and administrators firsthand experience in what the physician consultant can provide and what is not feasible to expect.

Table 8. — A Checklist*

State policies and programs

☐ Have you apprised yourself of state policies and programs related to comprehensive school health programs?

☐ Have you checked to see whether health outcome objectives exist, and, if so, how they are assessed?

Local policies and programs

☐ Have you apprised yourself of district policies and programs related to comprehensive school health programs?

☐ Have you determined what health curriculum, textbooks, and materials are actually being used in the schools?

☐ Have you ascertained:

- policies and programs that need strengthening?

- serious gaps or deficits?

- opportunities for health professionals to make a meaningful contribution?

Influencing local policies and programs

☐ Do you know how the local education system works? Who makes decisions? Who has authority? Who actually does the work?

☐ Do you know who supports and who is concerned with various aspects of comprehensive school health programs and their reasons for doing so?

☐ Have you contacted appropriate officials about your ideas and obtained their support for working with schools?

☐ Have you refined your ideas in consultation with key parties—teachers, administrators, school health professionals, public health professionals, school board members, and parents?

☐ Have you provided for periodic progress reports and made changes in direction or emphasis based on their results?

*From National Association of State Boards of Education.[2] Reprinted with permission.

Finally, a formal contract should be executed that details the expectations and objectives of a consultation agreement. This can serve as a basis for determining adequate compensation and can assure the school of a dependable source of consultation.

Table 8 provides a checklist for anyone considering initiating a consultative relationship with a school. Additional resources include the AAP Section and Committee on School Health. Once it becomes clear how schools work, how to integrate key aspects with community resources, and how to work with schools, it is possible to move ahead and overcome obstacles in achieving effective school health programs.

Remember that school health is a cooperative affair. No single professional or discipline is more important than another. Keeping this in mind will make the school health team, no matter how small or extended, better able to function to improve health and educational outcomes for children.

References

1. Nader PR. A pediatrician's primer for school health activities. *Pediatr Rev.* 1982;4:82-92
2. National Association of State Boards of Education. *How Schools Work and How to Work With Schools.* Alexandria, VA: National Association of State Boards of Education with support from the Division of Adolescent and School Health, Center for Chronic Disease Prevention and Health Promotion, Centers for Disease Control; 1989

PART II

IMPLEMENTATION OF
SCHOOL HEALTH PROGRAMS

CHAPTER 4

THE DEVELOPMENTAL CONTEXT FOR HEALTH AND EDUCATION PLANNING

One of the guiding principles for implementing a school health program is that the program, activity, or project be in tune with the developmental needs and characteristics of the children who are to be the major recipients of the activity. The school health program can also ensure that other school programs keep child development in mind when planning and carrying out educational activities. The school health program can be the resource in the school responsible for initially assessing the children's developmental strengths and weaknesses, and determining how these may relate to academic and social achievement.

The development of a child is both dynamic and interactional, determined both by neurophysiological and social growth, and both intrinsic and environmental factors are important. Development consists of more than moving along a schedule of milestones at a particular age. All areas of development—physical growth, and acquisition of gross motor, fine motor, language, and personal/social skills—are interrelated. Development is not necessarily continuous; it may be slowed or sped by various influences such as nutrition, emotional nurturance, illness, hospitalization, family crisis, or community or political events. While the school alone cannot influence or ameliorate the effects of developmental variability, it can be sure that it does nothing to impede or adversely impact the developmental process of physical, cognitive, and socioemotional growth required for the eventual emergence of a healthy and adjusted adult.

Psychosocial Development

Most educators and health professionals utilize a synthesis of existing child developmental theories. Psychoanalytic formulations of child development have centered on the conflicts arising between basic inner needs or drives and the demands of the external world. Tables 9 and 10 outline the major stages of development according to Freud and Erikson. Piaget (Table 11) saw children as active learners and explorers of their environment. His theories have important relevance to educational pro-

Table 9. — Psychoanalytic Theory*

Stage	Age	Erogenous Zone	Central Activities	Interpersonal Focus
Oral	Birth–1½ yr	Mouth	Feeding; sucking; biting	Self (primary narcissism); separation from mother
Anal	1½–3 yr	Anal area	Elimination	Rebellion vs compliance with parental demands; fear of loss of parental love
Phallic (oedipal)	3–6 yr	Genitals	Genital exploration; imitating adult roles	Sexual attraction opposite sex parent; identification with same sex parent after a period of rivalry
Latency	6–11 yr	None (?)	Increased control of sexual and aggressive drives; socially accepted activities	Self among same sex peers; identification with powerful or effective heroes
Genital	Puberty to adulthood	Genitals	Taking "flight" from the family; denial of pleasures; intellectualization	Separation from parents; successful extrafamilial relationships

*From Dixon and Stein.[1] Reprinted with permission.

gramming, especially in the early educational context. Cognitive social learning theory (Bandura) takes into account the mutual influences of the individual, the physical and psychosocial environment, and the task to be learned. This formulation stresses the importance of modeled behavior and mastery of skills to the development of a sense of competence in an individual. Familiarity with these theories of child development will assist the school health professional in interpreting a given

Table 10. — Erikson's Stages of Development*

Stage	Age	Issue
1	Birth–1½ yr	Trust vs mistrust
2	1½–3 yr	Autonomy vs shame and doubt
3	3–6 yr	Initiative vs guilt
4	6–11 yr	Industry vs inferiority
5	Adolescence	Identity vs role confusion
6	Young adulthood	Intimacy vs isolation
7	Adulthood	Generativity vs stagnation
8	Old age	Ego integrity vs despair

*From Dixon and Stein.[1] Reprinted with permission.

child's developmental status and needs, and will serve as a framework for evaluating the developmental appropriateness of proposed educational or health interventions.

Infancy and Preschool

Schools are increasingly responsible for programs that target infants and preschool-age children. As younger and younger children are grouped together, the special needs and requirements for a safe and hygienic environment that meets the physical and emotional needs of the youngsters become an important program area for school health. A developmental approach to the examination of infants and children is shown in Table 12. School health personnel serving these populations need to be skilled in assessment and interpretation of growth charts and the use of standardized developmental screening tests such as the Denver Developmental Screening Test and the Early Language Milestone Scale. Awareness of nutritional needs and practices will assist school health personnel in counseling and guiding the sometimes young and inexperienced parents of the infants and children enrolled in these programs. Constant updating of information concerning immunization recommendations and the importance of locating a regular source of medical care for the child are central objectives.

In addition to formalized developmental screening, observation of young children can provide a wealth of information on the

Table 11. — Piagetian Stages of Development*

Stages	Approximate Age	Ways of Understanding	Basic Concepts to Be Mastered
1. Sensorimotor	Birth–2 yr	Through direct sensations and motor actions	Concepts of object permanence, causality, spatial relationships, use of instruments, etc
2. Preoperational	2–6 yr	Mental processes that are governed by the child's own perceptions and linkage of events; no separation of internal and external reality	Sense of animism; egocentrism; transductive reasoning; idiosyncratic associations
3. Concrete operational	6–11 yr	Child can reason through real and mental actions on real objects; can reverse changes to the world mentally to gain understanding; can reason using a stable rule system	Concepts of mass, number, volume, time
4. Formal operations	12 yr	Abstract thought; can reason about ideas, impossibilities, probabilities, broad abstract concepts	Mastery of ideas and concepts

*From Dixon and Stein.[1] Reprinted with permission.

Table 12. — Pediatric Examination: A Developmental Approach*

Age (Approximate)	Developmental Stage	Approach to Examination
0–6 mo	Symbiotic (not fearful of strangers)	Usually easy to examine infant on table; start with least invasive parts of examination (abdomen, cardiac, pulmonary, nodes, etc)
6 mo–3 yr	Separation–individuation (fear of strangers initially followed by the toddler clinging to parent)	Examine while standing parent holds the child or while infant is in parent's lap; approach the child gently; use of toys, peek-a-boo games, keys, flashing otoscope may be helpful
3–6 yr	Preschool age: age of initiative (a period of fantasy play and increasing verbal ability)	Communicate with child in simple language; explain procedures and ask child to participate in examination; make use of child's interest in fantasy, eg, superheroes
6–12 yr	School age: age of industry (a period of cognitive growth; growing interest in and ability to understand cause and effect)	Recognition of child's ability to understand procedures leads to cooperation
12 yr	Adolescence: age of identity (heightened awareness of body and its perceived effect on others)	Respect privacy during examination; careful explanations help

*From Dixon and Stein.[1] Reprinted with permission.

progress of development. Table 13 illustrates the use of play materials that can be utilized in assessment of development and behavior.

School staff and young parents may need assistance in understanding that young children do not naturally share toys and

Table 13. — Suggested Play Materials and Their Potential Value in Assessing Development and Behavior*

Play Material	Potential Assessment Value	Appropriate Age Level		
		Infant	Toddler	Preschooler
Human figures: miniature doll and family house; hand puppets; doll with clothing and blankets	Functional and symbolic play; child's understanding of family dynamics and peer interactions; role identity; facilitate communication and expression	−	+	+
Miniature cooking utensils and tea set	Sensorimotor, functional and symbolic play; fine motor skills; eye-hand coordination	+	+	+
Car/truck	Functional and symbolic play; realistic play	−	+	+
1-in colored blocks	Sensorimotor, functional and symbolic play; fine motor skills and coordination, ie, reach and grasp, stacking; spatial orientation; organizational skills; object permanence; attention span and persistence	+	+	+
Toy telephone	Functional and symbolic play; fine motor skills; speech and language skills; facilitate communication and expression; glean child's insight into experience	−	+	+
Crayons and paper	Functional and symbolic play; fine motor skills; sensorimotor integration and perception; allow nonverbal child to express feelings; body image; family dynamics; intellectual functioning; cognitive milestones	−	+	+
Soft foam ball	Gross motor skills; object permanence; vehicle for give-and-take with clinician	+	+	+
Cardboard books	Fine motor skills; coordination; speech and language; cognitive abilities	+		+

Table 13. — Suggested Play Materials and Their Potential Value in Assessing Development and Behavior* (continued)

Play Material	Potential Assessment Value	Appropriate Age Level		
		Infant	Toddler	Preschooler
Mobile: unbreakable, out of reach	Ability to attend, tune in; visual capacity; distraction during physical examination	+	+	+
Mirror: unbreakable, next to examining table, on wall	Visual capacity; mirror play (5–6 mo); distraction during physical examination	+	+	−
Chalkboard: attached to wall, low enough for toddlers	Fine motor skills; cognitive skills	−	+	+
Posters: cheerful, related to the child's world, eg, Sesame Street, encased in plastic frame and cover, on walls and ceiling	Cognitive skills; speech and language; facilitate communication with provider; distraction during physical examination	−	+	+

*From Dixon and Stein.[1] Reprinted with permission.

play nicely with one another in group settings. Possessiveness and physical aggression are common. So-called short attention span needs to be recast in the context of normal behavior. Educational toys are toys that are simple, safe, have bright colors, and stimulate the child's imagination. School health personnel must watch for safety aspects of equipment and furnishings, such as blunt corners or rocking chairs that might tip over.

Parental support and involvement are mandatory for early childhood programs. Typical age- and stage-related characteristics of children and families are outlined in Table 14. Specific

Table 14. — Summary of Typical Stage-Related Characteristics of Child and Family (Ages 1 Through 5 Years)*

Age of Child (yr)	Growth, Nutrition, and Health	Body Control	Relate to World	Self-Awareness	Communication	Peer Relationship	Adult Relationship	Sexuality	Family Tasks
1–2	Slowing growth rate and decreased appetite; foot and leg "problems"	Runs, builds tower with blocks	Sensory motor, curiosity, points to named pictures	Says own name, recognizes self in mirror	Words, transient stutter	Solitary or parallel play, aggression or withdrawal	Separation problems, frequent adult contacts, stubborn, temper, whine	Handles genitals	Adaptation of family routines to small children
2–3	Frequent coughs and colds; high fevers	Toilet trained, eats with spoon, climbs small ladder	Symbolic thought, egocentric, animistic	Gender identity, awareness of differences in skin color	Short sentences, uses pronouns, transient stutter	Little sharing, some interactive play	Frequent help-seeking from adults	Curious about sex differences	Socialization of children
3–4	Looks skinny	Dresses self, copies a circle, rides tricycle	Egocentric, understands "tomorrow," counts to five	Pride in accomplishments, self-evaluation, verbalizes feelings	Understandable speech, uses plurals	Cooperative play, definite friendship	Separates easily, less adult dependency	Interested in where babies come from	Meeting increasing vocational demands, coping with frequent childhood illness Maintenance of adult relationships
4–5		Draws recognizable person, buttons buttons, cuts with scissors, skips, walks on balance board	Egocentric, distinguishes reality from fantasy, knows colors	Evaluates self	Articulates most beginning sounds, understands prepositions, communicates well with others	Sustained dramatic play	Mostly peer interaction in group settings, can use adults for help	Sex play with other children	Maintenance of individual interests, participation in community activities

*From Dixon and Stein.[1] Reprinted with permission.

Table 15. — Language Problems*

The following list may be used as a guideline for professional personnel working with young children and their parents. These landmarks may help personnel to estimate the speech and language development of a young child and to know when to refer a patient for speech evaluation:

The child is not talking at all by the age of 2 years.

Speech is largely unintelligible after the age of 3 years.

There are many omissions of initial consonants after age 3 years.

There are no sentences by age 3 years.

Sounds are more than a year late in appearing, according to developmental sequence.

There are many substitutions of easy sounds in child's speech.

The child uses mostly vowel sounds in speech.

Word endings are consistently dropped after age 5 years.

Sentence structure is noticeably faulty at 5 years.

The child is embarrassed and disturbed by his/her speech at any age.

The child is noticeably nonfluent after age 5 years.

The child is distorting, omitting, or substituting any sound after age 7 years.

The voice is a monotone,, extremely loud, largely inaudible, or of poor quality.

The pitch is not appropriate to the child's age and sex.

There is noticeable hypernasality or lack of nasal resonance.

There are unusual confusions, reversals, or telescoping in connected speech.

There is abnormal rhythm, rate, and inflection after age 5 years.

*From Dixon and Stein.[1] Reprinted with permission.

health and educational programming based on developmental principles will yield optimal results (see also chapter 5).

Language Development

Language and cognition are linked. No area of development is as important to eventual success or difficulties in learning than that of language development. Speech and language professionals are often available in schools and should be consulted frequently, and without hesitation. Table 15 lists language problems that require evaluation. Table 16 is a summary of receptive

Table 16. — Clinical Evaluation of Language Skills*

Age	Receptive Skills	Expressive Skills	Specific Indication for Referral
0–1 mo	Recognizes sound with startle; turns to sound and looks for source; quiets motor activity to sound; "prefers" human speech with high inflection	Differentiated crying; body language of positive and negative response	No response to pleasing sound when alert
2–4 mo	Prolonged attention to sounds; responds to familiar voice; watches the speaking mouth; enjoys rattle; attempts to repeat pleasing sound with objects; shifts gaze back and forth between sounds	"Ee, ih, uh" (hindmouth vowels); cooing, blows bubbles; enjoys using tongue and lips; reciprocal cooing; play dialogues; loudness varies	No response to pleasing sounds; does not attend to voices
5–8 mo	Seeks out speaker; localizes sounds; understands own name, familiar words; associates word to activity (eg, bath, car)	Pitch varies; babbles with labial consonants ("ba, ma, ga"); uses sounds to get attention, express feeling; sounds directed at object	Decrease or absence of vocalizations
9–12 mo	Responds to simple commands: "point to your nose," "say bye-bye"; knows names of family members; responds to a few words, ie, words associated with specific objects	First words, vocabulary of 5-6 words: "mama, dada"; inflected vocal play; repeats sounds and words made by others: "oo, ee" (foremouth vowels)	No babbling with consonant sounds; no response to music

Table 16. — Clinical Evaluation of Language Skills* (continued)

Age	Receptive Skills	Expressive Skills	Specific Indication for Referral
13–18 mo	Some understanding of words; single element commands; identifies familiar objects	Points to objects with vocalization; vocabulary of 10–50 words, pivot and open class words, rate and content varies; jargon with proper stress and intonation, monologues and dual monologues	No comprehension of words; does not understand simple requests
18–24 mo	Recognizes many nouns; understands simple questions	Telegraphic speech; vocabulary of 50–75 words; 2-word sentences, phrases; stuttering very common	Vowel sounds but no consonants
24–36 mo	Understands prepositions; can follow story with pictures	Vocabulary of 200 words; dependent on phrases, 2-word sentences; uses words for expressive needs; pronouns; uses action verbs	No words; does not follow simple directions
30–36 mo	Understands some syntax (difference between car hit train and train hit car); understands opposites; understands action in pictures	Sentences 4–5 words, 3 elements; tells stories; uses questions: what, where; uses negation; uses progressive and past tense, all regular form; uses plurals, regular form	Speech largely unintelligible to stranger; dropout of initial consonants; no sentences
3–4 yr	Understands 3-element commands	Grammar by own rules; vocabulary 40-1,500 words; speech intelligible to strangers; "why" questions; commands; uses past and present tense; spontaneous speech; nursery rhymes; colors, 1–4, numbers up to 5; tells sex, full name; articulation: "m, n, p, h, w"; 4-word sentences	Speech not comprehended by strangers; still dependent on gestures; consistently holds hands over ears; speech without modulation

Age	Receptive Skills	Expressive Skills	Specific Indication for Referral
4–5 yr	Understands 4-element commands; links past and present events	2,700-word vocabulary; defines simple words; auxiliary verbs: "has, had"; conversationally mature; "how and why" questions in response to others; articulation: "b, k, g, f"; 5-word sentences; "normalizes" irregular verbs and nouns	Stuttering; consistently avoids loud places
5–6 yr	Understands 5-element commands; can follow a story without pictures; enjoys jokes and riddles; can comprehend 2 meanings of word	Correct use of all parts of speech; vocabulary 5,000 words; articulation: "y,ng,d"; 6-word sentences; corrects own errors in speech; can use logic in recounting story plots	Word endings dropped; faulty sentence structure; abnormal rate, rhythm, or inflection
6–7 yr	Asks for motivation and explanation of events; understands time intervals (months, seasons); right and left differences	Articulation; "l, r, t, sh, ch, dr, cl, bl, gl, cr"; has formal (adult) speech patterns	Poor voice quality, articulation
7–8 yr	Can use language alone to tell a story sequentially; reasons using language	Articulation: "v, th, j, s, z, tr, st, sl, sw, sp"	
8–9 yr		Articulation: "th, sc, sh"	

*From Dixon and Stein.[1] Reprinted with permission.

and expressive skills from ages birth to 1 month to 8 to 9 years, along with indications for referral. If a parent is concerned about a child of any age, referral can be extremely helpful. General principles also apply; in a child of any age, a marked decrease in verbalization or a marked consistently loud verbalization may indicate an acute hearing loss. Language delays are often associated with delays in other areas of development. Therefore, assessment should always be comprehensive rather than narrowly focused. No child should undergo language development evaluation without a careful audiologic evaluation.

Entering the Formal School Environment

More and more children have preschool and child care experiences that provide the opportunity for them to begin to learn to adjust to a more formal educational environment. By age 5 to 6 years, depending on the state, all children are legally entitled to a public school education. Recent concern about the so-called readiness of children to enter formal schooling has led to controversy and lack of uniform opinion on the various options open to parents and schools. From a developmental perspective, it is clear that there are major variations in a "normal" designation that must be recognized among children of this age. School health programs should work to enable the school system to be able to meet the tremendous variability among entering students. This can be partly accomplished by interpreting the developmental needs of this age group, and of specific children, to the parents and to the school personnel.

The developmental tasks facing the child at school entry include separation (if not already accomplished), increasing individualization, compilation of the cognitive skills required to learn to read (if child is not already reading), formation of relationships with other children and with adults outside of the family, participation in group activities, following rules and directions, and the gradual strengthening of a sense of identity or self, both within and independent from the family.

Most severe or pronounced developmental delays will already be detected by parents and the health care system by the time children are 5 or 6 years old, at which point they will be eligible for and enrolled in special education programs. Difficulties arise when there is a mismatch between the particular level of development the child brings to the schooling situation and what is expected of the child by parents or teachers. More flexible educational settings, such as transition grades, grouping K-2 students, and modified programs, seem to hold promise for providing more developmentally appropriate early education.

The 6 Year Old: Learning to Use Symbols

The primary school tasks require children to decode reading, learn to spell, write, and solve simple addition and subtraction problems. While these skills are generally taught to all children at about age 6 years, there is wide variability in the cognitive, fine motor, and visual motor skills available to the child to perform these early learning tasks with ease and success. Any mild delay in one of the critical areas of development can have major implications in the development of a poor self-image and the child's awareness that learning is difficult for him/her. That is why early recognition of difficulty with early learning tasks is so crucial. Children with such difficulties may attempt to avoid failure by withdrawing, by acting out (to get attention from teachers or peers), or by becoming aggressive. At times, this behavior is viewed by teachers and parents as a manifestation of attention deficit disorder.

It should be recalled that a positive history of attention deficit disorder provides evidence for hyperactivity, inattention, and impulsivity beginning before age 7 years and lasting at least 6 months. Attention-related learning and behavior problems are one of the most common presenting in children of this age group and older. This topic is discussed in detail in chapter 14.

Table 17 illustrates some questions for children and parents that can be used to assess cognitive, social, and emotional development of the early school-age child.

The 7 to 10 Year Old: Growth and Competence

If the chief early school task is learning to read, the later school tasks include reading to learn. Mastery leads to a sense of competency in the child. Curiosity and a desire for novelty stimulate learning and a sense of industry. In addition to the mastery tasks associated with academic schoolwork, interactions with peers, family, teachers, the larger environment, and the media all offer opportunities for the child to develop a sense of competence, or a sense of failure and frustration.

Children of this age are able to think more like adults and to undertake more complex tasks involving reasoning and insight. They respond quite well to programs that stress their own skills in decision making, ideas, and self-responsibility. They become

Table 17. — Cognitive, Social, and Emotional Development*

Cognitive Development: Questions	Objective
For Children	
Where do you go to school? What grade are you in? What are you learning in school? Are there some things you do at school that you really like? Are there things about school that you don't like?	The 6 year old should be able to provide acceptable answers to nearly all of these questions. Such answers may suggest that the child is having difficulty in particular areas. When the child is reluctant to talk about school, or provides very little information, one should invite the parent to enter the discussion.
Which town do you live in? On which street? Do you know your address? Do you know your telephone number?	To assess the child's attention to basic information important to his well-being as he spends increasing amounts of time away from his family; to assess visual or auditory memory skills.
Ask the child to copy a cross (4 year old), a square (5 year old), a triangle (6 year old), and a diamond (7 year old).	To observe the child's handedness, his ability to grasp and control a writing instrument, and his competence in increasingly difficult fine-motor and visual-perceptual tasks.
Ask the child to draw a person while you are interviewing the parent.	An estimated mental age may be obtained by using Goddenough's scoring criteria. In addition, information may be obtained about the child's attentiveness, tendency to cooperate, compulsivity, and even emotional health if the drawing is atypical.
What makes the sun come up in the morning? What makes the clouds move in the sky? How can you tell if something is alive?	To assess the child's beliefs regarding causality and to help parents understand that the child remains in a transitional period relative to his cognitive abilities. Most 6 year olds, regardless of intelligence, will respond to these questions with magical thinking characterized by animism and egocentricity, for example, "the sun comes up in the morning so that I can play" or "it's alive because I see it and talk to it."

Cognitive Development: Questions	Objective
For Children	
How do you get to your house from school?	Children at this age continue to be highly egocentric in their ability to give directions and will often leave out important details. This may be interpreted to parents as normal developmental stage and will also help parents understand why it is difficult for children to reverse directions or see the world from another person's perspective.
Do you ever have dreams? Do the dreams ever really happen? Where do the dreams take place? What really happens to the people on television who fly or get hurt?	To assess the child's capacity for distinguishing between reality and fantasy, which should be well developed at this age.
Do you know the name of the team that plays baseball or football in our city? What is your favorite movie? What is your favorite television show? Where did you go on your vacation?	Such questions assess both the child's general fund of information as well as the child's interest in and retention of information about events that occur outside the home.
Who are your good friends?	By this time a child should have formed several close relationships outside the home. The child should name one and preferably more friends close to his age. A child who names nobody, or an adult, a family member, or a much younger child requires further evaluation. The parent may be asked to comment on the child's response.
What games do you like to play?	Assess the child's preferences for solitary vs peer activities. Is he comfortable with the give-and-take of peer group activities? Does he understand the necessity for and the nature of rules? Is he involved in organized community-wide activities such as team sports or a religious-based peer group?

Table 17. — Cognitive, Social, and Emotional Development* (continued)

Cognitive Development: Questions	Objective
For Children	
Who lives at your house? What do you think about your brother/sister/the new baby?	To assess the child's capacity to express both positive and negative effects relating to family members, and the degree of sibling rivalry that may be present.
For Parents	
How is school going? Have you had a conference with the teacher? How does (name) fit in with the classroom? What are the teacher's expectations for (name)?	To assess the parent's understanding and involvement with the school; to model the expected close interaction between parent and school personnel.
To the parents: How long is (name) in school? What does (name) do after school? What jobs does (name) do around the house? How much TV does (name) watch each day? What programs?	To assess the overall demands on the child's and family's circumstances, arrangements for care, and family responsibilities that the child shares.

*From Dixon and Stein.[1] Reprinted with permission.

quite sensitive to comparisons with others, peer opinions of their appearance or skills, and perceived evaluations by adults. They may utilize similar defense mechanisms as adults, with even more tenacity. When being teased about being overweight, a child may steadfastly refuse to admit such comments are of any concern. A child may also convince himself/herself and others that he/she understands a new arithmetic concept, only to show on closer examination a lack of having understood or mastered the concept.

One pitfall of the zeal to investigate and actively explore in the child in this age group is the "hurried child syndrome," noted by Elkind. The dangers of overscheduling free time, to the exclusion of allowing the child his/her own "space and time," may be reflected in somatic complaints or resistance to schoolwork.

School health professionals are aware that the child of this age is frequently able to clearly communicate feelings and relate aspects of personal, social, and health history. However, it is mandatory to also establish open communication with parents, so that important and crucial information can be gotten from the parents' perspective as well.

The 11 to 14 Year Old: Middle School, Junior High, and Early Adolescence

Early adolescence is a period of active exploration, both in fantasy and in reality. Recent research indicates that youth in this age group begin to experiment with many forms of health risk behaviors, including smoking, trying drugs, becoming sexually active, and taking risks that place them in danger of accidental injury. The onset of biologic changes associated with puberty make the period seemingly one of unexpected and rapid bodily changes, inducing reactions among children and youth as well as adults who interact with them on a daily basis. "Why don't you act more grown up?" is an admonishment frequently heard, rather than, "I guess you are acting like an adolescent." Variation in maturation is large, both between girls and boys, and among peers of the same sex. These differences do not go unnoticed and may cause significant feelings of embarrassment, envy, despair, or depression. All young adolescents are concerned about bodily changes, and the school health program must ensure that adequate education about puberty is available to young persons in this age group. Figure 2 illustrates the patterns of pubertal development for boys and girls.

Separation from parents and adults becomes prominent, and identification with the peer group is paramount. This may manifest in dress similarities, meeting together at specific places and times with religious regularity, and even identification in gangs with required initiation rituals. Health programs have capitalized on the importance of the peer group in approaches toward prevention of smoking and other health risk behaviors. Attempts to influence the social environment may hold promise as a health promotion technique with this age group.

Cognitive development is marked by a change from concrete thinking to more abstract reasoning during this period. This permits the young person to "think about thinking," to imagine a perfect person or concept, to find fault with adults' behavior, and to assess moral situations. These changes progress over time in

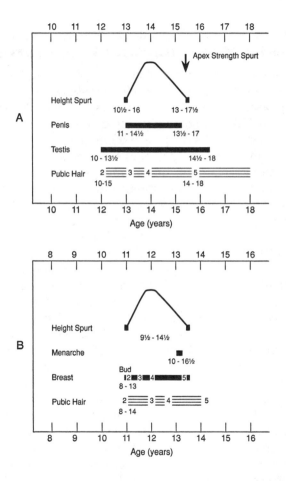

Fig 2. A, sequence of growth in boys at adolescence. An average boy is represented. The age range for each event is given directly below its start and finish. **B**, sequence of growth in girls at adolescence. An average girl is represented. The age range within which some of the events may occur is given directly beneath them. (From Tanner JM. *Growth at Adolescence*. ed 2. Oxford, England: Blackwell Scientific Publishers; 1962. Used with permission.)

this age group, and there is variation. This may present challenges to those interacting with this age group, and individualization in approach is never more relevant than with persons of this age.

Social and sexual development is also variable in this age group, but sexuality and sexual concerns are present in all adolescents. Exploration of self, fantasy life, and beginnings of interpersonal intimacy occur with same sex and opposite sex peers. Awareness of erotic impulses and physical sexual drives begins to manifest itself. Sexuality education (see chapter 26) can provide an important resource for youth searching for an understanding of their own sexual urges and interpersonal attractions.

The 14 to 18 Year Old: Senior High

The further transitions from mid-adolescence to young adulthood, with optimistic plans for integrating further education or work experience into the life goals of persons in this age group, provide the school health programs with an exciting substrate to strengthen positive health habits and decision making. Sexuality, while still important, begins to be integrated with other aspects of self and interpersonal relationships. The tasks of identity ("Who am I?" "What am I going to be in life?"); independence; and exploration of limits, values, and altruistic pursuits continue to be manifest during this age period. Literal arguments over minor deviations from rigidly interpreted rules signal the constant search of the young person for a balance between externally imposed and self-regulated limits.

This period represents the last available routine access to young people regarding life-style decisions, responsible use of drugs and alcohol, sexual practices, and attitudes toward preventive health measures. It is often difficult to match the need to communicate these issues to young people, with their prevailing attitude of invulnerability, denial of the relevance of a topic to their own situation, and their capacity to see the inconsistencies of adults telling them how to act but not adhering to their own advice. The best strategy is to be as honest and forthright in communication as possible, acknowledging the shortcomings of society, and strengthening young persons' confidence in their own control over their life.

Youth in this age group are beginning to live away from the home in which they were raised. Transition to a situation with little or no externally imposed limits may require preparation. The school health program can advocate for courses and learning experiences in the high school that target life skills. Some of these courses may need to be introduced early in the high school experience if they are to reach students who, for various reasons, drop out of school before graduation. The school may also remain a resource in some communities for school dropouts, for whom special programs, alternative education, and work/study programs have been developed. The school health programs have a special need and opportunity to serve such populations.

Reference

1. Dixon SD, Stein MT. *Encounters With Children. Pediatric Behavior and Development*. 2nd ed. St Louis, MO: Mosby Year Book; 1992

Suggested Readings

Bandura A. *Social Learning Theory*. Englewood Cliffs, NJ: Prentice Hall; 1977

Elkind D. *The Hurried Child: Growing Up Too Fast, Too Soon*. Reading, MA: Addison-Wesley; 1981

Erikson EH. *Childhood and Society*. 2nd ed. New York, NY: WW Nortan; 1985

Flavell JH. *Cognitive Development*. Englewood Cliffs, NJ: Prentice-Hall; 1977

Freund A. *Normality and Pathology in Childhood: Assessments of Development*. New York, NY: International Universities Press, Inc; 1965

Gesell AL, Amatruda CS. *Developmental Diagnosis*. 2nd ed. New York, NY: Harper and Row; 1969

Gesell AL, Ilg FL. *Child Development*. New York, NY: Harper; 1949

Maccoby EE. *Social Development: Psychological Growth and the Parent-Child Relationship*. New York, NY: Harcourt, Brace, Jovanovich, Inc; 1980

Patterson GR. *Living With Children: New Methods for Parents and Teachers*. Champaign, IL: Research Press; 1976

Piaget J, Inhelder B; Weaver H, trans. *The Psychology of the Child*. New York, NY: Basic Books; 1969

CHAPTER 5

PRESCHOOL HEALTH ISSUES

Grouped education programs for children under the age of 5 years are more common now than in previous decades, partially because of the increasing prevalence of working mothers. "Preschools" and "child day care" are common terms describing these programs. Their primary goals range from custodial to educational. The largest proportion of children with working parents are placed into family child day care. These are settings where a provider offers care in his/her own home. They aim to provide a safe alternative for children in their parents' absence, leaving education as an important, but secondary objective. In contrast, preschools generally promote themselves based on curriculum. They exist to provide education for children aged 3 to 5 years. Child care centers are in the middle of this continuum; they have "care" as a primary objective, but are apt to have written educational curricula and goals as part of the program. Boundaries for these definitions of "preschool" and "child day care" remain loose, with as much variation within, as there is between, categories.

Preschool health issues also vary with the type of program. Child care settings that have infants and toddlers grouped in close proximity to preschoolers have special problems in disease communicability and injury prevention. Exclusion policies for sick children vary with the relative emphasis on education vs child care.

Government willingness to take a role in ameliorating the effects of low income and other risks to later academic success accounts for a significant proportion of preschool programs. There are programs within many school districts for children of low-income families and other disadvantaged groups, such as children of teenage mothers who attend school. Presently, more than 27 states fund full-day and part-day preschool programs for children from low income families. Federal programs such as Chapter One prekindergartens serve more than 50,000 such children nationwide. Head Start serves almost 10 times that number. In most cases, children from middle class families do not qualify for public preschool education. However, many private preschools enroll some pupils who qualify for government subsidy. This helps to desegregate preschools and provides a more diverse ethnic and economic level student population.

Philosophies of Preschool Education

More often than not, until a child enters school, the physician providing pediatric care is the only child professional a parent has chosen to consult with on any matter. In contrast with school health matters of older children, it is often standard practice for health professionals to consult with parents of preschool-age children about issues that may seem as much educational as they are health related.

Educational philosophies of preschool programs vary greatly and can be a source of consternation for parents. It is worthwhile for health professionals to be familiar with the basic goals of these programs.

Traditional nursery schools are based on a behaviorist philosophy. There is an emphasis on training children through forming good habits (ie, repeating songs, learning handwashing routines, obeying the teacher, learning shapes through worksheets). The educational philosophy is sometimes referred to as cultural transmission. Often, prizes and punishments are used to motivate and control children. In all cases, the primary goal is to get children ready for the demands of an academic classroom.

Most of the nontraditional nursery school programs have an educational philosophy that supports either the theories of Piaget or another "developmentalist." A critical look at such programs can be found in DeVries and Kohlberg's *Constructivist Early Education: Overview and Comparison With Other Programs.*[1] These preschool educational philosophies share a common central objective: to achieve developmental progress for each child and to deemphasize achievement of academic progress. As such, these programs are often termed "child-centered." The premise is that a child at a given developmental stage is only capable of understanding the environment in a certain way. For instance, Piaget demonstrated that the young child perceives 10 mL of water in a tall, thin cup as "more" fluid than 10 mL in a regular cup. The theoretical basis of developmentalists is to enhance children's experience with such elements in their environment with the goal of facilitating progressive reorganization of their understanding of it.

Children's activities in these schools are not out of the ordinary. For instance, preschoolers play with paint and sand indoors and on slides and swings outdoors. Practically, what differs in these programs is the extent to which a child is directed toward activities, the nature of a teacher's response to a child's behavior, and the degree of interaction between children in the classroom.

Within the "child-centered" philosophy there are some differences. Montessori's method is one of the most popular in the United States and the world. Montessori schools foster progression in children's knowledge by allowing children to choose those games designed to enhance cognitive development that interest them. While there is some direction from the staff, children progress through self-motivation and the program enhances independence. The High/Scope preschool curriculum (also known as Perry Preschool model or Weikart model) is another popular program in the United States and elsewhere. High/Scope teachers have more interaction with children. They foster children's abilities to plan sequences of different activities and encourage the preschoolers to classify objects in their environment. The goal is to support the growing cognitive awareness of the preschool child.

The Bank Street and Constructivist early education models are less well known to the average consumer, but they bear similarities to the Montessori and High/Scope programs. Bank Street offers additional emphasis on emotional assistance to children who at this developmental stage are trying to manage conflict between dependence on adults and independence. The Constructivist curriculum emphasizes activities that foster cooperation, but it also deliberately includes activities that have potential for discussion or conflict so that conflict resolution can be learned.

The Health Professional as Advisor on Preschool Programming

Developmentally Appropriate Tasks for Preschoolers: The preschool years are marked by rapid growth in language, social, and motor skills (see chapter 4). Developmental tasks that are commonly achieved during the preschool period are outlined in

Table 18. — Developmental Milestones of Average 3 to 5 Year Olds*

Age	Gross-Motor Skills	Fine-Motor Skills	Socioemotional Skills	Language Expression	Language Comprehension	Language Articulation	Cognitive Skills
3	Walks up stairs, alternating feet; walks well on toes; rides tricycle; jumps from a step; hops 2-3 times	Builds 10-cube tower; strings beads; cuts with scissors; buttons	Feeds self well; knows own sex; dresses with supervision; washes and dries hands; plays associatively with others; dresses and undresses doll; separates easily from parents; relates experiences verbally; is toilet trained; takes turns consistently	Knows 300-500 words; 3-word sentences; relates simple experiences	Understands 800 words; follows 2-step commands; understands 2 prepositions (on, under); uses plurals	80% intelligibility in context; physiologic dysfluency	Copies circle; copies bridges with cubes; repeats 3 digits; matches forms; recites nursery rhymes; draws person's head
4	Walks down stairs, alternating feet; tandem walks forward; hops 5 times; balances on 1 foot, 5 sec; throws ball overhand; broad jumps	Opposes thumb to fingers; laces shoes	Dresses without supervision; tells fanciful tales; plays imaginatively; has imaginary friends; plays cooperatively with others; follows rules	Knows 600-1,000 words; 4-word sentences; speech is functional for communication	Understands 1,500 words; follows 3-step commands; understands 4 prepositions	100% intelligibility in context; physiologic dysfluency subsiding	Copies square; copies gate with cubes; knows basic colors; draws person (head and body)
5	Tandem walks backward; skips alternating feet; hops 10 times; balances on 1 foot, 10 sec	Ties knot in string; grasps pencil maturely; prints letters	Dresses totally without assistance; does simple chores; conveys feelings verbally; plans and executes projects; traverses neighborhood unattended	Knows 1,000-1,500 words; 4-5 word sentences; few errors in syntax/structure; no longer omits articles; uses correct pronouns; fully conversant	Understands 1,500-2,000 words; follows 3- to 4-step commands	100% intelligibility out of context; occasional sound substitutions; physiologic dysfluency resolved	Copies triangle; copies steps with cubes; repeats 4 digits; draws person, including arms and legs

*From Yale Child Study Center Revised Developmental Schedules, Gesell Institute of Human Development Preschool Test. In: Illingsworth RS, ed. *The Development of the Infant and Young Child.* Edinburgh: Churchill-Livingstone; 1980. Reprinted with permission.

Table 18 for ages 3, 4, and 5 years. Activities that allow children to practice and develop these skills should be the basis of traditional and child-centered programs. Parents should look for preschool programs that are designed to tolerate wide variations in children's acquisition of these skills. Programs should provide more than developmentally appropriate activities. The activities should be seen as the means to helping children attain new skills. A child who has not learned to wait his/her turn during a game should be seen as a child who will learn most from that activity, not as a "difficult" child.

Children between ages 3 and 5 years are naturally active, fidgety, and restless. They have limited attention spans. The duration of each activity should take this into consideration. Children at this stage are excellent observers, and they will imitate adults and other children with surprising accuracy. The adult's manner of communicating (both with language and with social skills) sets a certain standard for preschoolers. Children at preschool age begin to learn by observing how other children's behavior is rewarded or punished. Frank competition, however, is inappropriate at this stage. It is better to have children competing against their previous record than the achievements of a peer. Preschoolers should be taught to set their own goals as this has been shown to improve both effort and performance.

The Effects of Preschool Education: A small amount of research on this question has been done to settle the argument between proponents of preschool and those who believe children are best left with their parents until they reach the age of school entry. Not surprisingly, the answers are not simple and vary with the type of preschool, with the type of home environment that is being compared to preschool attendance, and with the characteristics that are being measured. Different parenting styles make it difficult to study the pure effect of preschool attendance vs home care of children.

Nevertheless, there are findings that deserve consideration by health professionals. Socially, preschool attendees may have more positive peer interactions, communicate better, have more advanced levels of play, be more assertive and aggressive, and be less cooperative with adults than children who remain at home with a parent. Cognitively, preschool education has been shown in some studies to decrease the likelihood for special education and grade retention in later years. However, in other studies, like the evaluation of Head Start, evaluators found that despite many other benefits of the program, academic advantages of Head Start attendance were no longer measurable after 2 years in elementary school.

Helping Parents Decide on a Preschool Enrollment: Depriving a child of a preschool experience is a common concern among those parents who have the option of staying home with their children during the day and those who can afford private in-home care for their children. Families who prefer these arrangements to child-care centers and preschool enrollment wonder if their children are going to be academically or socially lagging behind preschool attendees. Parents who cannot afford arrangements with comprehensive educational components have similar concerns.

Although there is no single good response to these concerns, health professionals can respond by taking into account the nature of the family environment, the characteristics and developmental stage of the child, the researched effects of preschool education, and the options available in the community. Health professionals can help parents identify ways to enrich a preschooler's environment around the home. Parents who have difficulty providing a rich environment at home and who can either afford preschool tuition or are eligible for publicly funded preschool enrollment can be advised to consider preschool for at least part of the week. Parents who stay home with a preschooler should be encouraged to provide a wide range of activities and toys to stimulate a child's interest and curiosity. If there are not many neighborhood playmates or playgrounds, concerned parents may, on occasion, enroll their preschooler in a local child group activity, such as library readings or play groups in community centers. This allows children the opportunity to socialize with others their age and to become comfortable with the structure of nonparental supervision.

Recent disruption in family harmony, such as birth of a new sibling, will make some children less emotionally ready for an academic setting and more comfortable in a small, coddling environment. A suitable family child care home, rather than a large preschool, may be recommended in that case. Alternatively, if a child's behavior is unruly, a highly structured preschool program may provide the consistency and predictability that is lacking at home.

Parents trying to decide between "traditional" nursery school vs a "child-centered" program, such as Montessori, should be reassured that most children can adapt to and benefit from either environment—although perhaps in different ways. Parents should be encouraged to visit the preschool before enrolling their child, and again after their child is attending the preschool. An adjustment period often exists for the first few weeks, and parents should be encouraged to give any new setting a chance before deciding to enroll a child in yet another new setting.

Licensing criteria vary from state to state. Some states require provider training in child development and in prevention and control of infectious diseases. The National Association for the Education of Young Children (NAEYC) has set its own standards that are more stringent than those of most states, and parents should be encouraged to compare the policies of the preschools available to them with these (standards available by writing to NAEYC; 1834 Connecticut Ave NW, Washington, DC 20009-5786). Numerous checklists and guidelines are available to parents of preschoolers who are evaluating a program. Sample observations are listed in Table 19.

The environment parents provide for their children outside of a preschool structure will be different from what is provided in a good preschool, but need not be inferior. Listening to stories, learning to draw and cut, helping to take care of a younger sibling, and similar home-based experiences are all part of a natural education. Parents need to understand that each child comes to kindergarten with individual strengths and weaknesses.

School Readiness: Parents feel pressure to have their children academically and developmentally "ready" for the first day of kindergarten or first grade. Formal school readiness assessments have occasionally acted as an unintentional hurdle to school entry, resulting in many children having been unnecessarily held back from school.

A worthwhile purpose of school readiness assessments is to help parents and educators understand a pupil's weaknesses and strengths so that a school entry program can be tailored to the

Table 19. — Examples of What Parents Should Be Observing When Assessing a Preschool

Teachers

Is the teacher sensitive to the needs of children (patient, warm, and accepting)?

Does the teacher display an understanding of child development and enjoy the job?

Is the teacher caring in relationships with the children, yet also consistent and firm?

Does the teacher encourage natural curiosity and exploration as well as the desire to learn?

Are there enough adults with the children to ensure the basic safety of the group and to help the individual child who needs it?

Preschool

Are the rooms and play areas large enough for the number of children and for the activities offered?

Are the areas planned for good supervision and visual contact with the children?

Is the preschool clean enough for health standards, but relaxed enough that children do not feel restrained?

Is there a safe and inviting outdoor play space?

Is the preschool licensed?

Equipment/Materials

Is there a variety of materials and equipment that will allow the child many different experiences, and are there enough to allow a child several choices at any time?

Are the materials and equipment appropriate for the age level?

Are the materials and equipment stored in an appealing way and easily accessible to the children?

Does the equipment show signs of neglect or wear and tear that may constitute a safety hazard?

---

student's needs. This can serve to lower the risk of overexpectations or underexpectations for children entering first grade.

Great variations in children's developmental readiness for school can be expected regardless of preschool experience. Achievement of developmental milestones in one area does not necessarily reflect the developmental level in other areas. For example, a child with less than average maturation of language skills does not need to be held back from school entry if gross-

and fine-motor skills and emotional development are on a par with chronological age. Even though language development may be the best predictor of later learning problems, a child who is slow with expressive language may still have better-than-average communicative skills for his/her age at maturity. Generalizations cannot be applied in individual cases.

An understanding of a child's behavior, emotional development, and classroom skills can be partially ascertained by a preschool physical examination and interview. Characteristics that constitute readiness for school are listed in Table 20. To augment this assessment, a number of screening tests have been developed. The Pediatric Examination of Educational Readiness (PEER) and the Denver Developmental Screening Test (DDST) are screening tests of different comprehensiveness and purpose that can be used by health professionals. Such tools identify strengths and weaknesses; screen for learning disabilities, developmental delays, and mental retardation; and can serve as indicators for more comprehensive evaluations. Their applications should be limited to the uses for which they were designed. Too often, they are used as the only measure of school readiness and as a gateway to school entry.

In order that all children can receive developmentally appropriate education, including those children with mixed levels of maturity, a criterion for determining school entry is whether the child has reached the legal chronological age of school entry. Health professionals can participate in the process of keeping schools responsive to the wide variation of young children's learning needs.

Children With Special Needs in Preschool

Public Laws: Most professionals involved with school systems are familiar with Public Law 94-142 (1975), which provides public education and related services for handicapped children, aged 5 to 21 years. Public Law 99-457 (1986) has expanded the eligibility to include children, aged 3 to 5 years. States also have the option of adopting part H (birth to 3 years) of this public law, which allows them to receive federal funds for early childhood intervention services for handicapped infants and toddlers. Health professionals in the schools and elsewhere in the com-

Table 20. — Predicting Adaptability to the Classroom Environment

Look for the following characteristics in the child:

Has good physical health

Lacks visual or auditory impairment

Has had successful preschool experience

Is completely toilet trained

Has self-care skills (dressing, washing)

Separates readily and for prolonged periods from parents

Follows direction

Shares and takes turns

Understands and follows routines

Has good interpersonal and friendship skills

Accepts adult supervision and assistance

Makes transitions easily

Tolerates frustrations and failure

Works independently for short periods of time

Has general fund of knowledge (days of week, coins)

Has good attention span

Has age-appropriate language skills

Articulates clearly

Has eye-hand coordination skills (cutting, drawing)

Has visual discrimination skills (letters of the alphabet, draw-a-person, copies geometric forms)

Has auditory discrimination skills (discriminates similar sounds, words)

Understands quantitative concepts (size, counts to 10)

Prints letters of alphabet and of first name

munity have a distinct role to play in the schooling of the population (see chapter 6).

Identification of Eligible Disabled Children: A small number of states have public mass screening programs for all preschoolers in order to identify those with need of early educational intervention. In the vast majority of states, however, pediatricians, nurse practitioners, other primary health care workers, and certain pediatric specialists are responsible for identifying eligible preschoolers. Health professionals suspicious of a developmental delay should either do a full evaluation or refer the child to an evaluation center. Underreferral by health professionals would be a problem in many states, resulting in lost opportunities for early intervention.

Eligibility criteria to receive services vary somewhat from state to state and to some extent even among school districts in one region. In general, children with *either* physical or cognitive handicaps are candidates. Children without a demonstrable handicap but with a diagnosis known to be associated with a handicap later in life (such as certain chromosomal abnormalities) are eligible. Isolated delays in speech/language, psychosocial, and self-help skills are also examples of eligibility criteria, depending on their severity. In some districts, children at risk for developmental disabilities based on biological or environmental risk factors (ie, poverty, intrauterine drug exposure) are provided with preventive services.

There is a great need for health services among this population. A far larger proportion of children of preschool age with identifiable developmental delays have health conditions requiring medical attention than children requiring special education services at an elementary or high school age.[2] The medical issues most frequently encountered by these preschool educators are recurrent seizures, gastric tube feedings, and chronic infectious diseases. Medically fragile and technologically dependent students are also overrepresented in this population.

The Consultative Role of the Health Professional: For each child under 3 years receiving public education because of PL 99-457 funding, there is an Individualized Family Service Plan (IFSP). It is a requirement of the IFSP that each student have a case manager; that a written plan target the family, and not merely the child, for intervention; that each "special need" of the child be described; and that each need be accompanied by a care plan or educational goal. Although a health professional can participate in the development of the IFSP or be the case manager, this is not required, even when a medical problem is the most relevant need. As such, it is important that school health professionals and students' personal physicians be involved to the extent that they are satisfied that all medical needs are addressed. After age 3 years, the traditional Individualized Educational Plan (IEP) is used in place of the IFSP. The medical contribution to this plan is equally important.

Specific contributions of school health professionals and community practitioners are to help collate and interpret all medical information on a given student and to assist in the process of modifying medical procedures and medication plans so that school attendance and safe transportation to the school site are optimal. Health professionals must provide health education to educators who find themselves on the front lines of urgent management situations. Decision for classroom placement cannot rest solely with special educators when there is a significant medical handicap. Sometimes, proximate availability of nursing services and, less frequently, access to physician consultation are required (see chapters 16 and 17).

Other Children With Special Needs: Many children with special needs who are ineligible for public funding also attend preschool; this includes children with seizure disorders, asthma, speech problems that do not qualify for publicly funded services, and certain physical handicaps. The health professional can help preschool educators with plans for these children, based on models similar to the IFSP. If the physical setting, staff ratio, or specialized expertise of the preschool educator does not adequately meet minimum safety, educational, or health standards, the health professional has a responsibility to notify the parent. Often, consulting with the preschool director and additional community resources will correct the situation.

Labeling: Preschoolers often have specific diagnoses that are considered responsible for their "special need." For example, Down syndrome and prenatal exposure to illicit drugs are two common diagnoses associated with developmental delay. It is not unusual for professionals in both health and education to refer to these children by the assumed cause of their handicap (eg, "crack babies"), rather than by the nature of the developmental delay (eg, "speech delay" or "mental retardation"). This is sometimes a convenient method of characterizing children because categorizing gives educators immediate understanding of the children's problems and prognoses. It allows educators to follow and compare different interventions given to children with similar problems. However, early labeling can also incur prejudice and cause self-fulfilling prophecy. Health professionals have a role in discouraging unnecessary labeling. They should explain what is known and unknown about the relationship of the underlying disease or condition with the demonstrated developmental delay.

Health and Safety for Preschoolers in Group Settings

Communicable Diseases: The pathogens causing infectious diseases in preschoolers are frequently the same microorganisms spread among older children (see chapter 19). However, just as children are not simply small adults, preschoolers are not simply smaller children. A number of factors account for increased disease communicability.[3] Preschoolers have poor hygiene; they have limited independence with toileting. Food preparation is a common group activity in preschools. Thumb sucking and biting occur relatively frequently. Preschools that combine toddlers and infants in a single physical setting further exacerbate the risk of disease communication.

Hygienic procedures applied universally to all children in preschool, regardless of known carrier states, is the basis for disease containment. Handwashing protocols and precautions with blood and other body fluids in preschool do not differ from those described in chapter 20. The impact of failure to comply is likely to be more quickly evident. Hygienic technique, together with close and continuous observation of staff compliance, has been shown to reduce diarrheal rates in these settings. Preschools should document that children have updated immunizations to diphtheria, pertussis, tetanus, polio, measles, mumps, rubella, hepatitis B, and *Haemophilus influenzae* type b.

Exclusion criteria for preschoolers do not differ from those of older children with rashes and respiratory, gastrointestinal, and other potentially infectious diseases. However, the likelihood that a young child will have difficulty containing loose stools is greater, so that a higher proportion of preschool children with diarrhea are excluded. It is probable that preschools more commonly accept mildly sick children than elementary schools. In elementary school, where the goal is to educate, any child not feeling well enough to keep up with the class stays at home. Those preschools with the philosophy that they are caretakers as much as educators often accommodate a mildly sick child by modifying the curriculum and increasing staff observation. School health professionals must be certain that the health expertise and staffing of preschools is adequate to accommodate mildly sick children.

Respiratory Diseases: Young children have little previous exposure to numerous pathogens. Young children attending preschool have higher rates of respiratory tract infections and otitis media than those remaining at home. Health professionals can help parents weigh the benefits of preschool with the increased risk of earlier exposure to certain pathogens. Most infections contracted during preschool are not a serious detriment and may be associated with fewer infections later in childhood. There are cases in which the impact of frequent infections for a preschooler must be considered more seriously. Severe asthma exacerbated by upper respiratory tract infection and certain immunodeficiencies are examples.

Haemophilus influenzae type b and *Neisseria meningitidis* are more common infections among preschoolers than in older age groups. However, unless there are children under the age of 2 years included in the preschoolers' environment, managing the spread of these organisms is the same as for groups of school-age children.

Enteric Diseases: Hepatitis A, *Giardia lamblia*, and rotavirus can be relatively difficult to eradicate in preschools, not only because of poor hygiene but also because these infections are commonly asymptomatic in young children. Immune globulin (IG) is recommended for all children and employees in the same room as an index case of hepatitis A. If the preschool includes children under 2 years of age or children who are not toilet trained, new employees and children arriving within 6 weeks of the last diagnosed case should also receive IG. Persons infected with *G lamblia* who have diarrhea should be treated. However, examining stools of asymptomatic contacts or treating asymptomatic carriers is unnecessary.

Other Diseases: There is a typically high prevalence of cytomegalovirus (CMV) excretion in the urine and saliva among children of preschool age. Teachers and mothers of children attending preschool are more likely to acquire primary CMV infections than other women of the same age. Infants born to mothers who acquire primary CMV during the first half of their pregnancy are at an increased risk for significant neurological impairment. Close adherence to universal hygiene precautions serves to protect against transmission of CMV from known and unknown carriers. However, many obstetricians advise their patients on the basis of their CMV serology results. The role of the school health professional is to provide education about these preventive practices.

Parvovirus B19 (cause of erythema infectiosum) is another pathogen infecting preschoolers that is of concern to pregnant caretakers. Primary infection has been reported to induce spontaneous abortions. As with CMV infection, the management of this illness rests with reassurance, routine hygiene practices, and elective serologic testing (when available) for evidence of previous infection.

Preschool attendees infected with human immunodeficiency virus (HIV) or who have acquired immunodeficiency syndrome (AIDS) have not been found to communicate this virus to their peers. Persistent biting behavior and staff contact with blood-containing body fluids may be a problem.[4] Therefore, the inclusion of an HIV-infected child in a program and the disclosure of the diagnosis to selected school personnel should be decided on an individual basis.

Safety: The rate of injuries requiring medical or dental attention for children at each year of age between birth and 5 years is lower than the rate for school-age children. Studies indicate that preschools and child care centers are as safe as home and other community sites. Nevertheless, the type of injuries that young children incur and the measures necessary to prevent them are different. By the time children reach preschool age, injuries related to biting and unstable locomotion are no longer frequent. Depending on the developmental maturity of the preschooler, there may be a relative inability to anticipate danger. Poisoning and misuse of foreign bodies are characteristics of children, aged 2 to 4 years. Preschoolers spend less time writing, reading, and listening quietly and more time exploring their environment through the use of various interactive toys than school-age children. Therefore, injuries in younger children are not as limited to specific times of the day.

Aside from the recommendations on play equipment, playground surfaces, and responses to emergencies that also pertain

Table 21. — The Preschooler's Environment: Additional Safety Measures

Nonskid surface floors

Nontoxic art supplies

Covered outlets, hidden extension cords

Inaccessible radiators and hot water pipes

Nonpoisonous plants

Unbreakable toys

Toys too large to aspirate

No nuts, hard candy, other aspiratable foods

Syrup of ipecac on hand

Separate play areas for children of markedly different developmental abilities

Electric-powered toys—battery only

to school-age children (see chapter 31), there are additional preventive practices useful for the younger population. These are summarized in Table 21.

Other Health Issues: Sleep, bladder control, stress, and nutrition are examples of health-related childhood problems with which preschool educators deal. Circumstances tend to constantly challenge policy for such matters, necessitating that ongoing health consultation be available. A school nurse, psychologist, pediatrician/physician, or other professional often can act as a bridge between the school and the family and develop solutions that take into account both the routines at home and preschool.

Preschoolers differ from older children and from each other in their need for rest and sleep during the day. Many require naps. Some cannot sleep during the day. Some will sleep, but then have difficulty falling asleep at night. Educators' expectations of children must vary widely.

Toddlers and preschoolers are notorious for having particular food likes and dislikes and for limiting their diets to very few foods. Most have not yet developed the maturity to try new food items. Communication between parents and preschool educators on daily intake and on likes and dislikes is important for ensuring that these young children have a well-balanced daily intake of nutrients.

Bowel and bladder control are achieved early in the preschool years, if not accomplished earlier. Control is lost easily when the child is in a new, unfamiliar environment or is otherwise stressed.

Stress is common during the period of separation from a parent. Depending on a child's personality, temperament, and developmental stage, enjoyment usually begins soon after the parent has departed, particularly if the teacher tries to engage the child in an activity. Reassurance on the developmental normalcy of this is helpful to parents. Under no circumstances should the parent leave without saying good-bye. The parent should not weaken once he or she has decided to leave. Allowing parents to play with their child for a short while in the center may decrease the child's reluctance to separate and allows the child to take note of the parent's acceptance and approval of this "out-of-home" environment.

References

1. DeVries R, Kohlberg L. *Constructivist Early Education: Overview and Comparison With Other Programs.* Washington, DC: National Association for the Education of Young Children; 1987

2. Taras HL, Martino J. *Medical Disability and the Need for Child Day Care Among Children With Developmental Delay.* Presented at the Centers for Disease Control International Conference on Child Day Care Health; Atlanta, GA; June 15, 1992

3. American Public Health Association, American Academy of Pediatrics. *Caring for Our Children: National Health and Safety Performance Standards for Out-of-Home Child Care Programs.* Washington, DC: American Public Health Association; 1992

4. American Academy of Pediatrics, Task Force on Pediatric AIDS. Pediatric guidelines for infection control of human immunodeficiency virus (acquired immunodeficiency virus) in hospitals, medical offices, schools, and other settings. *Pediatrics.* 1988;82:801-807

Suggested Readings

Hendricks CM, ed. *Young Children on the Grow: Health, Activity, and Education in the Preschool Setting.* Washington, DC: ERIC Clearinghouse on Teacher Education; 1991

Kagan SL. Readiness past, present, and future: shaping the agenda. *Young Children.* 1992;48(1):48-53

CHAPTER 6

SPECIAL EDUCATION

Historical and Legislative Underpinnings

Special education in the United States is an important component of the school environment. The passage of Public Law (PL) 94-142 in 1975 created a new emphasis on the rights of children with handicapping conditions and on the importance of child health functioning.

The Education for All Handicapped Children Act (PL 94-142) grew out of concerns that children with developmental handicaps were not receiving the same level of services as nondisabled children. Several lawsuits, including *Mills vs the Board of Education*, and *The Pennsylvania Association for Retarded Citizens vs Pennsylvania*, had established precedents for the civil rights of children with disabilities.

Public Law 94-142 codified these precedents in a sweeping piece of legislation. It mandated a free, appropriate public education for children with disabilities. Moreover, PL 94-142 laid down the principle that children should be educated within the least restrictive environment possible and created the notion that school systems must remove barriers to educational opportunities for children with handicapping conditions. To do this, PL 94-142 established schools as the locus of the provision of "related services," including transportation, physical therapy, occupational therapy, speech and hearing services, counseling (for both child and family), and physician services (for diagnosis only).

Two important new developments include the enactment of PL 99-457 (the amendments to the Education for All Handicapped Children Act of 1986) and the Supreme Court case *Tatro vs the Irving Independent School System*. These two recent developments have expanded the role of the school with regard to the provision of more than educational services. Both have implications for practitioners of school health.

Public Law 99-457 can be thought of as the "early intervention" law. Based on an acceptance of the literature hailing the success of early intervention programs, Congress passed PL 99-457 and thereby encouraged states to develop systems for the early iden-

Table 22. — Comparison of PL 94-142 and PL 99-457

PL 94-142	PL 99-457
Mandates "equal education for all"	Encourages early identification and intervention
Provides mandate for related services and sets standards	States have option to interpret eligibility and implement
Focus on *school*/placement in least restrictive environment	Requires *family* involvement in intervention process
Individualized Education Plan (IEP)	Individualized Family Service Plan (IFSP)

tification of and early intervention for children from birth to 3 years and to establish preschool programs for children with disabilities. Public Law 99-457 differs in some ways from PL 94-142 in that PL 99-457 is only an incentive to states, rather than a mandate; it is not a strict requirement to establish such services. Public Law 99-457 also differs from PL 94-142 in that the children covered include children with biologic handicaps, established handicaps, and "at risk" status. Also unlike PL 94-142, PL 99-457 leaves it to the discretion of the state to determine eligibility criteria and to establish the extent of services that will be provided. Finally, PL 99-457 explicitly involves families in the intervention process, which is a significant expansion of the scope of the service.

The other important recent development has been the Supreme Court case *Tatro vs the Irving Independent School System*. In 1984, the Supreme Court heard the case of Amber Tatro, a child with meningomyelocele, who required clean intermittent catheterization (CIC) every 3 to 4 hours. The Irving Independent School System argued that schools should not be required to provide such services. The Supreme Court found unanimously in favor of the child and family, basing their response directly on the legislation and regulations. The court indicated that it was the clear intent of the drafters of PL 94-142 that all barriers to education be removed and that a nursing procedure such as CIC was just such a removable barrier.

The *Tatro* case is extremely important for pediatricians and school health practitioners, because within it the Supreme Court documented that not only was CIC to be provided on a routine basis, but that any nursing procedure required by a child must be provided by the school system. With *Tatro*, the Supreme Court widened the purview of schools to include the explicit requirement for providing nursing care in the school setting (school care).

Each state has established special education procedures and plans, and defined the nature of services as well as the categories of children eligible for them. Children's and parents' rights are protected by due process procedures that are carried out under legal mandate. Table 23 lists the overall process of special education. These procedures are discussed in the following text, but state-specific information will supplement the physician's ability to interact knowledgeably on attempting to utilize special education services.

Identification/Referral

Inherent in both PL 94-142 and PL 99-457 is the notion that children's developmental problems and handicaps will first need to be identified by professionals. Moreover, there is the strong presumption that the earlier these problems are brought to attention, the more benefit the children can derive from special education. A heavy emphasis on identification is now articulated in PL 99-457, but was also a strong component of the initial legislation, called "Child Find."

Pediatricians are considered to be one of the major professional groups who may identify children who could benefit from special education. The authority regarding such early identification now rests in some states with the public health, education, or social service departments. Physicians may feel more comfortable interacting with departments of public health about such issues, but children will receive fewer services if linkages with education are not made in those states in which it is appropriate. The challenge from special education to pediatrics at this time is significant. Can we, in a routine way, identify those children most in need of services and for whom early intervention will be most effective? It is still largely conceded that developmental screening, whether through the use of questionnaires or guided observations, is still a flawed procedure. Nonetheless, the availability of early services now challenges pediatricians to define mechanisms for early identification within the practice situation.

Table 23. — Process of Special Education

Identification/referral
Evaluation
Designation/labeling
Placement and review
Services/intervention
Due process

Evaluation

Central to the special education process is the Individualized Evaluation Program (IEP). For young children under PL 99-457, this has been expanded into the concept of the Individualized Family Service Plan (IFSP). Both the IEP and IFSP are designed to have professionals put together as much information as possible about an individual child in order to come up with an appropriate plan of action. The notion, which was unique with PL 94-142, is that services within special education should be tailored to the specific needs of the child. Much of the success of PL 94-142 can be attributed to this philosophic commitment.

Depending on the child's problem (or suspected problem), different types of evaluations may be appropriate. Policymakers in education and pediatrics have struggled with this inherent problem for some time. Should all children have all evaluations (a very expensive proposition) or should a particular set of evaluations be used for particular categories of children? The problem with the latter is that a child may be misdiagnosed or misclassified by this use of an exclusive set of tests. Within different states, physicians and policymakers have come up with a variety of formulas to address these problems. In general, all children receive basic psychological testing, some form of family history taking, and then specialized evaluations regarding the presumed deficit or difficulty.

Physicians in many states are required to provide input into the IEP. This information may be requested in various forms. The most extensive information requested would include a recent history and physical and developmental observations by the physician. The most minimal information might include the name of the physician to contact at a later date.

Because of the increasing number of children with chronic illness who require ongoing health care provision, it is essential that a health care plan be drawn up for each child receiving health care services within the school (school care). Health professionals taking care of the child and school health professionals should advocate strongly that this health care plan be reviewed at the time of the IEP meeting with the same emphasis and importance as is placed on the individualized education program. This will allow for the training of appropriate staff and the priority rating of the health care issues.

Designation/Labeling

Based on the teams' evaluation, in most states children will be categorized as having one of the following: speech impairment, specific learning disabilities, emotional disturbance, mental retardation, visual impairment, deafness, and/or physical disability. In some states, a category of "other health impaired" is also included. There is considerable controversy as to whether it is useful to have such "labels." Those who argue for "labels" feel that using such terminology helps to define a package of services most appropriate for children and helps to alert professionals to the needs of the child who has been labeled. The countervailing argument is that children often cannot be pigeonholed into a particular category. For instance, a child with learning disabilities also may have components of an emotional disturbance; and labeling or categorizing the child leaves out the possibility of receiving services in the other area. Of particular poignancy now is the issue of whether attention deficit disorder (ADD) will be added to PL 94-142 as a specific label. Currently, if a child has ADD but no learning problem or other emotional disturbance, services may be denied under PL 94-142. This issue currently is being debated in the Department of Education and ultimately will go to Congress for a decision.

Placement and Review

The precipitant for the passage of PL 94-142 was the concern of parents of children with disabilities that their children were being isolated from the mainstream of public education. As a result, special education has placed a heavy emphasis on the normalization of educational placement for children with developmental disabilities and other handicapping conditions.

Within special education there is now a so-called "cascade" of placement options available for children with disabilities. Rarely, are children placed within *institutions*, but even in those rare cases, educational interventions are performed through the public school system. *Special schools* are generally reserved for children whose disabilities are extremely severe or who require large amounts of therapeutic intervention. Even in these cases, however, efforts are made to involve the children in integrated activities for recreation and other community activities. Going up the "cascade," the next option is a *special classroom within the regular school*. This option is generally determined as a percentage of time from 10% to 100%. Within the *regular class*, intervention for children with disabilities also can be provided. In some cases, *aides* will assist children with handicaps in their normal, daily routine. In other situations, the teacher may be given *special training* in how to work with a given child, or modified curricular materials may be provided. Finally, within the regular classroom, there are options for *monitoring* a child's situation before resorting to placement in a specific special education arrangement.

"Mainstreaming" is an issue that also has occasioned considerable debate. On one hand, it is clear that the opportunities available to a child in the mainstream setting resemble those offered to children without handicaps. This often allows a child a wide range of educational options. However, when services are not provided in tandem with the placement, it has been argued that the normal setting may sometimes be more restrictive than the specialized placement.

School health practitioners facing the decision as to how to advocate for a particular child with regard to placement in or out of the mainstream need to be cognizant of the needs of the child and the resources available within the school system. Every effort should be made to integrate children as fully as possible, and an awareness of local philosophy and resources may occasionally aid in coming to the optimum solution for a particular child.

Services/Intervention

One of the consequences of the passage of PL 94-142 is the fact that special education programs have distinct structure and authority within most public school systems. Often, the director of special education for the school system is a deputy superintendent with a direct reporting relationship to the superintendent. As a result, special education programs have received a certain autonomy and often operate somewhat independently of the regular programs. However, there must be overlap, particularly for those children who are in regular class placements.

The major service provided through special education is, of course, education itself. For the purposes of PL 94-142, education includes any "leading out" of a child from one level of functioning or knowledge to a higher level. Therefore, education is construed extremely broadly, and services that help mentally retarded children with daily living activities are considered to be part of the educational purview. In addition, services that help children to learn how to organize their work and prepare their assignments are included within the educational services of special education. Within most school systems, specialists in the teaching of children with mental retardation and learning disabilities are available both to provide direct services and to assist teachers in incorporating special educational interventions into their regular teaching plans.

In addition, within many school systems, there is now extensive experimentation with new teaching techniques, including the use of computers, both for children with serious physical disabilities and for children with learning disabilities. Moreover, the use of sign language is being explored for children with mental retardation as well as for children with hearing and speech problems. Other experimental work is using "peer teachers," pairing children within the same classroom for conjoint learning. These experiments have been extremely successful and are continuing to show real promise.

In addition to educational services, within special education there is now extensive provision of so-called related services. In many districts, school nurses/practitioners receive financial support from special education funds. These adjunct services are considered those interventions necessary to allow children with disabilities to attend school and to benefit most fully from special education. The school health team may be called upon in a variety of ways regarding "related services." The team may be asked to comment on the best package of services, or the school health physician may be asked to "order" and monitor these services. Every effort should be made to consider the efficacy and effectiveness of the services and to keep high quality of service provision as a priority.

Due Process

A core aspect of the special education program is the fact that parents have the right to agree or disagree with the educational plan established for their children. This due process right includes parents' ability to call for second opinions regarding the service plan for their child. Often, physicians who have shown an interest in school health will be called on to carry out the second opinion consultation.

Pediatricians also may become involved in the due process procedures if they choose to serve in their community as hearing officers. If the parents are dissatisfied with the plan proposed by a school system, a hearing may be held. A knowledgeable but unbiased observer, such as a community pediatrician, may be asked to serve as the hearing officer. This is an avenue through which physicians can provide an extremely important community service. As a hearing officer, the physician needs to be fully aware of the child's needs as well as the practical aspects of the school's situation. The school, however, cannot deny particular services on the basis of cost or actual availability of those services.

Health Care Providers and Special Education

Opportunities for pediatric and school health involvement exist at all levels of special education. With the advent of PL 99-457, physicians interested in school health are often being called on to serve on the Interagency Coordinating Councils (ICC). Physicians are being asked to develop systems for the coordination of pediatric identification with referral to early intervention programs.

Physicians have an extremely important role to play in the evaluation of children with disabilities. School health physicians often may be asked to become involved with this aspect of the program. Having intimate knowledge of the school resources, the physician can be an important communicator between the family and the schools, and can provide the schools with realistic information about the child's limitations and potential. Likewise, the physician can provide the families with knowledge of the resources that can be reasonably expected from the school.

Physicians serve as a continuity link for families. Because of the longitudinal nature of their interaction with families, pediatricians often have much more historical information regarding a given child than is available within a school system. This is particularly true at school entry. Now, with PL 99-457, which mandates separate programs for children aged birth to 2 years, 3- to 5-year-olds and school-age children are at important transition points; a pediatrician or a family physician can be extremely helpful in easing the transition. This is also true when a child moves from elementary school into junior high or high school. One of the frustrating moments for families and for physicians is at the final transition into adulthood. Increasing attention now is being placed on this important stage.

Another critical role for pediatricians in conjunction with special education is involvement in training programs for special education providers, such as special education teachers, physical and occupational therapists, speech and hearing providers, psychologists, and counselors. Through the various university-affiliated facilities (UAFs) throughout the United States, pediatricians and others working in the developmental disabilities field have shown a leadership role in such training programs for school professionals.

Moreover, pediatricians can join other specialists in providing input into curricular and programmatic planning for school systems, particularly when major changes may occur, as with the building of a new school or new community facility.

Pediatricians have a new role to play in the schools vis-a-vis the new population of children who are termed "medically fragile" (see chapter 17). This group of children needs extensive evaluation before placement within school systems and careful planning so that the services they require are in fact available from the moment they enter the school system.

A particularly challenging group of children who fit the definition of "medically fragile" are the increasing number of children with human immunodeficiency virus (HIV) infection (see chapter 20). School physicians are increasingly being called on to suggest policy within school systems regarding children with HIV. To date, issues regarding confidentiality have been of paramount concern. As increasing numbers of children with HIV infection are presenting to schools, another major issue will be the availability of necessary nursing involvement and psychological counseling for the children and their friends as they encounter the complications of this life-threatening condition.

The School Health Team in Special Education

The special education process requires a multidisciplinary approach to children with educational handicaps. It is absolutely essential that professionals from different backgrounds work together and that they incorporate parents and children in the process. Often, pediatricians are not trained in working in this vein. Increasingly, training programs must emphasize the importance of this type of interdisciplinary work.

The IEP format, which requires exchange of information and, if possible, a meeting among the involved professionals, the family, and (when appropriate) the child, can help to break down communication barriers. Unfortunately, physicians rarely are able to attend IEP meetings. A problem that frequently occurs is that a physician's report will be read without thorough knowledge of the child or of the issues involved. This makes it mandatory to clearly, and in nonmedical terms, state the nature of the problems, their educational implications, and any limitations or requirements placed on the child as a result. Financial barriers continue to make it difficult for physicians to involve themselves directly in the IEP meeting. Nonetheless, the involvement that can occur through telephone calls and exchange of reports is very valuable.

Since both the school health providers and the special education team work with the child and family as a common constituency, the two groups have important opportunities to provide comprehensive health and developmental services for children with developmental disabilities and educational handicaps.

CHAPTER 7

SCHOOL HEALTH SERVICES

Organization and Staffing of School Health Services

School health services as traditionally delivered in a school building are under the authority and ultimate supervision of the school principal. In school-linked or school-coordinated care systems, the school health services may operate under the jurisdiction of a health department or other health care provider. The day-to-day management of these services is usually organized by a school nurse. The school nurse may in turn have reporting and consultative supervision by other nurses at the district level. The nurse also may supervise and delegate responsibilities to others, such as aides, health clerks, and volunteers, in carrying out activities. If the nurse is also a nurse practitioner, or the district has so arranged, physician backup and consultation may be available to the local school health team.

Assignment of nurses, aides, and clerks is determined by local specialized needs of students in a particular school and availability of resources in the school district. Recommendations have included having a full-time school nurse in every school. While this might be optimal, it is rarely found. A differentiated school staffing pattern with aides, nurses, clerks, nurse practitioners, and physician backup could have an aide for each school, a nurse for about 800 to 1,000 students, and a nurse practitioner for about 1,500 to 2,000 students. One physician should be available for backup consultation for a district, assuming that no actual primary care services are being delivered on-site, and not including other extensive aspects of school health program consultation in addition to the backup activities. These estimates are just that, and require revision upward or downward depending on local needs and resources.

Various nurse staffing patterns have been utilized by schools. Obviously, the extent of services desired is reflected by the pattern employed. A minimal staffing pattern assures minimal services within a school. If additional services are readily available and accessible to school students and staff, utilization of outside

Table 24. — Nursing Staffing Patterns for a School Health Service*

Model	Advantages	Disadvantages
Nurse aide alone	Cost: with appropriate back-up, systems might be able to meet basic and required needs (eg, immunization records and first aid).	Requires outside resources: special education needs will not be met.
Aide with nurse	Frees nurse to meet more important needs.	Increases costs if ratio too "rich."
Nurse/teacher	Potential for increasing integration of health services and health education.	Costs may be difficult to justify; half of job usually sacrificed.
School nurse	Readily available resource for children, teachers, parents.	Costs for services may be difficult to justify in traditional programs.
Public health nurse	Costs to district may be lower than district-supplied nurses.	Services to schools diluted by other tasks.
Nurse practitioner	Cost for service obtained may be cost-effective; meets more special education needs on site (potentially decreases unnecessary referrals); better problem definition; potential for generating income for services provided.	Should have some form of physician back-up (may increase costs); role change difficult; requires time, training; expanded services may conflict with existing sources of care.

*From Nader.[8] Reprinted with permission.

school resources may be the choice made (for example, a neighborhood health center or health clinic is able to provide school health services). Table 24 illustrates advantages and disadvantages of various school nursing staffing patterns.

Staffing the school health service depends on the desired goals and objectives. Utilization of multiple levels of expertise should result in the most efficient delivery system.

Assuring Access to Primary Care

Asking parents (and recording the information) about their regular source of health care for their child, and when and for what reason they last contacted that source of care, is a good initial step in defining the linkages required to bridge the gap between the school and the health care system. If there is a physician or clinic designated, record the name, location, and phone number. Determine if parents will agree to have this provider be the source of medical care if the need for referral is agreed on by the parents. Studies have indicated a much higher referral completion rate if the nurse knew the provider of care to whom the referral was directed. Some children will not have a regular source of care. All available resources—public, private, and charitable—need to be sought for such children and active steps taken to enroll each student with an ongoing source of care somewhere in the community.

Some geographic areas may find it necessary to establish primary care resources in or near the school building. As much as possible, these efforts must examine, at their onset, the mechanisms of long-range funding and support. They also will have to be tied into existing systems of care in order to provide backup, specialty or emergency care, or care when the school-based facility is not available.

Provision of Emergency Services

Students, teachers, other school employees, and visitors may have medical emergencies at school or off the school premises (eg, on the school bus or on field trips). School personnel and selected students in all schools should be regularly trained and be able to provide first aid in emergencies and know how to perform cardiopulmonary resuscitation (CPR). All personnel should know how to access 911 or other community emergency medical systems.

While most emergency situations encountered in schools are not life threatening, the possibility exists that they may be. Therefore, appropriate plans must be in place for immediate treatment and mobilization of emergency services. Table 25 illustrates a triage plan developed for schools by a Connecticut AAP School Health Committee.

Table 25. — Triage Plan*

Category	Emergency Plan
I. Immediate treatment and mobilization of emergency medical services needed	
A. Acute airway obstruction	Immediately notify administrator. Get nurse or trained staff person to victim. Initiate ambulance call. Notify nurse if not with victim. Administrator or nurse notifies parent.
B. Cardiac or respiratory arrest	
C. Near drowning	
D. Massive external hemorrhage and internal hemorrhage	
E. Internal poisoning or external poisoning	
F. Anaphylaxis	
G. Neck or back injury	
H. Chemical burns of the eye	
I. Heat stroke	
J. Penetrating/crushing chest wounds and pneumothorax	
II. Immediate evaluation and referral to treatment facility needed	
A. Internal bleeding	Immediately notify administrator. Get nurse or trained staff person to victim to evaluate condition. Initiate ambulance call, if necessary. Notify nurse if not with victim. Administrator or nurse notifies parent.
B. Coronary occlusion	
C. Dislocations and fractures	
D. Unconscious states	
E. Heat problems	
F. Major burns	
G. Drug overdose	
H. Head injury with loss of consciousness	
I. Penetrating eye injuries	
J. Seizure—cause unknown	
III. Medical consultation desirable within an hour	
A. Lacerations	Contact nurse or, in nurse's absence, administrator. Nurse or trained staff person assesses extent of injury. Notify parent and refer to medical facility if necessary.
B. Bites and stings—animal, insect, and snake—(without anaphylaxis)	
C. Burns with blisters	
D. Accidental loss of tooth	
E. Acute emotional state	
F. Moderate reactions to drugs	
G. High fever (above 103° F)	
H. Asthma/wheezing	
I. Nonpenetrating eye injury	

Table 25. — Triage Plan* (continued)

Category	Emergency Plan
IV. Attention by a trained staff person with school nurse/parent consultation needed	
A. Convulsion in known epileptic	Contact nurse or, in
B. Insulin reaction in diabetic	nurse's absence,
C. Severe abdominal pain	administrator. Nurse
D. Fever 100° to 103° F	or trained staff person assesses extent of in-
E. Sprains	jury. Notify parent and
F. Frostbite	refer to medical facility if necessary.
V. Minor injuries/illnesses—can be handled by a trained staff person following standard procedures	
A. Abrasions	Refer student to
B. Minor burns	trained staff person.
C. Nosebleeds	Child may remain in school.

*Adapted from American Academy of Pediatrics (Connecticut Chapter), Committee on School Health.[9]

Most schools operate emergency first aid procedures on accepted procedures sanctioned by Red Cross and nursing or physician groups. A physician's standing order may be utilized in certain instances. An example is given in Table 26.

In addition to specific procedures for specific situations and mechanisms to continually update training of school health and school staffs in first aid and CPR, there is a need to develop programs for monitoring and preventing school accidents, for making plans that may be specific to the needs of a particular child's condition or illness, and for educating students in self-care and management of minor accidents, abrasions, and minor trauma.

Problem Identification/Solving

Most school-age children are relatively physically healthy. The reasons that children visit school health rooms are generally due to minor trauma and self-limited illnesses. The major morbidities of school-age children and youth have to do with accidents, the effects of family violence and dysfunction, school

Table 26. — Example of a Physician's Standing Order

Standing order for anaphylaxis
A. An allergic reaction that may be triggered by an insect bite,
   a drug allergy, or a food allergy (rarely).
   1. For emergency medical service.
   2. For assistance/ambulance: DO NOT wait for symptoms to
      appear if sensitivity is known.

B. Assess patient for symptoms of shock/allergic reaction.
   1. Skin: cold to touch, may be clammy and moist, itching, hives
      may be present.
   2. Color: pale at first, then mottled or bluish.
   3. Respiration: may be wheezy, may cease.
   4. Pulse: rapid at first, may be faint.
   5. Blood pressure: low or unattainable.
   6. Other: restlessness, severe headache, severe nausea,
      vomiting and diarrhea, unconsciousness.

C. Monitor airway: give artificial respiration if indicated

D. Administer epinephrine per the following instructions if patient
   is in shock and no other physician order is available:
   1. First dose:
      Weight <40lb   0.1 mL Epinephrine 1:1000, SC
      Age 3 to 5 yr   0.2 mL Epinephrine 1:1000, SC
      Age 6 to 18 yr   0.3 mL Epinephrine 1:1000, SC
   2. Repeat the injection as above in 20 minutes if child's condition
      has not improved or has deteriorated and ambulance/EMT
      has not arrived and heart rate is below 180 beats/min.

E. Other measures to be used, depending on severity of symptoms:
   1. Lie patient down flat, elevate feet 8 to 12 inches unless leg is
      site of insect bite.
   2. For insect bites:
      a. If bee sting, look for the stinger and carefully scrape it out.
         Do not push, pull, squeeze with tweezers, or further embed
         the stinger.
      b. Apply constricting band (in Anakit) above insect bite if on
         arm or leg (between the bite and heart). Do not apply tightly;
         you should be able to slip an index finger under the band
         when in place.
      c. Keep affected part below level of victim's heart.
   3. Provide only enough insulation to keep patient from losing
      body heat.
      DO NOT ADD EXTRA HEAT.

learning and adjustment problems, and life-style decisions about healthful behaviors and habits.

However, a consistent 10% to 25% of parents indicate that their child has had some problem in school, and failures and dropout rates, especially among disadvantaged populations, are an alarming 40% to 50% in some areas. Ten percent to 15% of children have identifiable learning difficulties, and an additional 5% to 10% must deal with the long-term stress of a chronic medical problem or handicapping condition.[1-3] Children also get acquired immunodeficiency syndrome (AIDS), are physically and sexually abused, show the effects of maternal drug abuse, and have asthma, seizures, pneumonia, anemia, and other health problems. Many of these specific health problems are discussed in later chapters in this manual.

It is not difficult to discover problems, although school health programs have been criticized for expending personnel and time on relatively minor problems while ignoring serious long-term educational problems, such as low achievement. Table 27 lists some of the routine ways of problem identification utilized by many school health services.

An innovation in student-identified referral is the system of self-initiated care, piloted in several school districts.[4] This system permits free access to the health room whenever the child feels it is necessary. This free access, when coupled with health-care decision-making interactions in the health room and reinforced by classroom and home teaching programs, could be a way to begin to have children learn appropriate use of health care services.

If school health programs rely solely on referrals from others, they will miss potentially needy children. Routine review of frequent health room visitors is likely to detect problems needing intervention (see chapter 13). Similarly, those children with frequent repeated, short periods of absence or longer periods of not attending school need investigation. A mid-school year review of the lowest achieving students may reveal unknown medical, social, or cognitive problems that are impacting adversely the ability to benefit from the learning environment. Doing this routinely at the kindergarten, first, second, and third grades might go a long way in reducing later dropouts and casualties of the educational system.

Table 27. — Methods of Problem Identification

1. Student identified
  A. Visits to the health room
  B. Self-initiated care
  C. Systematic review of frequent health room visitors

2. Teacher referrals
  A. Health room referrals
  B. Result of regular teacher conferences
  C. Systematic review of students with achievement at lowest 10%

3. Parent referrals
  A. Calls and visits initiated by parent(s)
  B. Result of systematic review of annual survey of parents to detect previously unknown medical problems.

4. In-school referrals
  A. From administration
  B. From counselors, special education personnel, school pupil services teams, absenteeism offices

5. Out-of-school referrals
  A. For information/follow-up/management of students who are clients, patients of community sources of care (health and mental health)
  B. Social services referrals

6. From review of school records
  A. Cumulative health record review of new students
  B. Review of school health records

Problem Resolution

The school health service cannot resolve or solve students' problems by itself. Cooperative and collaborative efforts with parents, teachers, counselors, psychologists, social workers, physicians, lawyers, administrators, caseworkers, and speech and language specialists may be necessary. Many times problems cannot be completely resolved. A system should be in place to facilitate follow-up and tracking of problems once they are identified. Thus, it makes no sense to dutifully record that a referral for a failed vision test was sent to the child's parents, if there is no reminder or "tickler" system in place to check on the outcome

Table 28. — Methods of Tracking Problems

1. Health room encounter forms/log.
2. SOAP forms (see text).
3. Referral form with copy to reminder file.
4. Quarterly or bimonthly review of incomplete referrals.
5. Assign outreach worker to assist families in accessing systems of care.

of that referral. A school health service might wish to set criteria for minimum standards of allowable time to elapse for completion of a straightforward referral for eyeglasses or treatment for a skin infection. Such criteria not only will set standards but will assist in evaluation of the quality of services provided and point out areas of deficiency in systems of care that need to be addressed.

Many school health rooms utilize a log or form for recording the child's name, date of the visit, reason for visit, and disposition. Such data may be useful for later tracking of frequent visitors, as well as for documenting common problems that present to the health room (Table 28). Once the most common problems are identified, simple protocols can be developed for efficient handling and disposition. These protocols can be used by aides under the direction of the nurse, which frees the nurse to attend to more involved problems or those requiring more professional expertise. For problems that cannot be capsulized in several word phrases, the SOAP format has been utilized in some services. This notation permits recording, by problem list, for each problem: Subjective (historical) data; Objective (examination, observation) data; along with an Assessment of the nature of the problem; and a Plan for what is to be done. Included in each plan should be the time and manner in which follow-up of the problem will be accomplished. This frequently involves education of school staff, including teachers, principals, and others, regarding management issues. Since follow-up is time consuming, the service may wish to specify the types of problems for which follow-up might be the most productive. Means also exist for developing formats, checklists, and automated processing of this information to ease the burden of paperwork on busy school health professionals.

Table 29. — Categories of Problem Resolution

1. Problem unresolved, follow-up indicated.
2. Problem unresolved, work initiated, in progress.
3. Problem resolved, temporarily, follow-up indicated.
4. Problem resolved, permanently.
5. Status of problem unknown.

Table 29 gives a simple classification system for codifying the status of referrals or problems identified. Each unit (eg, school building) should routinely review the status of all active problems. A year-end review will indicate one measure of program effectiveness and will flag problems that need to be followed up over the summer or reinvestigated during the next school year.

Since many students' problems involve families, and families often have more than one child in a given school district, there may be a need to organize intervention and services on a family basis, not on an individual or multiple child basis. This will require designation across schools of one health team member taking the lead with a given family in order to coordinate the services required and to reduce duplication and confusion for the family. Several social experiments are taking place in which a school catchment area (elementary-middle-secondary) becomes the focus for a cooperative agency approach to serving the needs of the families in that area. These experiments require policy and procedural changes in all cooperating agencies in order to facilitate resolution of the multiple problems besetting many families. The school health service can be a key link in facilitating such coordinated programs and services.

Provision of Mandated and Optional Screening Procedures

Health screening is the process of using a relatively simple test to sort a population into those who do or do not have a particular health problem. Health screening in schools became popular in the 1950s and 1960s as an efficient means of detecting health problems in schoolchildren without having to do a complete examination on all children. Unfortunately, screening programs are themselves subject to a number of inefficiencies that can significantly reduce or eliminate their utility. The value of a particular screening program should be regularly reassessed to ensure that it is worth the valuable school resources that are being devoted to it. Table 30 shows eight specific criteria that are essential features of a successful screening program. Failure in any one of these criteria is likely to reduce or eliminate the benefit of the program.

Immunizations: The laws of each state will determine when and how schools will document student compliance with immunization requirements. Schools usually are required to review student records to identify those not in compliance with the law, setting a deadline when proper documentation must be produced to remain in school.

Vision: The most significant visual abnormalities develop before or around the time of school entry. These include strabismus, hyperopia, and amblyopia. Infantile esotropia and exotropia are the most common forms of strabismus, but they usually occur early in life and should be detected and treated well before school begins. Accommodative esotropia is the result of excessive ocular convergence in farsighted children when they accommodate for near vision. This occurs most commonly in toddlers but may arise as late as age 7 years. Mild hyperopia is normal in children up to age 7 years and should not be confused with more severe hyperopia of +2.5 diopters or more, which may be progressive and also lead to accommodative esotropia. Amblyopia is the progressive loss of visual acuity in one eye, usually as a result of strabismus or a unilateral refractive error. If left untreated in children under age 7 years, the acuity loss frequently will become permanent.

Most of these visual problems should be detected well before kindergarten, but some may develop during the first two years of school. Visual screening for strabismus, hyperopia, and amblyopia should be done just prior to or early in kindergarten to identify those children whose problems have gone undetected in the preschool years. Further testing late in first grade would pick up problems that had developed during the first two years of school. Distant visual acuity testing of each eye separately is fairly sensitive and specific for these problems, but testing with the Titmus Stereo Fly test and the cover, uncover test improves

Table 30. — Criteria for a Successful Screening Program

Disease: Undetected cases of the disease must be common (high prevalence), or new cases must occur frequently (high incidence). The disease must be associated with adverse consequences, either physical or psychologic (morbidity).

Treatment: Treatment must be available that will effectively prevent or reduce the morbidity from the disease. There must be some benefit from this treatment before the disease would have become obvious without screening; that is, there must be an early intervention benefit.

Screening test: The ideal test detects all subjects who have the disease (high sensitivity) and correctly identifies all who do not (high specificity). Low sensitivity results in missed cases (false-negative results), and low specificity yields many false-positive results. Another measure of effectiveness is the positive predictive value, or the number of true positive results divided by the total number who fail the test. A good test is simple, brief, and acceptable to the person being screened. The test must be reliable, that is, repeated testing will yield the same results.

Screener: The screener must be well trained; experience is important, particularly if judgments must be made.

Target population: To reduce inefficiency, the screening should be focused on groups in which the undetected disease is most prevalent or in which early intervention will be most beneficial.

Referral and treatment: All those with a positive screening test must receive a more definitive evaluation and, if indicated, appropriate treatment. The ultimate measure of effectiveness is the reduction in morbidity that results from early intervention among those with positive screening test results. This depends on the successful treatment of those in need.

Cost/benefit ratio: Cost includes all expenses of screening, referral, and treatment, including administrative costs and the cost plus anxiety that result from false-positive results. The benefit is the reduction in morbidity from early intervention among those with true-positive results who are in need of treatment. This benefit is hard to quantify in dollars and may vary among communities. Greater efficiency at any level will improve this ratio.

Program maintenance: Need for improvements in program efficiency is determined by periodic review of research on the value of each screening program and an assessment of program effectiveness within the community. Local review also allows community leaders to make reasonable decisions as to the allocation of limited resources for screening. Local politicians can also be influenced to increase those resources when it can be shown that monies are being spent wisely.

the detection of strabismus. Significant hyperopia is best detected by testing distant vision through a +1.5 diopter lens and failing all those who *can* read the 20/30 or 20/20 line correctly.

The most common visual abnormality that develops during the school years is myopia. Binocular myopia of 20/70 or worse rises in prevalence from 1% in 6 year olds to 20% at age 16 years. This defect can be detected by a simple Snellen chart examination. Peckham et al. studied myopic 11 year olds and found that they academically outperformed their normal-sighted peers even before their myopia had been detected, suggesting that failure at early detection of this problem might not adversely influence school performance.[5] Snellen chart testing should be done two or three times in elementary and middle school. High school students usually are tested by the motor vehicle department, and school vision screening can be reserved for referrals, or to be sure that youth having school problems do not have untreated vision problems.

Hearing Screening: Hearing problems in the school-age child can be divided into two categories: (1) sensory neural hearing loss, and (2) conductive hearing loss. Sensory neural hearing loss has its origins either before birth or as a result of subsequent illness or injury. Although all such sensory neural hearing loss should be detected prior to school entry through regular health maintenance, some children may reach school without this condition being diagnosed. Although their numbers should be very small, one of the purposes of hearing screening at school entry would be to identify these few children. However, one of the difficulties is distinguishing these children from children with the far more common conductive hearing loss.

At any one time, between 5% and 7% of children aged 5 to 8 years will have a 25 dB hearing loss.[6] This prevalence decreases significantly with age. The vast majority of these are the consequences of middle ear effusion, which will resolve spontaneously over a period of a few months. Fluid in the middle ear is a very common consequence of respiratory or middle ear infections and may affect as many as 50% of normal 5- to 8-year-old children.[6] Few of these children have any significant hearing loss.

Children found to have sensory neural hearing loss need a thorough evaluation and institution of an appropriate treatment. It is somewhat less clear what needs to be done for those children whose persistent hearing loss is due to middle ear fluid. Close follow-up with treatment with antibiotics and possible consideration of tympanotomy tubes is appropriate. School personnel need to monitor the follow-up of those children referred for hearing test failure, to ensure that they receive a further, more definitive evaluation and appropriate treatment. Only a small number of those referred ultimately should receive tympanotomy tubes, and most would agree at this time that tonsillectomy and adenoidectomy are not appropriate treatments for this problem.

Fluid in the middle ear can be detected reliably using tympanometry. However, the vast majority of children who fail tympanometry have normal hearing and are not in need of any treatment. This is therefore inappropriate for mass screening and is not a substitute for pure tone audiometry.

It is recommended that at, or soon after, school entry, children whose hearing has not been tested during a recent medical examination should be screened with pure-tone audiometry at 25 dB over at least three frequencies. Those who fail should be retested 6 to 12 weeks later, and, if the numbers of failure remain large, a third screening might be carried out 6 weeks following the second. All those who fail these tests should be referred, and the outcomes of the referrals should be monitored to ensure proper follow-up without overtreatment. Evaluation will include an adequate examination of the ears and referral for appropriate treatment, when indicated.[6,7]

Scoliosis: Some degree of lateral curvature of the spine occurs in 1% to 5% of children in early adolescence. However, the prevalence of scoliosis in need of bracing or surgery is found in only 5 per 1,000 girls and 0.5 per 1,000 boys in adolescence. The purpose of screening for scoliosis is to identify those with significant curvature who would benefit by wearing a brace to prevent progression of the curvature, and thus avoid surgical intervention. Randomized controlled trials testing the efficacy of bracing have yet to be carried out, and some recent studies have suggested that many curves in the 20- to 35-degree range do not progress significantly with or without a brace. Some also progress despite bracing. Therefore, the number who benefit by early detection and bracing, and thus avoid surgery, may indeed be very low.[6,7]

If screening is carried out, the target population should be girls near the beginning of puberty, ie, fifth or sixth grade. Only then will the condition be detected before progression has proceeded during the growth spurt. Those with scoliosis detected later are least likely to benefit from bracing. Because the forward bending test requires experience in judgment, those persons carrying out the test should be carefully trained and screen a large enough number of children to gain adequate experience. A second screening by an experienced clinician will significantly reduce overreferrals.

New Screening Programs: School systems are asked to consider new forms of screening programs on a regular basis. Blood pressure, cholesterol, and sickle cell disease are but a few examples. Proposals for new screening programs are frequently the result of the development of some new technologies that gain political support through influential members of the community. The school health committee should carefully review such proposals using the eight criteria in Table 30 to determine the scientific basis and the efficacy of screening.[6,7] Health resources are very limited in the school system. Therefore, the value of every screening test should be weighed carefully against the valuable resources required to effectively carry out the program. The schools must carefully determine their priorities for the use of those limited resources.

Relation of School Health Services to Health Education/Health Promotion Programs

In most schools, there is a wide schism between health services and health education. This is often due to separate administrative and professional views of responsibilities and strengths. Many individual teachers and nurses have overcome this natural schism and cooperated to provide interesting and relevant health instruction to students on an individual and group basis. However, there are very few examples of system-wide, planned integration of health services with the health curriculum, or other related curriculum offerings in the school.

Several possible opportunities present themselves for consideration for joint program development. One principle of health instruction involves opportunities to practice a health behavior. The previous example of a child-initiated care system would permit classroom discussion of methods of decision making regarding seeking health services, as well as principles of self-care and coping and managing daily stresses that might result in a tension (or "math") headache or stomachache.

The school health service might be involved or even coordinate a community effort in sexuality education. Parents and others in the community may respond better to efforts in education in this area if health professionals as well as educators are visible participants. The demonstration to students of the various roles and personal counseling availability of the school nurse may facilitate additional health counseling that might be needed by a student in the future.

School nutrition programs and school physical activity programs are increasingly oriented toward health objectives. The school health service also could provide invaluable consultation to these efforts.

School Health Records

In many states, the school health record is considered part of the pupil's cumulative record, and some information is included in the mandated permanent record. This record may contain:
1. Information identifying the pupil (name, birth date, sex).
2. Month, day, and year of mandatory immunizations.
3. Health information relevant to the pupil's education or physical exercise program.
4. Medically related elements of physical, developmental, emotional, or behavioral problems that may be used in evaluating pupils for special education.
5. Recommendations for referral and follow-up.
6. Clinical information, when appropriate (medical history, relevant positive and negative physical findings, growth charts, medications taken regularly, and treatment plans).
7. Copies of reports of serious school injuries.
8. Copies or notation of child abuse reports.
9. Record of screening test results.

Information to be used in emergencies is frequently considered part of the school health record. However, this information should be kept separately, filed in the school office where it is available to all school personnel, and updated annually. In schools with a high degree of transiency, this information should be updated twice a year. Emergency information should include:

1. The pupil's name, birth date, and sex.
2. Parents, guardians, or adult(s) with whom the child resides, their names, addresses, home and office telephone numbers, and places of employment.
3. The name, address, and telephone number of a relative or neighbor who may be called in an emergency.
4. The name, address, and telephone number of the pupil's pediatrician and dentist.
5. A letter stating parental consent for treatment at a local emergency hospital if parents, legal guardian, or personal physician cannot be reached.

Unless school health records are reviewed periodically, they may lose their relevance and value. School health records should be reviewed annually, particularly those of students with identified health problems. All data relevant to diagnosis and treatment should be recorded.

Confidentiality

Information in school records is easily misused. Private information about pupils and families or inaccurate, prejudicial, and/or inappropriate statements can be extremely damaging in the wrong hands.

School personnel may be inhibited, through fear of violating confidentiality, about completely and accurately recording information that could be of value to other persons working with a student. It is becoming increasingly more common in the United States to copy recorded information, and copies of school records may be requested by colleges, employers, the military, and law enforcement agencies.

Laws requiring parental or student consent for release of records may give false assurance that confidentiality is maintained. Consent to release information may constitute a blanket release rather than a strictly limited one. Once released, information can be stored indefinitely in data banks such as those maintained by health insurers or state government registries of drug abusers, psychiatric hospitals, and social agency contacts. Long-term information storage (and accessibility by unknown persons) can adversely affect employment, eligibility for insurance, and other activities.

School health records, as well as written records provided by a physician to elementary and secondary schools receiving federal funds, are required by federal law to be open to inspection by parents and can be subpoenaed as court evidence. Under the provisions of the Educational Rights and Privacy Act, parents (or students on reaching 18 years or older or in postsecondary school) may:

1. Review their child's (or their own) educational records on request.
2. Challenge the accuracy of any entry, seek its correction or expungement, or, barring this, insert their own rebuttal statement.
3. Have sole authority to release records to a third party for a stipulated purpose.

School board members and others (particularly federal funding officials) may have access to school records, without parental or student consent, to determine funding eligibility, *but not for individual student review.*

Written records are subject to misinterpretation, and school personnel or health professionals cannot rectify inappropriate interpretations if they do not know who will be reading the records or their reasons for doing so. Data entered on official school health records or sent to schools by health care providers should be factual and selected with concern for the possible consequences of the record's being made available to the pupil, the parents, or to persons outside the school. For example, an educational diagnosis of "emotionally disturbed," "handicapped," or "mentally retarded," may affect later graduate school acceptance.

The fact that the school health record is open to inspection by parents may create another area of concern. Persons working with problem families sometimes make observations that are pertinent to a particular situation but may not be appreciated by family members, eg, suspected neglect or emotional or physical abuse. This information is best kept on informal notes (sometimes called "nurses' notes") not considered part of the pupil's school health record. Such notes are classified as memory aids developed by an individual for the sole purpose of remembering pertinent facts from discussion, records, or observation. They should not be available or revealed to any other person and should be stored in a location accessible only to the writer. Informal notes can include a pupil's name, birth date, sex, grade, and subjective observations.

Because of the health record's value to various members of the school staff, a workable means for sharing school health records without violating confidentiality must be established. At times, both school and private health professionals may need access to records kept by other school professionals (eg, social workers, psychologists, and teachers); in turn, these other professionals may need to inspect school health records. By law, health records are not available for inspection by third parties without the permission of parents or eligible pupils. They should be kept in locked files. Persons within the school system using health records should be informed of their confidential nature. Each school district should have written rules governing accessibility of school records in conformity with existing privacy regulations.

Data Processing Systems

In recent years, computer data processing systems have been increasingly used in schools. This represents an advantage to school health programs. Computers can be programmed to call attention to children with incomplete immunization records, physical growth deviations, specific health problems, high absence rates, academic failure, or other factors associated with health problems. Computers have been used to compile monthly or annual statistical reports, to make classroom printouts of nurses' worksheets, and to print immunization records on gummed labels to attach to health records.

A data processing system for health services programs alone probably would not be cost-effective. Including health services programs in the overall district data processing system, however, has proved both time efficient and cost-effective.

References

1. Kaufman P, Frase MJ. Dropout rates in the United States: 1989. *Resources in Education*. March, 1990. (ERIC: ED 325561)

2. The Annie E. Casey Foundation, Center for the Study of Social Policy. *Kids Count Data Book*. Washington, DC: Center for the Study of Social Policy; 1992

3. Chavez EL, Edwards R, Oetting ER. Mexican American and white American school dropouts' drug use, health status, and involvement in violence. *Public Health Rep.* 1989;104:594-604

4. Lewis CE, Lewis MA, Lorimer A, Palmer BB. Child-initiated care: the use of school nursing services by children in an "adult-free" system. *Pediatrics.* 1977;60:499-507

5. Peckham CS, Gardiner PA, Goldstein H. Acquired myopia in 11-year-old children. *Br Med J.* 1977;1:542-544

6. Cross AW. Health screening schools: part I. *J Pediatr.* 1985; 107(4):487

7. Cross AW. Health screening schools: part II. *J Pediatr.* 1985; 107(5):653

8. Nader PR. A pediatrician's primer for school health activities. *Pediatr Rev.* 1982;4:82-92

9. American Academy of Pediatrics (Connecticut Chapter), Committee on School Health. *Providing Emergency Medical Care to Students in Connecticut Public Schools.* Madison, CT: American Academy of Pediatrics (Connecticut Chapter); 1984

CHAPTER 8

SCHOOL HEALTH EDUCATION

Health education has been defined as the lifelong process by which individuals acquire knowledge, attitudes, and behaviors that promote health and foster wise decisions for solving personal, family, and community health problems. Health education begins with parental interaction with an infant. Attitudes and health practices are learned early in childhood as parents act as models of behavior. Pediatricians can capitalize on this naturally occurring phenomenon by using periodic health evaluations for health instruction of parents.

Formal health education is appropriately begun in child care programs and continued through kindergarten and secondary school. Physicians can make a significant contribution to the health of the community by assuring that a planned sequential and comprehensive course of study in health education has been initiated in the public schools and, ideally, in private schools.

Educators, health professionals, and three presidential commissions have supported the need for health education as a necessary and distinct subject within the school curricula.[1] According to data from *School Health in America*, a survey of state policies to protect and improve the health of students, 31 states and the District of Columbia require that health education be taught at sometime during kindergarten through 12th grade; 13 other states require a combination of physical education and health education.[2]

Health Education Components

As defined by the National Professional School Health Education Organizations,[3] a comprehensive health education program should include:

1. A planned, sequential prekindergarten to 12th grade curriculum based on students' needs and current health concepts and societal issues.
2. Instruction intended to motivate health maintenance and promote wellness and not merely to prevent disease or disability.

3. Activities to develop decision-making skills and individual responsibility for one's own health.

4. Opportunities for students to develop and demonstrate health-related knowledge, attitudes, and practices.

5. Integration of the physical, mental, emotional, and social dimensions of health as the basis for study of 10 content areas including the following: (1) community health, (2) consumer health, (3) environmental health, (4) family life, (5) growth and development, (6) nutritional health, (7) personal health, (8) prevention and control of disease and disorder, (9) safety and accident prevention, and (10) substance use and abuse.

According to the most current information available, the topics most frequently mandated by state policy are drugs and alcohol abuse prevention, tobacco-use prevention, and nutrition.[2]

Teaching Health Education

There are three basic opportunities for teaching health education:

1. *Direct instruction*, which involves the organization, coordination, and presentation of material to students in an organized course in health education.

2. *Integrated instruction*, which involves the organization, coordination, and presentation of material to students in the course of study of subjects other than health education. Ideally, both direct and integrated instruction occurs, particularly in biology, social science, and home economics classes.

3. *Incidental classroom health education*, which is a personalized and spontaneous method through which health issues are discussed in response to students' questions or educators' initiatives. Random incidental instruction occurs at a "teachable moment." Planned incidental instruction can occur during a community immunization program, a clinic visit, or school club meetings in which the students become personally involved in a learning experience.

Health Education Content

Determining the content for a health instruction program may be based on state mandate or locally developed curriculum. It always should be based on the developmental and health education needs of students. Determining the health education needs of students has been facilitated by the discovery that the cause of premature morbidity and mortality can be traced to the following four major factors: (1) heredity (20%); (2) environmental factors (20%); (3) health care delivery system (10%); and (4) personal life-style (50%).[4] Because life-style plays a critical role in health, helping individuals adopt a health enhancing lifestyle should contribute significantly to reducing premature illness and death.

Specific behaviors that would contribute to reducing premature illness and death were identified in 1980 by a national public/private initiative entitled *Promoting Health, Preventing Disease: Objectives for the Nation*. Of the 226 specific objectives that should be the target of all health promotion efforts, a third focus directly or indirectly on children and youth.[5] Public schools can contribute significantly to the attainment of these national objectives through the health education course of study. Specific educational strategies for health education as well as other disciplines within the school are outlined in a document titled *Achieving the 1990 Health Objectives for the Nation: Agenda for the School*, which is available from the American School Health Association (see Resource Agencies listing at the end of this chapter).

In 1990, a new set of objectives, which once again emerged from a nationwide consensus development, was published by the US Public Health Service.[6] Those objectives that target children and youth can, once again, be used by curriculum planners as the basis for the content of the course of study in health. Health instruction will play a critical role in meeting our nation's health objectives for the year 2000 in specific target areas, such as nutrition, physical fitness, tobacco use, alcohol and drug use, sexual behavior, and violent and abusive behavior.

Health Education Curriculum Materials

Resources for quality school health programs are many and varied. Suppliers include private companies, nonprofit organizations, federal agencies, and professional associations. A number of national curriculums are used extensively. Several of the more common ones include:

1. Growing Healthy: Primary Grades Health Curriculum Project (kindergarten through 3rd grade) and the School Health Curriculum Project (fourth through seventh grades). The School Health Curriculum Project is designed to teach students that the body is each person's greatest natural resource, and that its well-being is affected by personal choices made throughout life. Address: School Health Programs, National Center for Health Education, 30 E 29th St, New York, NY 10016. Phone: 212/689-1886.

2. The Michigan Model (kindergarten through 8th grade): The model consists of 40 lessons at each level, focusing on the 10 topical areas of health. Features of the curriculum are the parent component and a series of take-home worksheets that reinforce classroom instruction. Address: Michigan Department of Public Health, Division of Health Education, 3500 N Logan, Lansing, MI 48909. Phone: 517/335-8390.

3. Know Your Body (1st through 8th grades): This promotes wellness by making health education personal and individually relevant. Students are taught the significance of personalized health data, such as blood pressure, pulse, height, and weight measurements, and are encouraged to monitor their own health behavior patterns. Address: American Health Foundation, 320 E 43rd St, New York, NY 10017. Phone: 212/953-1900.

4. The Teenage Health Teaching Modules (8th through 12th grades): Provides adolescents with knowledge and skills that enable them to act responsibly toward their health now and in the future. The curriculum features health skills, self-assessment, communication, decision making, health advocacy, and health self-management. Address: Education Development Center, 55 N Chapel St, Newton, MA 02160. Phone: 617/969-7100.

5. Quest (8th through 12th grades): Designed to assist pupils and their parents in developing the skills needed to communicate more efficiently with themselves and others, with an emphasis on self-esteem and problem solving. The core

of the program is its "skills for living" curriculum and the companion book for students. Its theme is "you are somebody special." Address: Quest International, 537 Jones Rd, Granville, OH 43023. Phone: 614/587-2800.

Many national voluntary health organizations have superb health educational materials, curricula, special projects, films, and videos. A listing of the available material from the voluntary associations can be found in a publication titled *Coalition Index: A Guide of School Health Education Material*, which is available from the American School Health Association (listed in Resource Agencies at the end of this chapter).

The federal government operates a number of clearinghouses and information centers, most of which focus on a particular topic, such as food and nutrition or smoking and health. Their services vary but may include publications, referrals, or answers to consumer inquiries. There are more than 35 such government clearinghouses. A listing of these agencies, their services, and phone numbers can be obtained through the US Department of Health and Human Services' National Health Information Center.

Integrating School and Community Programming

A health education curriculum can be enhanced by integrating programming with that of the community. There are a number of ways in which this can be accomplished:

1. Bring community resources into the classroom. (Physicians can be invited to discuss various health issues that correspond to instructional units. In addition, they can provide in-service training to school staff and serve on curriculum committees planning health instruction.)
2. Send students into the community to participate in health service projects. (Students might volunteer at the local hospital, blood bank, or hospice.)
3. Take the classroom into the community via field trips. (Visits to hospitals, clinics, ecological organizations, and voluntary health agencies could be arranged.)
4. Engage health and community agencies in the joint planning and delivery of events. (There are a number of national health observances, such as American Heart Month, that

could become the focus for events planned by the school and the community.)

5. Initiate a school-community interagency network to help prioritize approaches to health education in the school. (A coalition of agencies and individuals could be formed to address such critical issues as preventing the spread of the human immunodeficiency virus [HIV] infection in adolescent populations, teen pregnancy, violence, suicide, or drug abuse.)

Effectiveness of School Health Education

It has been demonstrated that school-based health education programs improve targeted health knowledge, attitudes, and skills, and inconsistently improve targeted health behaviors. The effectiveness of interventions in changing behaviors is dependent on specificity and quality of the intervention, sufficient time for the intervention, parental or peer support for the targeted behavior, degree of implementation, and reinforcement of the intervention over time.[7] A landmark study in the field of school health, the School Health Education Evaluation, provided evidence that the key factors related to a successful program are: (1) teacher fidelity to curriculum, (2) amount of time students are exposed to the curriculum, and (3) extent to which that exposure is accumulated year to year.[8] In this three-year study, which compared four different health instruction programs for grades 4 through 7 and involved 1,071 classrooms in 20 states, it was found that success is predicated on administrative support and commitment, as well as adequately prepared and motivated teachers.[9]

Recent results from an evaluation of Teenage Health Teaching Modules (THTM) affirmed that teachers trained before teaching the THTM curriculum implemented it with greater fidelity and had greater positive effects on the health knowledge and attitudes of their students when compared to teachers who received no in-service training.[10]

Health Education Providers

While the teacher responsible for health education teaching serves as a primary source of health instruction, it is important to recognize that the classroom is only one element of a health education program. Health education providers for school-age children also include physicians, nurses, dentists, counselors, psychologists, and other health care providers. By virtue of their individual contact with students, these providers interact with students in situations ideal for providing new information and reinforcing the instructional process that occurs in the classroom. One of the essential components of a health education program is the participation of qualified personnel. Health care providers can help ensure quality health education by supporting a planned course of study and planned initiatives that target specific high risk behaviors. Further, health service providers can supplement classroom instruction during local initiatives that correspond to national health observances and during clinic visits.

Health Educators

Certification requirements for teachers are established by state certifying agencies. Typically, different standards are established for teachers in elementary and secondary education. In many states specific certification in health education is available, but not mandated by law. It also is often available either as a separate health certificate or in combination with physical education.

In 1989, the National Task Force on the Preparation and Practice of Health Educators established a process for credentialing health educators. The credentialing process, spearheaded by health education professionals, identified the role competencies of the entry-level health educator. These include: (1) assessing individual and community needs for health education, (2) planning effective health education programs, (3) implementing health education programs, (4) evaluating effectiveness of health education programs, (5) coordinating provision of health education services, (6) acting as a resource person in health education, and (7) communicating health and health education needs, concerns, and resources.[11]

It remains unclear how this credentialing process will influence the state certification process for health education teachers. The credentialing process certifies the individual's attainment of the competencies described above, and could serve as an additional requirement for state certification to teach health education.

Because of the critical need, more health education principles and methods should be included in requirements for certification of *all* teachers, elementary through high school.

Personal Physicians

Pediatricians can incorporate health education into patient visits by providing information about causes, mechanisms, and consequences of health problems to patients and their parents. Pediatricians and other health providers can also play an important role as medical advisors, members of school health committees, consultants to health education curriculum committees, occasional classroom teachers, and spokespersons in the community, to stimulate interest in comprehensive health education.

Comprehensive School Health Education

The primary goal of health education, one component of a comprehensive school health program, is to provide students with the knowledge, skills, and behaviors to choose a health-enhancing life-style. While instruction plays a primary role in determining the behaviors students incorporate into their life-style, it is important to recognize that a healthy life-style is not achieved through individual instruction alone. Instead, the behaviors that contribute to one's life-style are a result of a complex interplay of psychological, social, intellectual, and physical factors. Thus, a health promotion model that solicits environmental support for healthy behaviors through policy mandates, environmental changes, direct intervention, media, access and availability of health services, parental support, and peer involvement is more likely to achieve and maintain individual behaviors that contribute to a healthy life-style than is a program that relies entirely on health instruction.[12]

Using multiple strategies extends and reinforces the impact of the instruction that occurs in the classroom. For example, nutritional content incorporated into the kindergarten through 12th grade health education course of study is reinforced if the school has a policy that candy will not be used as a fundraiser, sold at lunchtime, or be available in vending machines located in the school. A variety of media channels are useful in reinforcing nutritional messages including: (1) messages on the bulletin boards that students can view from the cafeteria line, (2) labels showing the nutritional content of cafeteria choices, (3) use of "table tents" with nutritional messages, and (4) inclusion of brief nutritional messages in cafeteria menus that are sent to student's homes or published in the local newspaper.

Multidisciplinary Effort

The establishment of a comprehensive health education program is best accomplished by an interdisciplinary team composed of the health teacher, the school nurse, the physical education teacher, the guidance counselor, the administrator, and teachers. This school team can be enhanced by active participation of parents, pediatricians, and other professionals from the community. The team can coordinate the development and implementation of the curriculum, policy mandates, direct intervention, environmental changes, social support, and peer involvement. Further, parents, physicians, and other professionals can assist the school in the integration of school and community programming.

Resource Agencies Involved in Health Education

American Academy of Pediatrics
PO Box 927
141 Northwest Point Blvd
Elk Grove Village, IL 60009-0927
708/228-5005

American Alliance for Health, Physical Education, Recreation, and Dance (AAHPERD)
1900 Association Dr
Reston, VA 22091
703/476-3461

American Association of School Administrators
1801 N Moore St
Arlington, VA 22209
703/528-0700

American Cancer Society
19 W 56th St
New York, NY 10019
212/586-8700

American Dental Association
211 E Chicago Ave
Chicago, IL 60611
312/440-2500

American Heart Association
7320 Greenville Ave
Dallas, TX 75231
214/706-1446

American Lung Association
1740 Broadway
New York, NY 10019
212/315-8700

American Medical Association
Department of Health Education
515 N State St
Chicago, IL 60610
312/464-4690

American Public Health Association
1015 15th St NW
Washington, DC 20005
202/789-5600

American School Health Association
PO Box 708
Kent, OH 44240
216/678-1601

Association for the Advancement of Health Education
1900 Association Dr
Reston, VA 22091
703/476-3437

Centers for Disease Control and Prevention
Bureau of Health Education
1600 Clifton Rd NE
Atlanta, GA 30333
404/639-3311

National Association of State Boards of Education
1012 Cameron St
Alexandria, VA 22314
703/684-4000

National Cancer Institute
9000 Rocksville Pike
Bethesda, MD 20892
301/496-1771

National PTA
Health Education Project
700 North Rush St
Chicago, IL 60611-2571
312/787-0977

National School Board Association
1680 Duke St
Alexandria, VA 22314
703/838-6722

US Department of Education
400 Maryland Ave SW
Washington, DC 20202
202/708-5366

References

1. Coalition of National Health Education Organizations. The limitations to excellence in education. *J Sch Health*. 1984;54(7):256-257

2. Lovato CY, Allensworth DD, Chan M. *School Health in America: An Assessment of State Policies to Protect and Improve the Health of Students*. 5th ed. Kent, OH: American School Health Association; 1989

3. National Professional School Health Education Organizations. Comprehensive school health education. *J Sch Health*. 1984; 54(8):312-315

4. US Department of Health, Education and Welfare. *Healthy People: The Surgeon General's Report on Health Promotion and Disease Prevention*. Rockville, MD: DHEW (PHS) Publication No. 79-55071. 1979

5. Iverson DC, Kolbe LJ. Evaluation of the national disease prevention and health promotion strategy: establishing a role for the schools. *J Sch Health*. 1983;53(5):294-302

6. US Department of Health and Human Services. *Healthy People 2000: National Health Promotion and Disease Prevention Objectives.* (conference edition). 1990

7. Kolbe LJ. Why school health education? An empirical point of view. *Health Education.* April–May 1985:116-120

8. Connell DB, Turner RR, Mason EF. Summary of findings of the School Health Education Evaluation: health promotion effectiveness, implementation, and costs. *J Sch Health.* 1985;55(8):316-321

9. Fors SW, Doster ME. School health education evaluation. Implication of results: factors for success. *J Sch Health.* 1985;55(8):332-334

10. Gold RS, Parcel GS, Walberg HJ, Luepker RV, Portnoy B, Stone EJ. Summary and conclusions of the THTM evaluation: the expert work group perspective. *J Sch Health.* 1991;61(1):39-42

11. National Task Force on the Preparation and Practice of Health Educators. *A Framework for the Development of Competency-Based Curricula for Entry Level Health Educators.* New York, NY: National Task Force on the Preparation and Practice of Health Educators, Inc. 1985

12. Allensworth DD, Kolbe LJ. The comprehensive school health program: exploring an expanded concept. *J Sch Health.* 1987;57(10);409-412

Suggested Reading

American School Health Association: Healthy People 2000, National Health Promotion and Disease Prevention Objectives and Healthy Schools. *J Sch Health.* 1991;61(7):292-330

CHAPTER 9

PROVIDING FOR A HEALTHFUL SCHOOL ENVIRONMENT

Positive reinforcement for healthy behaviors based on acquired knowledge, skills, and values is a powerful method to improve health outcomes in children and youth. The school environment is rich with opportunities to implement such a model. A school's curriculum, faculty, physical plant, and support services each offer opportunities to have impact on students.

A healthful school environment, by our definition, is one that protects students and staff against immediate injury or disease and promotes prevention activities and attitudes against known risk factors that might lead to future disease or disability.

A healthful school environment emphasizes disease prevention and health promotion for both students and staff. Subject areas that especially lend themselves to creating a healthful environment include sound nutrition, regular physical fitness, safe work and play habits and sites, recognition and management of stress, periodic medical and dental health maintenance and practices, and strategies to avoid use of harmful substances (ie, tobacco, alcohol, drugs).

A Strategy for Creating a Healthful School Environment

Because most school districts have a full cup and little time or energy to take on new projects related to health, the most common opportunity to improve the school health environment will occur around a crisis, a serious accidental injury, a sudden death (ie, suicide or homicide), or a school bus accident. Other opportunities may occur as a result of interest in the release of local or national studies or reports (eg, Fitness in the Schools, Obesity in Adolescents), as a result of an effort in another segment of the community that relates directly to children and youth (ie, drug abuse prevention programs), or during the creation of a school district's 5- or 10-year plan.

At these times, faculty and/or administrative staff may solicit or be receptive to suggestions. First, the problem must clearly be identified: characterized by frequency, severity, and both direct and indirect consequences considered. The initial inquiry may provide detail, or it may be vague. For instance, "We seem to have too many accidents on our playground. Is it safe?" However, if there is only an enhanced general interest, such as in preventing drug and alcohol problems, further assessment may be needed to define the perceived problem and further characterize its nature.

If it is possible, when generating potential solutions, identify interventions and approaches used in other districts for which there is some evidence of effectiveness. If there hasn't been any experience locally or regionally, it might be wise to review the *Journal of School Health* for articles on such interventions. Last, try to ensure some form of monitoring or follow-up that will provide the district with results and progress or lack thereof. This step is particularly important in providing credibility to the community and school decision makers to be able to continue such interventions in the future.

Opportunities in the School Environment to Impact on Health

Teachers as Role Models for Health

Few persons do not remember the powerful influence classroom teachers had on our lives in early school years. If these influences were positive, we continued to identify with and emulate our teachers throughout our school years. School districts are in a unique position to influence the health of the faculty and, thus, the role models provided to students. In addition, benefits that accrue to the district are increased employee retention, decreased absenteeism, and enhanced performance. Districts can hold health fairs, faculty retreats, and seminars to increase their faculty's understanding of the risk factors that affect health (ie, diet/weight, stress management, physical fitness, regular medical and dental checkups, and options for dealing with tobacco and alcohol use and other unhealthy habits). School facilities can be used for classes in aerobics, yoga, smoking cessation, and diet, and to provide nutritious and healthy breakfasts and lunches. Continuing education classes on child development, problems of children with chronic illness, behavioral disorders, and learning problems, can also be provided, thus enhancing a teacher's understanding of child factors influencing classroom management techniques. Financial incentives for health club memberships can be offered for regular attendance and cost reductions provided in health insurance plans (ie, for nonsmokers, designated drivers, seat belt users). The demonstration of a healthy faculty, both on school grounds and events and in the community, can serve as an important reinforcement for a healthy school environment.

The School as a Model for Physical Safety

The prevention of intentional and unintentional injury has become a major focus in health promotion for children and youth today. Increasingly, we are faced with violence in schools (see chapter 30). Past problems, limited to occasional schoolyard or sports events scraps, have turned into gang and drug distribution violence, resulting in death and injury. Random violence as a way of life closely follows these life-threatening behavioral patterns. In order for schools to be safe, there must be low tolerance for and high vigilance against physical assault. The school can provide a specific setting for nonviolent conflict resolution and require its use to settle differences. Adequate school security, including comprehensive intelligence and appropriate, quick disciplinary responses, as well as intimate cooperation with law enforcement agencies, is essential. However, in districts in which these problems are surfacing, even more is needed. Seminars involving the community are needed to provide skills for defusing violence if we are to avoid the development of "war zones" and promote a nonviolent environment. Security personnel and law enforcement officers, like faculty, can be influential role models and develop positive relationships with students if appropriate educational and integrational models are used (see chapter 30).

Clearly, the violation of students' basic human rights and physical abuse through corporal punishment convey the wrong messages; these approaches should be abandoned.

A dramatic example of an intentional injury that a school district can control is exposure to tobacco smoke. School districts have modeled smoke-free schools for a number of years, and it is estimated that 17% of school districts have developed smoke-free policies. Not only do such policies protect students and staff from passive smoke exposure, but they also send smokers and potential smokers a powerful statement about the health values of the school environment.

The prevention of unintentional injuries in schools addresses more traditional areas of accident prevention, and these usually are identified by site. The playground is the site for the highest number of student injuries. Fortunately, most of these accidents are minor in nature, but a triage system should be in place to appropriately address minor to the most severe of injuries (see chapter 18). What is more important, the factors contributing to the largest number and most severe injuries on the playground should be reviewed and addressed (eg, replace or redesign playground equipment, provide more direct supervision). Other common sites for unintentional injuries include vocational education/shop classrooms, art classrooms, and laboratories. In order to significantly reduce the risks of these hazardous sites, it is necessary for school districts to have a regular review of all of these areas. Each of the areas should be evaluated for risks and for the safety precautions taken to avoid these risks, and an accounting of how consistently the use of these precautions should be carried out. As a classroom exercise, students can participate in each of these evaluations, thus learning the steps to creating a safe environment and coming to understand the importance of prevention's role in safety.

The message that the school environment is safe and healthful also needs to be sent to the school district's faculty and staff. The most common activities or sites for unintentional injury include the handling of materials (especially lifting), ladder safety, and food safety as well as the safe use of electrical appliances and outlets (see chapters 19 and 31, which address communicable diseases and environmental hazards).

Nutrition Messages in the School: What Are the "Values"?

Because the consequences of poor nutrition often are chronic in nature and occur over the long term, many practitioners today overlook the daily importance and consequences of sound nutritional practices. Thus, the health-promoting quality of our school breakfast or lunch programs is often ignored. Budgetary changes in these programs often go unnoticed, but may have a significant impact on the content of food value. Important nutritional messages associated with school meals can be linked to immediate values that students appreciate (ie, appearance, hair, complexion) as well as to long-term consequences.

If junk food is readily available, if school policies encourage students to purchase low nutritional value fast foods at lunchtime, and if the quality of the food provided by the school doesn't adhere to nutritionally sound standards, there is a loud and clear message to students that nutritional consequences are of little or no importance. We all recognize how difficult it is for schoolchildren to plan for tomorrow, much less for 30 years from now. Conversely, if only healthy foodstuffs were available through the school food services and included attractive—but powerful—messages to students, over time the students may come to understand the relationship between lifetime habits that are healthy and their positive consequences.

Transportation Safety: A Missed Opportunity

Vehicular-related accidents cause more morbidity and mortality than any other single vector for children and youth. Although the controversy over the cost-effectiveness of placing seat belts in school buses to prevent death and injury continues to rage, what is the message for schoolchildren riding the bus? On the other hand, if school buses had seat belts and children were provided with an annual education program on their use and importance, would there not be a more powerful message applied daily on the necessity of using seat belts? (See Appendix for AAP statement on School Bus Safety.) There are numerous health promotional activities related to transportation safety (ie, street crossing, getting off the bus, bicycle safety) (see chapter 29). For example, school districts could have a policy in which they would provide a safe lockup for bicycles to all students wearing bicycle helmets. With the possible exception of the student's home, there are few places, other than at school, where health messages and behavioral reinforcements can be applied systematically and repetitively to achieve improvement in healthy behaviors and subsequent health outcomes.

Is Fitness Part of Our Physical Education Curriculum?

A number of short- and long-term benefits have been associated with physical fitness, particularly in reducing cardiovascular morbidity and mortality. The American Academy of Pediatrics recently lamented the current and probable future decline of physical fitness for our children and youth. Among the reasons cited for this decline were the reduced budgets for physical education curricula as a result of financial strains on school districts and a return to the "basics" in education. Also, traditional physical education curricula have deemphasized physical fitness activities in favor of competitive sports. Perhaps one strategy to address this problem would be to establish physical fitness as "basic" in the school's health curriculum. By linking the components of physical fitness (ie, cardiovascular endurance, muscular strength and endurance, flexibility, and body composition) with health classes in carrying out these activities regularly each week, the school environment could reinforce the short-term benefits while helping students develop long-term physical fitness habits with valuable health consequences. Other strategies could include providing fitness activities before and after school for both students and faculty. The role modeling potential of this combination of students and faculty provides additional benefits. Finally, physical education curricula that have survived need to more intimately link their curriculum with physical fitness, since as a lifetime skill, or "basic," their curriculum will be less vulnerable to the fiscal variability that districts are experiencing.

In conclusion, there are a number of elements or characteristics of a healthful school environment. A basic requirement includes helping children and youth value human life, build their own self-esteem, and develop into good citizens. Disease prevention/health promotion makes no sense if children or adolescents do not value themselves or honor and respect the rights of fellow students. Conversely, in the presence of self-esteem, students can better understand why avoiding harmful risk factors and embracing healthy behaviors and habits greatly influences the quality of their future. Schools that employ the idea of multiple reinforcement use every opportunity with their facility, faculty, staff, and community to provide students with powerful health messages, resulting in healthier life-styles and behaviors.

Suggested Readings

Allegrante JP, Michela JL. Impact of a school-based workplace health promotion program on morale of inner-city teachers. *J Sch Health.* 1990;60(1):25-28

American Academy of Pediatrics, Committee on School Health. Corporal punishment in schools. *Pediatrics.* 1991;88:173

American Academy of Pediatrics, Committee on School Health and Committee on Accident and Poison Prevention. School bus safety. *AAP News*. February 1985

American Academy of Pediatrics, Committee on Sports Medicine and Committee on School Health. Physical fitness and the schools. *Pediatrics*. 1987;80:449-450

Blair SN, Tritsch L, Kutsch S. Worksite health promotion for school faculty and staff. *J Sch Health*. 1987;57(10):469-473

Falck VT, Kilcoyne ME, Jr. A health promotion program for school personnel. *J Sch Health*. 1984;54(7):239-243

Hawkins JD, Catalano RF. Broadening the vision of education: schools as health promoting environments. *J Sch Health*. 1990;60(4):178-181

Iverson DC, Kolbe LJ. Evolution of the national disease prevention and health promotion strategy: establishing a role for the schools. *J Sch Health*. 1983;53(5):294-302

McKenzie JF. Twelve steps in developing a schoolsite health education/promotion program for faculty and staff. *J Sch Health*. 1988; 58(4):149-153

CHAPTER 10

EVALUATION OF SCHOOL HEALTH PROGRAMS

The evaluation of ongoing school health programs and activities can add credence to the program and encourage support of the stakeholders in the community. Program resources are often in short supply, and the use of scarce resources for program evaluation may appear to be foolish. However, information gained through evaluation can increase awareness of the accomplishments of a school health program and the ongoing needs of the student population. This chapter describes steps in setting up and carrying out evaluation of school health activities.

For a locally funded school health program, most evaluation issues will focus on the determination of locally appropriate goals and objectives, the activities that lead to implementation of these goals and objectives, the specification of the target population, and the impact of the program on the health-related knowledge, attitudes, and behaviors of students, their parents, and school faculty and staff as they relate to the program goals and objectives. The evaluation needs to be designed to gather information that will facilitate decision making regarding change and continuation of school health components and activities. Sharing evaluation results can increase program visibility, elicit support through acknowledgment of involvement of key community individuals, maintain shared resources, and assure that the school health program is meeting the stated needs of the students.

A program evaluation cycle typically includes conducting a needs assessment, setting program goals and objectives, developing a documentation system to measure attainment of program goals and objectives, collecting information over a period of time, assessing results with feedback to staff and stakeholders, and implementing necessary changes in the program. The following sections describe these steps in detail.

How to Do a Needs Assessment

A needs assessment becomes important when scarce resources dictate that not all viable program opportunities can be addressed at once, and programmatic choices must be made. In addition to the information gained about student health needs, the process of designing and conducting a needs assessment can be used to develop and educate a core group of involved persons who will be interested in the success of the school health program.

Each community has the opportunity to configure its school health program uniquely to meet its needs. A needs assessment will help determine this unique configuration. The overall program goals and objectives can be based on these identified needs. Requests for resources can result from expressed needs. It is far more powerful to request funds based on data from the population to be served than on anecdote or conjecture.

Using a Needs Assessment to Gain Support in the Community and the School

To assure that the school health program will have school and community support, it is necessary to include various stakeholders in the development of the needs assessment and the analysis of the resulting information. Possible groups include school faculty and staff, students, parents, the medical community, school nurses, voluntary agencies, educational groups, and community groups working with youth, such as the YMCA. The child/youth health council discussed in chapter 1 can be an excellent vehicle for oversight of the needs assessment process.

Enlist the members of the group in reviewing questions and approaches to the needs assessment, in determining who will be surveyed or interviewed, and in reviewing the information gathered. Table 31 gives the steps to be taken in carrying out a needs assessment. A considerable portion of this assessment will focus on the students and their perceptions of needs. However, other important sources of data such as school records, teacher and counselor perceptions, parental perceptions, and those of other community groups working with children and youth will serve to present a more complete picture of student needs. Often, services are available but students lack the ability to access them. A needs assessment that focuses both on students and on agencies and youth service providers in the community will minimize the chances of possible duplication of services.

Table 31. — Steps to Carrying Out a Needs Assessment

1. Constitute the child/youth health committee or another group for oversight.

2. Develop list of possible survey subjects
   Students
   Parents
   Teachers
   Staff
   Community agencies

3. Formulate survey items to relate to specific areas of school health, such as access to primary care, healthful environment, and health concerns of adolescents (eg, birth control, smoking cessation).

4. Review and revise survey items to assure conciseness and clarity.

5. Administer survey(s).

6. Collate responses and present to child/youth health committee.

7. Determine those areas of greatest need that will receive emphasis.

Defining Goals and Measurable Objectives

The definition of programmatic goals and objectives will come after review of the needs assessment information and analysis of the availability of resources. For the school health program to succeed, this process must involve those who will be affected by the program: students (especially adolescents), parents, school administration and staff, the school board, those who will be working to meet the program objectives, and community stakeholders.

Program goals should be overarching, state the basis on which the program is developed, and remain constant over a period of years. Examples of school health program goals are given in chapter 2 and encompass such items as access to primary health care, systems for medical crisis response, and screening and health maintenance. Goals such as these facilitate evaluation because they are specific and translatable into measurable objectives.

Program objectives may be developed to be accomplished in a shorter time: a school year, perhaps. Objectives should be stated as specific to a goal and be measurable. A measurable objective is one that cites who, what, where, and when. Table 32 gives

Table 32. — Program Objectives for School Health

Goal 1: Access to Primary Health Care

Program Objective 1: School health service will work with the medical community to create a plan for an on-site primary care clinic for high school students. Plan complete by March.

Program Objective 2: Beginning in September, school nurses will provide instruction in all junior high and high school health and homemaking classes on how to access the community health care system.

Goal 2: Provide a System for Dealing With Crisis Medical Situations

Program Objective 1: By September, the school health service administrator will provide school first aid and emergency management policies for each individual school building.

Program Objective 2: By Nov 1, the school health service will have a data bank of information on all those students who may need emergency medical care during the school day.

Goal 3: Provide Mandated Screening and Health Maintenance Programs

Program Objective 1: By Oct 1, the elementary school nurses will ensure that 90% of incoming kindergarten children are fully immunized.

Program Objective 2: By April 1, the elementary school nurses will ensure that 90% of third graders receive a hearing and vision screen.

Goal 4: Provide Systems for Identification and Solution of Students' Health and Educational Problems

Program Objective 1: By Dec 15, each school nurse will have worked with the faculty to identify procedures by which individual teachers and counselors can express concern about a student to the school nurse.

Program Objective 2: By March 1, the school health administration will have developed record-keeping requirements for the school health room that will enable detection and management of health and educational problems.

Goal 5: Provide for Comprehensive and Appropriate Health Education

Program Objective 1: By April 1, the district administrator for curriculum will have reviewed all current health education requirements and offerings within the district.

Program Objective 2: By November, the school health program will have arranged to offer one series of smoking cessation classes in each high school each semester.

Goal 6: Provide for a Healthful and Safe School Environment That Facilitates Learning

Program Objective 1: The school health services administrative staff will work with the district facilities administration to provide an impact-safe surface under all play equipment at each elementary school by May 1.

Program Objective 2: The district food service will offer at least one "heart healthy" main dish each day in all cafeterias starting with the new school year.

Goal 7: Provide a System for Evaluating the Effectiveness of School Health

Program Objective 1: The child/youth health committee will develop and carry out a district-wide student needs assessment at the high school level, to be completed by Feb 1.

Program Objective 2: District records administration and the district school health administrator will develop a computer-based record system for the elementary school health rooms.

---

examples of measurable objectives for each of the school health goals discussed in chapter 2. These objectives are written to be accomplished over a school year. Note that each objective presents a specific avenue for addressing the program goal. The objectives are concrete. Taken together, they present a picture of the school health-related activities that will be undertaken in the district over the school year. These are the activities that will be subject to evaluation.

To ensure implementation of a comprehensive program, these objectives can be subdivided into action steps. Use the action steps to describe key points in the process of attaining the objec-

Table 33. — Action Steps to Accomplish the Objective of Provision of Smoking Cessation Classes in Each High School

Program Objective: Offer one series of smoking cessation classes in each high school each semester.

Action Step 1: Present data from needs assessment on the number of high school smokers who wish to stop to administration and staff. (July)

Action Step 2: Determine possible times and sites of classes, get school faculty sponsor if necessary. (July)

Action Step 3: Contact volunteer agencies for possible classes or materials. (July)

Action Step 4: Review possible school-based interventions that have been shown effective in other schools. (August)

Action Step 5: Make decision about program to be offered. (September)

Action Step 6: Design student evaluation form for program. (September)

Action Step 7: Schedule time and place, and notify students. (October)

Action Step 8: Implement program. (October)

Action Step 9: Ask students to complete an evaluation. (Last meeting of each class series).

tive. Accomplishing all the action steps listed for an objective will lead to the accomplishment of the objectives, and the accomplishment of all the objectives for a given goal can lead to the realization of that goal. Table 33 gives an example of action steps for the program objective: offer one series of smoking cessation classes in each high school each semester.

While the development of goals, objectives, and action steps may appear to be an extreme amount of work, these objectives will facilitate program description, help develop a consensus as to the direction of the school health program, and facilitate evaluation through the statement of desired accomplishments in concrete terms. The process of developing goals, objectives, and action steps with involved staff and the child/youth health committee will build a committed interest group.

Documentation Systems

Two types of documentation can be used for evaluation of the program: available existing record systems (eg, school health room logs) and archival documents (eg, faculty and school board meeting minutes), and information gathering tools designed for a specific objective (eg, participant survey, focus groups). Often, the persons collecting the information will not have data collection as their primary concern. Therefore, the program documentation system should be as unobtrusive as possible.

Many of the record systems currently in place in the school system can be used to monitor health program objectives. Daily attendance records, critical incident reports, sports-related reports, reports of the teachers and counselors, and school health room records are all sources of information that can be used to monitor a school health program and student needs over time.

On occasion, it is necessary to determine program standing at a specific point. Often, special measures can be constructed for use in such cases. For example, you may wish to know what students like or do not like about the school health services, what types of problems are seen early in the morning on a Monday, or what students really eat for lunch. These questions can be answered with a short survey, observation, or student focus group. Often these may be questions that arise from the child/youth health committee as a program progresses or at the end-of-the-year review, when evaluation data indicate less-than-desired implementation or use.

Determining Process and Outcome Indicators

A review of the objectives and action steps will elicit ideas on possible sources of evaluation information. Table 34 gives examples of possible data sources for the objective of providing smoking cessation classes in the high schools and related action steps to accomplish the objective. The collection of this data would enable a description of the decision to offer the classes (needs assessment), the process of developing and offering the class (archival records), and student response to the class (survey, focus group). Note that some of the desired information relates to the process of implementing the program and other informa-

Table 34. — Measurable Indicator and Data Sources for Evaluation of Objective to Provide Smoking Cessation Classes in Each High School

Data Source	Measurable Indicator
Needs assessment	Number of students who have tried to quit; desire of students to quit; availability of cessation classes for adolescents.
Archival records	
Faculty meeting minutes	Decision to offer class.
Class schedules	Time and frequency.
Attendance rosters	Number of students.
Student class evaluation	
Survey	Self-report on smoking cessation/reduction; student attitudes
Focus group	Reactions to class; suggestions to make more effective.

tion relates to the student response and outcomes. These indicators should be related directly to the activities required to accomplish the objective. Outcome indicators should relate directly to the program goal. For this objective, the process indicators can be the number of classes offered, the number of students attending, and the proportion of smoking students who attend classes. A good outcome indicator is the number of students taking the class who report stopping smoking.

A table such as the one constructed for the smoking cessation class objective can serve as a monitoring plan for any school health objective. Construction of such a table will ensure that the objective and related action steps have at least one measurable process and one measurable outcome indicator included in the evaluation. Use more if possible, as a greater number of measurement points will help with year-end administrative decisions.

Development of the Documentation System

Two major points to be considered in developing a documentation system are (1) that the data collected be based on the measurable indicators for the objectives, and (2) that those who will be using the system will be involved in the process of designing it.

Any documentation system to be used by school personnel should require as small an amount of additional time as possible. Systems must be developed with input from staff that will be responsible for documentation. The first step in developing the system depends on previous determination of measurable process and outcome indicators from the objectives and action steps as discussed in the preceding section. Once these indicators are determined, a review of current record-keeping procedures and documents can be done to determine if the information is currently available or, if not, where and how it might most easily be collected. For some objectives, such as those dealing with legal mandates and requirements, the documentation system may be in place or suggested by the regulatory body. Do not assume that because documentation is available it will automatically address the program objective. Review current records and implicit and explicit decision rules used by the staff to document items of importance to the evaluation.

As the documentation of school health program activities will impact on the school staff time, it is important to include review of new documentation systems and records by the school staff who will be using them. This step will minimize staff resistance to additional paperwork and make the final product more usable in the school. Finally, after initial implementation, schedule time with the staff for feedback and revision of records and collection procedures.

Program Review and Adjustments

As discussed in the preceding section, much of the information collected in the evaluation of school health program goals and objectives may be drawn from existing records; therefore, documentation is ongoing. Program objectives and action steps are written with explicit and implicit time lines. Evaluation of the program should recognize the need to measure accomplishment at given points. The information gathered can be used to provide

Table 35. — Examples of Negative Evaluation Results

Missed target population	School clinic implemented to meet access needs of lower income students, used only by upper income students.
No implementation	Educational program selected and provided but not implemented in classroom.
Competing priority	Measles epidemic occurs, and staff time and funds are taken from planned playground changes to prevent injuries.
No impact	Smoking prevention curriculum implemented in the 9th grade, and no change in smoking initiation detected.

feedback to the school administration and staff, the school board, and community groups who have specific interests in the issues examined. The information can then be used to make program adjustments and reset program priorities for the coming year. Consider providing an "end-of-the-school-year, state-of-school-health-in-our-community" review for the child/youth health committee, school health staff, school board, and any other funding sources.

Taking Action on Evaluation Results

The actions to be taken after an evaluation depend to a large part on the results. Of course, if the results are positive, few changes may be required. Often, however, evaluation results are equivocal or negative. Negative evaluation results include the following: (1) missing the target population, (2) reaching the correct population but without implementation of the intervention, (3) addressing a high priority unplanned for need, and/or (4) implementing the objective and no change seen. Table 35 gives examples from the objectives of what a negative evaluation might look like in these cases.

In all cases, and especially those with negative findings, two actions should be taken. First, reconvene the child/youth health committee and review needs of the student population. Did the program selected meet needs as revealed in the needs assessment? If the answer is yes, the next step is to review, with the staff, the activities of the past year. Questions to be answered include what activities occurred, where the problems were, and how these can be overcome. Finally, if the program objective related directly to an action to be taken by the students (eg, attendance at smoking cessation classes, selection of heart-healthy foods in the cafeteria), a student focus group can be convened to gather information on their reaction to the program.

The information gathered during the evaluation review can be used by the school staff and the child/youth health committee to reformulate the objective and related action steps for the coming year, thus completing the evaluation cycle.

PART III

SPECIFIC PROBLEMS AND ISSUES

CHAPTER 11

SCHOOL ATTENDANCE AND SCHOOL AVOIDANCE SYNDROMES

Children with school avoidance stay home from school or are sent home from school for emotional reasons. In the classic case, the child awakens with a stomachache on Monday morning, is allowed to stay home, and feels fine by midmorning. The terms "school refusal," "school avoidance," and "school phobia" are often used interchangeably. The term school phobia, however, has lost favor because the child usually fears growing up and being away from the parent rather than being fearful of something specific at school.

Frequency

School avoidance syndrome is the most common cause of vague symptoms in school-age children. Approximately 5% of children in elementary school and 2% in junior high school have this disorder. The reappearance of school refusal when youngsters enter junior high school is probably the result of the introduction of multiple teachers, the loss of a parent surrogate, and the hazing that commonly occurs there. The incidence of school refusal may be decreasing because of the increasing numbers of working mothers. This social change requires most children to master their separation fears before entering kindergarten.

Etiology

There are two basic types of school avoidance syndrome: the anxiety-related type and the secondary-gain type. In the anxiety-related type, a child is worried about something at home or school. Common examples are worrying too much about grades, catching up, or being liked by other people. Most of these children also have a persistence of the separation anxiety that normal children master by 3 or 4 years of age. Many of the children have a shy and sensitive temperament. The parent tends to be overprotective and worries too much about the child experiencing stress within the community and school. These children are good to excellent students and cause no behavioral problems in the classroom. Girls outnumber boys, and the onset usually occurs in kindergarten. Approximately 20% of this group also have an acute precipitating event (eg, being teased by someone at school).

The children with the secondary-gain type of school refusal do not manifest any symptoms of anxiety. Their poor school attendance often follows an acute illness that seems to stretch on and on. They tend to get behind in their schoolwork during the illness. The desire to stay at home is also perpetuated by the sympathy they receive and the amount of television they are allowed to watch. They often have a lenient parent who does not place much value in education. Boys outnumber girls in this group, and often they are poor students.

Presentations

Most children with school refusal experience physical symptoms at the time of departure for school. The child with the anxiety-related type usually has physiologic manifestations of anxiety (eg, diarrhea). The children with the secondary-gain type of school refusal usually fabricate symptoms (eg, sore throats). The foremost symptoms associated with this disorder are recurrent abdominal pains, sore throats, headaches, and leg pains (Table 36).

Differential Diagnosis of School Absence

Excessive or chronic school absence can have many causes (Table 37). School avoidance syndrome is just one of the subsets of etiologies. Some parents keep a child home for a prolonged period because of mistaken health beliefs regarding the need for bed rest or isolation (eg, keeping a child home 10 days for streptococcal pharyngitis). Children with chronic physical disease or learning disabilities may become reluctant to attend school because they are unable to adapt well to the academic environment or to the other children. A truant is a youngster who is neither at home nor at school during school hours. These children are at risk for becoming school dropouts. Other contributing factors to truancy are substance abuse, juvenile delinquency, depression, psychosis, or teenage pregnancy. A chaotic family life also reduces the child's commitment to daily school attendance.

Table 36. — Presenting Symptoms for School Refusal*

General: **Insomnia**, excessive sleeping, fatigue, "always tired," "fever," "always sick"

Skin: **Pallor**

Ear, nose, and throat: Recurrent sore throat, recurrent sinus problems, "constant" colds

Respiratory: **Hyperventilation**, coughing tics

Cardiovascular: **Palpitations**, chest pains

Gastrointestinal: **Recurrent abdominal pains, anorexia, nausea, recurrent vomiting, diarrhea**

Skeletal: Bone pain, joint pain, back pain

Neuromuscular: **Headaches, dizziness, syncope,** "weakness"

---

* Symptoms in boldfaced type can be physiologic manifestations of anxiety. The other symptoms may be fabricated or exaggerated.

Table 37. — Chronic School Absence: A Differential Diagnosis

School refusal
    Anxiety-related type (school phobia)
    Secondary-gain type (school avoidance)

Overresponse to minor illnesses

Chronic physical disease with poor adaptation

Learning disability with poor adaptation

Truancy

Substance abuse

Psychosis

Teenage pregnancy

Family dysfunction

Some children encounter an acute stress that makes it particularly difficult to attend school (Table 38). Most normal children who are also exposed to similar stresses, however, handle them well and continue to attend school. The most common cause of acute school avoidance is a change of schools or loss of a school chum. Some children react to family stresses, such as acute marital strife, the father's loss of work, a sick mother, or the birth of a new sibling. Others are troubled by stresses that

Table 38. — Acute School Refusal: Precipitating Events

Change of schools

Family stress

Travel stress

Academic stress

School environment stress

---

occur en route to school, such as encountering a bully at the bus stop. Academic stress may accelerate suddenly because of an impending test, a requirement to recite in class, or a poor report card. Other stresses occurring in the school environment include bathroom restrictions in children with small bladders, physical fitness requirements in overweight or clumsy children, or teasing or hazing on the school grounds.

Confirming the Diagnosis of School Avoidance Syndrome

School refusal is a diagnosis of inclusion that can be confirmed by demonstrating the following four diagnostic criteria: (1) The child complains of recurrent vague, mysterious physical symptoms. Symptoms of unknown etiology are the main reason a primary physician inevitably becomes involved with this problem. (2) No physical cause is found on careful evaluation, including a physical examination and appropriate laboratory tests. This discrepancy between how sick the child sounds and how well the child looks is one of the hallmarks of this disorder. (3) Physical symptoms predominate in the morning and are accentuated when the family tries to get the child to go to school. Often the symptoms clear by 10 am. This pattern is not found with any organic condition. (4) The child has missed 5 or more days of school because of these physical symptoms. In contrast, children with chronic physical diseases often have excellent school attendance records.

The diagnosis of school phobia is mainly confirmed through taking a thorough history. The child's symptoms must be reviewed in detail. However, their timing is of greatest importance. Not only do they usually occur in the morning, they also are worse on Mondays, during September, and following holidays. Usually the onset of symptoms dates to entering kindergarten or first grade. The health care provider must ask the crucial question, "How much school has the child missed for these symptoms?" It is a mistake to assume that the parents will mention poor school attendance; they often believe that everyone keeps "sick" children at home and in bed. Because parents may blame school absence on some acute event occurring during the current school year, the physician must inquire about school attendance during the previous school years. Special stresses (see Table 38) should be inquired about. Because these children often spend little time with their peer group, this area can be explored. An understanding of family functioning is obviously relevant to treating the problem. Close coordination between the school nurse and health care provider will provide essential information to the workup. Much of the evaluation could be accomplished in the school setting if the child is present, and cooperation to accomplish necessary laboratory tests is available. Parents often resist the diagnosis, regardless of where or how the workup is carried out.

Ten Steps in Convincing Parents of the School Avoidance Diagnosis

The main barrier to successful treatment is changing the family's focus from organic to nonorganic symptom origins. The following 10 steps usually are helpful to this process.

1. *Elicit Complete History:* Encourage the parents to talk and listen carefully. Mention both organic and psychologic causes on the first visit with the parents. Try to identify the parents' specific fears about what might happen if they send their child to school or what medical diagnosis they are worried about. For recurrent pain, have the child keep a diary of episodes.

2. *Perform Meticulous Physical Examination:* Parents place an inordinate amount of faith in the ability of the physical examination to uncover hidden disease. During the examination, discuss normal findings, rather than proceeding in silence.

3. *Order Sufficient Laboratory Tests to Convince Yourself of Child's Physical Health:* The primary health care provider

should become confident of the diagnosis as soon as possible. Get laboratory results as soon as possible. Laboratory tests should not be ordered on a delayed basis or as a routine.

4. *Tell Parents Diagnosis After Evaluation Is Complete:* If laboratory studies have been ordered, do not tell the parents your diagnosis until all results are known. If no laboratory work is needed, parents can be told the diagnosis during the initial visit.

5. *Clarify That the Child Is in Excellent Physical Health:* Pronounce the child unequivocally physically well. We must make up our mind. The parents should not be left hanging with statements such as "He probably has school avoidance, but we can't be certain." If a physician is unwilling to call the cause emotional, at least he/she should attribute the symptoms to a benign physiologic process such as gas pains, a sensitive stomach, growing pains, or tension headaches.

6. *Explain What School Avoidance Is, Namely, That Emotions Can Cause Physical Symptoms:* Explain the difference between physical symptoms and physical disease. Explain that pain is real, even when it has an emotional basis. Review that everyone's body has a certain physical way of responding to emotional stress.

7. *Tell Parents Reasons Why Symptom Is Not the Result of Physical Disease:* Justify the nonorganic diagnosis with the same reasons that have convinced you of the correct diagnosis. These include the timing of the symptoms, the age at onset that coincides with school entry, and the presence of the symptom during previous school years. Underscore that physicians know how to make this diagnosis.

8. *Reassure Parents About Any Specific Diagnosis They Fear:* The diagnosis may be one that someone else in the family has experienced. In other cases, another physician has previously mentioned the possibility of a serious diagnosis.

9. *Clarify for Parents That School Avoidance Occurs in Normal Children and Normal Homes:* This common condition affects 5% or more of children. Mention that it is a stress-

related problem and not a "psychiatric" problem. Support the parents' feeling of being good parents.

10. *Reassure Parents That the Condition Can Be Effectively Treated:* The health care provider can promise to provide a treatment plan that will reduce the symptoms in the majority of cases. The minimal goal of this discussion should be to get the parents to agree to regular school attendance pending additional observations, even if they cling to the idea that their child may have some rare disease.

Treatment of School Avoidance Syndrome

Talking With Parents

The primary care provider can manage the majority of children with school avoidance. The only treatment that is effective is regular school attendance. Being in school every day must be an ironclad rule. Once the family has been convinced that the youngster is physically well, the child must return to school immediately. Being in school is intrinsically therapeutic and breaks the vicious cycle that occurs when a child gets out of step with schoolwork and friendships. Parents will need to be extra firm in the morning for several weeks. On any morning that the child "has to stay home for illness," the condition should be reassessed and the child sent to school if the condition is minor or turns out to be a psychosomatic symptom. The primary goal is to know how to return a child to school.

Talking With Youngster

Reassure the youngster of his or her good physical health and that he or she is in no physical danger. Blame the symptoms on worrying too much about competition, grades, bad things happening, or catching up with schoolwork. Offer a face-saving way to accept the diagnosis. Emphasize that daily school attendance will help the child feel better. Clarify that this requirement is nonnegotiable. For the child with secondary-gain type school refusal, simply state that "you can't miss any further school because it is illegal to do so." This type is the easiest to treat and the child responds quickly to this warning and limit-setting by the parent. For the child with anxiety-related school avoidance, more sympathy is in order. If the child has severe symptoms at school, promise the availability of lying down in the nurse's office for 5 to 10 minutes. Clarify, however, that the child cannot go home because of these symptoms.

Contacting School Staff

Communication between the primary care provider and school personnel is essential. The school nurse is usually the best person to contact about physical problems. In some schools, the counselor, teacher, or principal may be more readily available. The primary care provider should be called if the child's attendance remains poor or if the child is in the nursing station and wants to go home. Then, the physician and school nurse can work together to decide whether the child should stay in school or visit the physician. School staff can also help to make the return to school as nontraumatic as possible.

Treating Contributory Stress Factors

Most of the stress factors listed in Table 38 can be dealt with by the parent, school principal, special education teacher, or the primary health care provider. Be forewarned that correction of most of these factors alone produces little improvement in school attendance, because they only partially account for the child's preference for staying home. Changing to a different class or a different school generally is of no benefit except in those rare situations in which an unstable teacher is mistreating one or more children.

Providing Follow-up Visits

Follow-up visits are essential for monitoring attendance. Children with school avoidance should have return visits in approximately 1 week, 1 month, and again approximately 2 weeks into the following school year. These children also need to call their health care provider on the first day of acute illnesses so that the family can be helped to decide whether the child needs to stay home. These contacts can help to identify patients who need referral because of treatment failure.

When to Refer to Mental Health Professional

The following patients with school refusal need to be referred to a child psychiatrist or psychologist: psychotic children, depressed children, children incapacitated with fear and anxiety (often due to a panic reaction or obsessive-compulsive behavior), and symbiotic parent-child relationships. Most children who have been on prolonged bed rest should be referred. Most of all, those patients who are unresponsive to pediatric counseling also need referral.

Occasionally, there may be a need to refer a family to child protective services because of educational neglect. In these cases, families are unable to send their children to school despite several medical evaluations and school conferences, and children are being deliberately kept home to do housework or to look after younger children. The juvenile court system may need to order the child back to school with the warning that the child will be placed in foster care if the family continues to be uncooperative.

Prognosis

With appropriate counseling, more than 95% of children are cured of their school avoidance in a matter of 2 or 3 weeks. It is important to warn the parents that during the first few days back at school, the child's physical symptoms may increase temporarily. Approximately 5% of these children have intermittent recurrences that respond to helping the family become firm in their resolve to send the child to school. Many of these children will continue to have homesickness when faced with slumber parties or camping trips, and these can be introduced gradually into the child's life-style. The children with anxiety-related type of school avoidance usually take longer to respond and have more recurrences than the secondary-gain type.

Summary

School avoidance is one of the major school problems with which school and health professionals need to become involved. In general, parents will only accept this diagnosis after evaluation by a physician or nurse practitioner considered by them to be an expert in physical disease. Unfortunately, sometimes this disorder is not included among the differential diagnoses of physical symptoms. School attendance should always be assessed whenever a child is evaluated for recurrent or persistent symptoms. Once considered, the diagnosis is easy to confirm. Intervention is also straightforward. The condition responds well to decisiveness about the physical health of the child, insistence on an immediate return to school, and monitoring of the student's progress.

Suggested Readings

Atkinson L, Quarrington B, Cyr JJ, Atkinson FV. Differential classification in school refusal. *Br J Psychiatry*. 1989;155:191-195

Blagg NR, Yule W. The behavioural treatment of school refusal—a comparative study. *Behav Res Ther*. 1984;22:119-127

Krugman RD, Krugman MK. Emotional abuse in the classroom. The pediatrician's role in diagnosis and treatment. *Am J Dis Child*. 1984; 138:284-286

Nader PR, Bullock D, Caldwell B. School phobia. *Pediatr Clin North Am*. 1975;22:605-617

Schmitt BD. School refusal. *Pediatr Rev*. 1986;8:99-105

Weitzman M, Klerman LV, Lamb G, Menary J, Alpert JJ. School absence: a problem for the pediatrician. *Pediatrics*. 1982;69:739-746

CHAPTER 12

PSYCHOSOMATIC COMPLAINTS

It is estimated that at least 20% to 25% of all school-age children experience physical symptoms that are largely caused by psychosocial factors. Most of these children are not seen by physicians, but instead are managed in school or at home. Some of the more common symptoms seen in school-age children that have a psychosomatic basis include the following: recurrent abdominal pain, recurrent headaches, chest pain, chronic back pain, limb pain, hyperventilation, fatigue, and dysmenorrhea. Effectively dealing with these symptoms presents a challenge to school professionals and the student's physician.

Definitions

There are four general categories of psychosomatic physical symptoms: psychosomatic symptoms, conversion symptoms, malingering, and hypochondriasis.

Psychosomatic symptoms are those symptoms for which psychological processes or psychosocial factors contribute to the development of the symptom (ie, tension headache, stress-related abdominal pain, or chronic fatigue as a result of stress) or for which psychosocial factors have influenced the course of the symptom or disorder (ie, anxiety worsening the course of an asthmatic attack). Psychosomatic symptoms usually involve the involuntary innervation of visceral organs (autonomic innervation). It is generally accepted that certain children have a physiological predisposition and a psychological predisposition to development of psychosomatic symptoms. When these children experience certain stresses or psychosocial events, they develop the involuntary symptoms. These symptoms usually have their onset in the early school years, and there is usually a predictable target organ.

Conversion symptoms develop when a psychological conflict or wish is expressed through a bodily symptom, rather than through verbal expression or through the development of mental symptoms. The symptoms are often a symbolic representation of the conflict manifested in a bodily function. Examples of conversion symptoms may include the inability to speak, hear, eat, swallow, defecate, walk, or move an extremity. It may also include symptoms such as vomiting, hyperventilation, or irregular breathing. Usually, the affected body parts are innervated by voluntary components of the central nervous system. The symptoms may not conform to anatomic distribution of motor or sensory innervation. For example, conversion numbness would be in a glove or stocking distribution as opposed to following the nerve distribution by dermatomes. There are no bodily structural changes. Conversion symptoms are uncommon in children younger than 7 or 8 years.

Malingering is the conscious fabrication of a symptom in order to accomplish a specific goal; for example, feigning a headache in order to get out of a test.

Hypochondriasis refers to the misinterpretation of a normal or physiologic sensation. The hypochondriacal child perceives a physiologic sensation as a potential threat or serious symptom. This may be caused by (1) vulnerable child syndrome; (2) hypochondriacal role modeling by parents; or (3) infantilization. The child's perception usually is learned from or reinforced by other family members.

Psychosomatic Symptoms

Incidence

The most common psychogenic symptoms among school-age children and adolescents are psychosomatic symptoms. Since many children with psychosomatic symptoms do not seek medical attention, it is difficult to ascertain the actual incidence of these symptoms. It is estimated that 10% to 15% of all school-age children and adolescents experience recurrent abdominal pain, and 5% experience recurrent headaches. An estimated 3% to 4% experience recurrent limb pain. Chest pain affects fewer than 1% of children. Periods of fatigue are common among adolescents, and may affect 10% to 15%.

Conceptual Model for Psychosomatic Symptoms

The sensory experience of pain has been extensively studied and is becoming increasingly better understood. Pain has a sensory component and a psychological/affective component. The sensory component is the result of the stimulation of nerve endings by physiologic or pathologic processes. The sensory component can be modified by a variety of psychological or affective experiences: secondary gain; temperament; cognitive style (dependent or independent); previous role modeling; stress in the environment; anxiety or depression; social or cultural background; developmental stage; level of understanding or intelligence; perception of the risks of pain; perception of one's control over pain; expectations; sense of support, empathy and understanding; level of self-esteem; and fears. It is presumed that psychosomatic symptoms other than pain likewise have both physical and psychological/affective components.

Psychosomatic symptoms occur in individuals who have a physiologic, involuntary, "functional" predisposition to developing the symptom and have a psychological, affective, or temperamental predisposition that enhances the likelihood of developing the psychosomatic symptom. In the context of certain precipitating social or environmental events, the symptom develops. The physical predisposition is often familial. Other family members often have psychosomatic symptoms affecting the same target organ. The psychological predisposition can take a variety of forms, but may include one or more temperamental characteristics, such as having high expectations; being sensitive to criticism or stress; having a tenuous self-image; or being "high strung," anxious, or fearful. The precipitating events might include one or more of the following:

- Loss or separation (real, perceived, or anticipated): death, divorce, desertion, reduced interaction between child and significant adult, entering school, moving, or placement out of the home. Fear of loss of love or acceptance.
- Illness in the family, child, or significant other.
- Low self-esteem, peer rejection, or embarrassment.
- Stresses associated with social or physical changes of adolescence or concerns about sexuality.
- Underachievement/learning disorders.
- Family stresses, including marital discord, alcoholism, financial difficulties, child abuse, parental depression, or anxiety.
- Parent/child interaction problems.
- High personal or parental expectations.
- Fear of injury, reprisal, or failure.

- Usual daily stresses can at times precipitate symptoms, particularly when associated with other precipitating factors.

Children who are predisposed to experiencing psychosomatic symptoms have different vulnerabilities depending on their developmental stage, previous life experiences, and role modeling. The symptoms can be modified as a result of positive or negative reinforcement.

There is often a family history of recurrent psychosomatic symptoms or diseases that involve a psychosomatic component. Common parental psychosomatic symptoms include tension headache, irritable bowel syndrome, dyspepsia, neck tension, or hyperventilation. The parents may refer to these symptoms in lay terms such as "stress headache," "nervous stomach," or "nervous diarrhea." Parents may have diseases such as peptic ulcer disease, Crohn disease, ulcerative colitis, or migraine headaches, or they may simply describe unexplained symptoms similar to the child's. The family history is an indication of familial predisposition to psychosomatic symptoms. It also may reveal a source of symptom modeling in the child's environment.

Evaluation Process

The evaluation process requires time and patience. It is important for the child and the parents to feel that the evaluation has been thorough and has considered all of the potential organic causes. A statement should be made early in the process indicating that symptoms may be caused either by physical diseases or by stresses, or sometimes by both, and the evaluation will assess all possible causes.

The focus of the history and physical should be twofold: to rule out organic causes and to identify those factors suggesting psychosomatic causes. The correct diagnosis is usually most evident in the history. It is essential to obtain a detailed description of at least two recent episodes of symptoms, in step-by-step (sometimes minute-by-minute) detail. A diary of symptoms that correlates the symptom, time, duration, associated activities, associated feelings, and preceding events may also uncover useful clues. It also is important to (1) clearly delineate the symptom in terms of location, intensity, temporal relationships, frequency, duration, quality, and modifying factors; (2) explore the meaning of the pain to the child and the effect of the pain on the child's life; (3) ask why help has been sought at this particular time; and (4) ask what the parents think the cause may be. Often, parents already suspect that the symptom is psychosomatic.

A thorough psychosocial history should utilize direct questions regarding predisposing events (such as those listed in the preceding section). It is also important to ask the parents to describe the child's personality. Their description often will help identify temperamental characteristics that may predispose the child to psychosomatic symptoms.

In many cases, the child's psychosomatic symptom closely resembles a symptom associated with a preceding illness (called a sentinel symptom). For example, the character of pain in recurrent abdominal pain often resembles the pain of a preceding episode of gastroenteritis. Psychosomatic chest pain may become a problem after the child has had an episode of costochondritis. The sentinel illness serves as a model or template for the subsequent psychosomatic symptom. This may cause the initial episode of the symptom to seem to be organic.

The family history is essential, since it is often possible to identify family members with psychosomatic complaints closely resembling those of the patient, and this information strongly supports the diagnosis of psychosomatic symptoms in the child. It also may serve to identify role models for the symptom within the child's environment. This information also becomes helpful later during management, as the physician or nurse can point out to the child and parent that both of them are "cut from the same cloth."

The nurse or physician should be aware of the complete differential diagnosis for the presenting symptom (including the many organic causes) and be aware of the common red flags for organic disease and the common indicators of psychosomatic causes. The physical examination must be thorough in order to rule out organic causes and to reassure the child and parents that the evaluation has been complete. Laboratory testing should be limited to those tests that are necessary to rule out likely organic causes. It is helpful to give feedback to the patient and parents during the physical examination, particularly to indicate the normality of the various organ systems.

Management of Psychosomatic Symptoms

The nurse or physician should take adequate time to (1) describe and interpret the information obtained during the evaluation; (2) describe the conceptual model for understanding psychosomatic symptoms; (3) list factors that make serious organic disease unlikely; (4) list factors that make psychosomatic illness likely; and (5) answer all questions and concerns. As many as one third of parents in this situation have a suspicion that their child's symptom may be psychosomatic. The health care provider can corroborate the parents' recognition of the possibility of psychosomatic symptoms and build on that early in the discussion of management. It should be emphasized that the child's symptoms are real, but the child can learn ways of reducing the symptoms. When there is a positive family history, the physician can draw on that family history, pointing out that many people have such symptoms and learn to adapt. The parents and child can work on their symptoms together.

It is important to encourage the parents to express their most feared diagnosis and equally important to be able to assure them that their child does not have the feared disorder. The child and parents need to be reassured that the child will come to understand the symptom and gain control of it over time. The child and parents will begin to recognize that the symptom is often a signal that something is stressful, worrisome, or otherwise bothersome to the child. Management then should be directed toward investigating the child's life with an eager, positive attitude in an attempt to identify the predisposing factors. The physician should attempt to generate enthusiasm within the family for learning to adapt to these predisposing factors.

Establishing follow-up visits is reassuring to the child and family and allows them to receive ongoing guidance in recognizing and adapting to the predisposing factors. The professional also can help the family identify sources of secondary gain and maladaptive coping and parenting styles. When the symptoms are severe or progress is slow, referral to a psychologist or psychiatrist may be needed. It is important for the patient and family to see the health care provider as an eager resource for insight and future help; this will allow them to cope in a more independent fashion.

Prognosis

At least half of the psychosomatic symptoms that develop in childhood persist in adulthood. For that reason, management should focus not on cure, but on understanding, adapting to, and coping with the symptom.

The Role of School Professionals

Communication between school personnel, parents, and the child's source of care is essential in management of psychosomatic complaints that occur in the school. The school nurse has a pivotal role in this communication. The school nurse can (1) gather information from teachers, organize that information, and provide it to the physician; (2) serve as an intermediary in coordinating the management plans with school personnel; and (3) provide information and education regarding illnesses and symptoms for school personnel. If the nurse is a nurse practitioner, evaluation and management can be undertaken with backup and supervision of a physician. The school teacher can help (1) in assessment, by providing useful classroom observations, and (2) in management, by reducing secondary gain for the student and by providing ongoing progress reports for the school nurse and physician.

An effective approach for the management of psychosomatic symptoms that interfere with school functioning or school attendance is to establish the expectation that the child whose symptoms interfere with participation in classroom activities should be assessed immediately, either by the school nurse or physician. If it is determined that the symptom is psychosomatic, the student is returned to the classroom. Later, the student can be assisted by a parent, psychologist, or other health professional to identify and adapt to the predisposing psychosocial factors.

Common Psychosomatic Symptoms in School-age Children

The following are brief discussions of selected common psychosomatic symptoms in students and helpful hints in their assessment and management.

Recurrent Abdominal Pain

Definition: Abdominal pain is defined as three or more bouts of abdominal pain severe enough to interfere with routine activity, occurring over a period of 3 months or longer.

Conceptual Model: The current conceptual model of recurrent abdominal pain identifies three main etiologies. The first category is "organic" and includes the gamut of organic causes. The second category is psychosomatic abdominal pain. Psychosomatic abdominal pain (1) is usually periumbilical or epigastric and often vague; (2) is associated with a reassuring history and review of systems; (3) includes a history that suggests a predisposing temperament and predisposing psychosocial factors; (4) often is associated with a positive family history for psychosomatic symptoms; (5) is associated with a normal physical examination except for mild to moderate abdominal tenderness (including a normal rectal examination and negative test for occult blood in the stool); and (6) includes normal screening laboratory testing.

The third category is dysfunctional pain, which refers to pain in that group of school children, usually between the ages of 5 and 10 years, who have vague abdominal complaints with many of the characteristics of psychosomatic abdominal pain, but for whom obvious stressors in the environment are not readily apparent. Physical examination, rectal examination, and laboratory tests are normal. It is believed that this group may have psychosomatic abdominal pain in response to the usual stressors of everyday life. With this group, it usually is not possible to identify the specific precipitating psychosocial factors.

Evaluation Process: The evaluation process should be directed toward ruling in or out organic causes and ruling in or out psychosomatic or dysfunctional causes. The following findings should increase the clinician's suspicion of organic pathology: abdominal pain away from the umbilicus; pain that is constant, well localized, or shows a consistent pattern; pain that interrupts sleep; fever; weight loss or poor growth; joint symptomatology; anorexia; jaundice or acholic stools; stools positive for presence of occult blood; anemia; or dysuria and/or frequency of urination. The following findings should increase the clinicians suspicion of psychogenic abdominal pain: secondary gain; declining school performance; school avoidance; depression; positive family history of similar symptoms; significant family psychopathology; evidence of poor parent-child interaction; abdominal pain that resolves for long periods between episodes; an undiscernible pattern or vagueness of symptoms. Children with psychosomatic or dysfunctional abdominal pain often have associated symptoms such as constipation, vomiting, mild diarrhea, headache, pallor, or dizziness.

The physical examination is usually normal in children with psychosomatic or dysfunctional abdominal pain, except perhaps for mild to moderate tenderness. Patients with organic disease may or may not have obvious abnormalities on physical examination. The rectal examination with test of the stool for occult blood is a key element in assessment. The presence of occult blood in the stool is an indication for further evaluation for organic pathology. Screening laboratory should include a complete blood cell (CBC) count, sedimentation rate, and urinalysis.

Either psychosomatic abdominal pain or dysfunctional abdominal pain is extremely likely if (1) there are historical findings suggestive of psychosomatic abdominal pain; (2) a thorough review of systems fails to identify findings suggestive of organic causes; (3) a carefully taken family history reveals other family members with either unexplained or psychosomatic gastrointestinal symptoms; (4) a normal physical examination is obtained, including rectal examination and negative test of the stool for blood; and (5) the CBC count, sedimentation rate, and urinalysis are all normal. For patients who meet these criteria, further testing can be kept to a minimum and management should commence for psychosomatic or dysfunctional abdominal pain.

If the history or physical uncovers the suggestion of organic causes, then further workup will be necessary. The common organic causes for abdominal pain that may be difficult to differentiate from psychogenic abdominal pain include: chronic constipation, inflammatory bowel disease, peptic ulcer disease, lactose intolerance, giardiasis, and occult renal disease (ie, current urinary tract infection, hydronephrosis, and obstruction). Table 39 lists additional organic causes.

Management: Management of psychosomatic abdominal pain should proceed as described earlier in the chapter (Management of Psychosomatic Symptoms). If the child is presumed to have dysfunctional abdominal pain (ie, symptoms suggesting psychosomatic abdominal pain, but without identifiable stressors in the environment), the thrust of management is to learn to ignore and cope with the pain.

Table 39. — Causes of Recurrent Abdominal Pain

Psychosomatic abdominal pain

Dysfunctional abdominal pain

Gastrointestinal
  Peptic ulcer disease
  Crohn disease
  Ulcerative colitis
  Foreign body
  Partial obstruction
  Lactose intolerance
  Giardiasis
  Bacterial enteritis
  Infestation
  Hepatitis
  Pancreatitis, pancreatic pseudocyst
  Cholecystitis
  Choledochal cyst
  Overeating, overdrinking
  Constipation
  Neoplasm

Urogenital
  Urinary tract infection
  Nephrolithiasis
  Obstruction, hydronephrosis
  Trauma
  Tumor

Gynecologic
  Dysmenorrhea
  Pelvic inflammatory disease
  Endometriosis
  Hematocolpos
  Rupture of ovarian follicle
  Ovarian cyst: rupture, bleeding, enlarged

Other
  Sickle cell anemia
  Collagen vascular disease
  Pelvic abscess
  Tumors
  Henoch-Schönlein purpura
  Familial ß- thalassemia
  Porphyria

Chronic or Recurrent Headaches

Table 40 lists the common causes of recurrent headaches in children and adolescents. There are many articles and texts to guide the clinician through the differential diagnosis. It is beyond the purview of this chapter to go into detail regarding the differential diagnosis.

Muscle contraction headache, or tension headache, is the most common cause of headaches and, in most instances, is psychosomatic in nature. This form of headache may be occipital, due to tension in neck muscles, or frontal, due to tension in facial and temporal musculature. The symptom is often described as "a tight band" or "a pressure from the outside." It can be mild to severe. Evaluation usually reveals (1) a reassuring review of systems, (2) a positive family history, (3) a temperamental or psychological predisposition, (4) a normal physical and neurological examination, and (5) often, with careful history, identification of precipitating psychosocial events. Management of tension headaches focuses on symptomatic relief and identification and modification of predisposing factors.

Migraine headaches present differently at different ages, and they are more atypical in their presentation prior to adolescence. Migraine headaches often fit the criteria of a psychosomatic illness in that there is a physiological/familial predisposition and they can be precipitated by psychosocial factors. Management of migraine headaches should include an attempt to address identifiable stressors in the environment.

When considering the extent of diagnostic workup for chronic or recurrent headaches, the health care provider should keep in mind those symptoms and signs suggesting organic pathology: vomiting without nausea; pain worse when the child is lying down at night or on first arising in the morning; pain worse with coughing, straining, sneezing, bearing down, or change of position; anorexia or weight loss; dizziness or vertigo; progressively worsening symptoms; neurological symptomatology that persists between episodes of pain; abnormalities on neurological exam; nuchal rigidity; head tilt; evidence of papilledema; slow pulse or high blood pressure; and onset before the age of school entry.

Table 40. — Causes of Recurrent Headaches

Tension/muscle contraction headache

Migraine headache

Post-traumatic

Traumatic (soft tissue, fracture)

Mass lesion: tumor, abscess, hematoma

Sinusitis

Dental disorder

Ictal or postictal headache

Hypertension

Ear disease

Neuralgia, neuritis

Hydrocephalus

Arteriovenous malformation, aneurysm

Temporomandibular joint syndrome

Eye strain, poor visual acuity

Hypoglycemia, anemia, hypoxia

Rare metabolic conditions

Encephalitis

Recurrent Chest Pain

Chest pain is less common than recurrent headache or recurrent abdominal pain. In our society, chest pain produces a high level of anxiety due to fears about serious heart disease. The majority of children with recurrent chest pain have minor musculoskeletal disorders or psychosomatic pain. Nevertheless, a thorough assessment is necessary and should include a thorough history and physical examination. When the diagnosis is not readily apparent and the degree of symptomatology seems significant, a chest x-ray and ECG should be performed.

It should be remembered that hyperventilation can produce chest pain, and anxiety about chest pain can produce hyperventilation. The differential diagnosis is presented in Table 41. The clinician should consider a serious cause if the following are present: severe distress; a sick appearance; syncope; reproduc-

Table 41. — Causes of Recurrent Chest Pain

Idiopathic

Musculoskeletal
  Costochondritis
  Rib fracture
  Soft tissue injury
  Chest wall strain
  Slipping rib syndrome
  Tussive trauma

Psychosomatic

Pulmonary
  Bronchitis, tracheitis
  Pneumonia
  Reactive airway disease
  Pleuritis, pleural effusion
  Pneumothorax
  Pneumomediastinum
  Foreign body in airway
  Pleurodynia

Gastrointestinal
  Esophagitis
  Hiatal hernia
  Gastroesophageal reflux
  Esophageal dysfunction

Cardiac
  Arrhythmias (most commonly supraventricular tachycardia)
  Idiopathic hypertrophic subaortic stenosis
  Aortic stenosis, pulmonic stenosis
  Mitral valve prolapse
  Anomalous left coronary artery
  Pericarditis
  Myocarditis
  Coronary arteritis
  Myocardial infection
  Cardiomyopathy

Neurologic
  Spinal cord tumor
  Epidural abscess

Neoplastic
  Variety of tumors or neoplasms in lung, chest wall, mediastinum, etc

Other
  Shingles
  Sickle cell anemia

ible pain with exercise; or associated respiratory symptoms. Management should proceed as described in the previous discussions when the clinician is able to rule out serious causes of chest pain and there is the following evidence suggesting a psychosomatic cause: (1) reassuring review of systems; (2) positive family history of psychosomatic symptoms; (3) predisposing temperament; (4) normal examination, chest x-ray, and ECG; and (5) precipitating events.

Limb Pain

Nonarticular lower extremity pains in the late day or evening, without a demonstrable physical finding ("growing pains"), are quite common in school-age children. They involve thighs, calves, or behind the knees, and are usually bilateral. They respond to massage, heat, and analgesics. Pain that occurs during exercise should be further investigated. Evaluation of limb pain should include an x-ray at a minimum. If the pain is (1) chronic or recurrent, (2) nonarticular, (3) without an apparent organic cause, (4) accompanied by normal x-ray findings, and (5) involves school absenteeism, it is often psychosomatic. Table 42 lists the common causes of recurrent limb pain in school-age children.

Hyperventilation

Hyperventilation is one of the frequent psychosomatic symptoms that can result in an exaggerated response in the school. A panic stricken student who states "I cannot get my breath" can result in excessive use of a community 911 emergency system. Once the symptom is diagnosed by an appropriate medical professional, the provision of a paper bag to the student, along with quiet reassurance, is the appropriate emergency management. If attacks continue, attention should be directed to dealing with anxiety in the student's life.

Other Recurrent Symptoms

Other symptoms should be addressed in a manner similar to that described above. This approach will serve the clinician well when applied to symptoms such as chronic back pain, fatigue, and dysmenorrhea.

Table 42. — Causes of Recurrent Limb Pain

Recurrent, nonarticular limb pains (growing pains)

Trauma
  Sprains
  Fracture
  Overuse injury
  Bruise, contusion,
    hematoma

Bone/joint
  Chondromalacia of the patella
  Osgood-Schlatter disease
  Slipped capital femoral
    epiphysis
  Osteochondritis dissecans
  Benign bone tumors

Neoplasms
  Bone tumor
  Leukemia
  Lymphoma
  Neuroblastoma
  Fibrosarcoma
  Synovial cell sarcoma

Collagen vascular disorders
  Juvenile rheumatoid arthritis
  Systemic lupus
    erythematosus
  Dermatomyositis
  Rheumatic fever
  Inflammatory bowel disease
  Henoch-Schönlein purpura

Muscles
  Myopathies
  Fibromyalgias

Infections
  "Toxic" synovitis
  Osteomyelitis
  Septic arthritis
  Pyogenic myositis and
    viral myositis
  Discitis
  Rubella arthritis (and
    postvaccination)
  Trichinosis
  Leptospirosis
  Poliomyelitis

Neurologic
  Guillain-Barré syndrome

Nutritional/metabolic
  Scurvy

Hematologic
  Sickle cell anemia
  Hemophilia
  Severe anemia

Endocrine
  Hypercortisolism
  Hyperparathyroidism
  Hypothyroidism
  Osteoporosis

Miscellaneous
  Hypermobility
  Shortened hamstring
  Tight Achilles tendon

Management of Conversion Symptoms

Most students with conversion symptoms are referred to pediatricians, psychologists, or psychiatrists for treatment and follow-up. Close contact between the health care professionals and school personnel is essential. The child will require help in dealing with the primary conflict. Parents and school professionals will need to do the following: (1) help the child handle that conflict and (2) reduce the secondary gain associated with the conversion symptom. A treatment plan that involves teachers, school administrators, school nurse and counselor, and parents is best communicated at a conference. Because of time constraints, it may be necessary to coordinate activities over the phone. The school nurse can serve as the intermediary in the exchange of information and development of the plan.

Management of Malingering

Malingering is often a "ticket of admission" for assistance with some perceived problem. Therefore, attempts should be made to assist the child in dealing with the conflict or concern in a direct manner. Ongoing help, usually from parents, physician, or school personnel (occasionally from counselors) is required to deal with similar conflicts in the future. When symptoms arise in the future, it is helpful for the teacher to assist the child in looking at recent events to identify the conflicts, fears, or concerns and assist the child in dealing directly with them. When the student claims to have symptoms, evaluation by the physician or the school nurse should be carried out. If malingering is suggested, every effort should be made to return the child to class.

Management of Hypochondriasis

Hypochondriasis is usually a problem that affects more than one generation in a family. The nurse or physician needs to assist the child and the parents in understanding the attitudes, fears, and concerns that may exist. Sometimes counseling is necessary. School professionals can be of help by providing reassurance and real world interpretations of bodily sensory experiences.

CHAPTER 13

THE FREQUENT VISITOR TO THE HEALTH ROOM

In an elementary school, about 10% of students will account for nearly half of all the visits to a school health office or school nurse. Excluding those students who are asked to come on a frequent basis for administration of medication or other health procedures, many of these students will have significant clusters of associated characteristics, including increased dependency, low self-esteem, learning or behavior problems, family dysfunctions, psychosomatic complaints, and poor peer relationships.[1] In addition, research suggests that frequent visits to the school nurse are also associated with increased use of health care services in the community. All of these findings suggest that the school health program should specifically target frequent visitors as a population that may need special attention and intervention.[2] This chapter reviews procedures and practices that can detect, evaluate, manage, and possibly prevent frequent and medically unnecessary use of the health office.

Detection

Without a system of logging of visits by student name, it will be impossible to pick out every child who might fit into the category of a frequent visitor, since the nurse or aide may not always be in the health room at all times and may not remember every child who comes in for a complaint. Such health room logs are commonly kept, but sometimes the student's name or ID number is not written down. If grade and teacher are also recorded, review is facilitated, and children with similar names are less likely to be confused. About every 1 to 2 months the daily logs should be reviewed.

How many times will the average student be expected to visit the school health room?[3] While there is some variation, based on available personnel, school policy, teacher referral, and parent referral, the average number is between three to five visits per school year, with girls tending to visit more frequently than boys and to have had more than several different complaints over the year. In one study of visits to the elementary school nurse during a period of more than 2 years, the top 10% of visits in each year were accounted for by about 8% of students, who each visited the nurse between 13 and 66 times during the year. There was no difference in the rank order of the types of presenting complaints between the high-frequency users and more moderate users: trauma, illness (usually fever or respiratory), stomachache, and headache. Interestingly, only 4% to 5% of the students made no visit at all in either school year. It was also found that frequent visitors tended to remain frequent visitors to the nurse's office the next year. Table 43 illustrates the major reasons for visits to the nurse's office.

If day of week and time of day are also recorded on the log sheet, interesting patterns of visiting may emerge. A student who visits the nurse on days when there is a spelling test or whenever math or reading is taught, may be attempting to cope with the stress of not being able to successfully complete the assigned work. While simple examination of the patterns of illness (eg, headaches every Monday morning following a weekend visitation to a divorced parent) may yield strong clues as to the etiology of the stressors in the child's life, usually more evaluation is needed to identify the underlying problem.

Evaluation

The first step after identification of the frequent visitor is to review the stated reasons for the visits. A preponderance of headaches or stomachaches may signal that this is the somatic "ticket" for the child to deal with an uncomfortable or stressful situation. It is important to not be confrontational at the student's next appearance with a similar complaint. Do not remove a crutch until it is clear that the child can function without it or that alternative sources of support are available. Remember that so-called malingering almost always represents a call for attention and help by the child for some real or perceived problem.

It is wise, however, once the suspicion is raised, to do a careful history and examination limited to the presenting problem, with opportunity for the child to comment on "what was the thing that most worried you about the pain," or to trace what feelings

Table 43. — Number and Percent of Boys and Girls Visiting the School Health Room for the Indicated Complaints During Two School Years*

Complaint	Boys (N = 350)		Girls (N = 313)		P Value
	No.	%	No.	%	
Trauma	270	77.1	258	82.4	.30<.50
Other Illness	230	65.7	231	73.8	.05<.10
Stomachache	130	37.1	146	46.6	<.001
Headache	120	34.3	132	42.2	.10<.20
Dental	74	21.1	76	24.3	.50<.70
Upper respiratory tract infections	56	16.0	72	23.1	.05<.10
Ear Complaints	35	10.0	51	16.3	.05<.10
Rash/infection	59	16.9	76	24.3	.05<.10
Social/family	32	9	22	7	.50<.70
Behavioral/learning	45	12	35	11	.80

*From Nader and Brink.[3] Reprinted with permission.

were experienced just before the child became aware of the pain. Negative findings from specific problem-oriented physical examination, if a nurse practitioner is available, or lack of general indicators of serious physical illness, such as fever, can be important adjuncts in responding to the student.

A specific evaluation should be scheduled for the child to be seen by the nurse or nurse practitioner. During this visit, the nature of the complaints and the frequency and timing of the visits are reviewed and explored with the student. Assistance is sought in helping to understand what is going on from the student's perspective. It may be helpful to supplement this interview with a discussion with the teacher and the parent. A clear picture of how the child functions in school, at home, and with peers should emerge from this evaluation. If physical symptoms form a part of the picture, appropriate examination and laboratory tests as indicated need to be performed.

Management

Once the underlying problem is identified, steps must be taken to resolve or ameliorate it. The child can be scheduled to be seen on a regular basis for ongoing brief counseling and support; it is hoped that this will obviate the need for frequent unscheduled visits. The goal of the brief sessions is to help the student identify the real sources of stress (not illness) and to practice strategies of coping with anxiety-provoking situations, such as taking tests (by being prepared) or fear of asking a teacher to explain a task not well understood (by rehearsing the situation with the nurse or counselor). Monitoring will assess the frequency of unscheduled nurse visits and progress toward problem resolution. Some problems will be too large or complex to be easily or completely resolved. In this event, ongoing support and coping still will be helpful.

Prevention

The school health service could, in concert with classroom and home support, create a "child-initiated care" system, along the lines described by Lewis et al.[4] Such a coordinated system (see chapter 7) could begin to teach children to utilize health services in an appropriate way and become more active consumers and more at ease in self-assessment of their physical complaints. The process includes free access to the health room at all times, when the child determines the need to go. Part of the interaction that initially occurs in the health office is an assessment of how that decision was reached and what major outcome of the visit is desired by the student. When assessments are made, the child is given the results and their interpretation and asked to suggest a disposition: return to class, call home, or rest in the office for a bit, and then return to class. If practical, the child's decision is followed and consequences discussed. These efforts will not result in changes in use of services unless efforts are reinforced by teaching decision making in the classroom and by involving parents in letting children assume responsibility for making initial judgments about their health and health care needs at home. Obviously, a child only can be given responsibility consistent with age and maturity. This applies to decisions about health maintenance as well as diseases and illness.

Such a coordinated approach to educating children to have the skills to become informed health consumers may be an important tool in decreasing unwarranted use of an already overburdened health care system. In addition, by concentrating on frequent visits to the school nurse more major health or disability problems may be averted.

References

1. VanArsdale WR, Roghmann KJ, Nader PR. Visits to an elementary school nurse. *J Sch Health*. 1972;42:142-148

2. Gilman S, Williamson MC, Nader PR, Dale S, McKevitt R. Task differentiation among elementary, middle, and high school nurses. *J Sch Health*. 1979;49:313-316

3. Nader PR, Brink SG. Does visiting the school health room teach appropriate or inappropriate use of health services? *Am J Public Health*. 1981;71:416-419

4. Lewis CE, Lewis MA, Lorimar A, Palmer BB. Child-initiated care: the use of school nursing services by children in an "adult-free" system. *Pediatrics*. 1977;60:499-507

CHAPTER 14

LEARNING PROBLEMS

Reasons for Learning Problems

More than 10% of US schoolchildren are receiving special education and related services for various learning problems. Learning problems are complex issues, defying traditional methods of pediatric assessment and management, and are of obvious multidisciplinary concern. Nonetheless, the pediatrician and school health program may assume critical roles in helping children with learning problems, including clarifying the reasons for school difficulties and facilitating appropriate evaluation and intervention.

A student's learning problems may result from a wide variety of causes. Such causes may be simplistically regarded as either intrinsic characteristics of the child (eg, specific learning disabilities, mental retardation, sensory impairment) or as adverse external influences, such as ineffective schooling, family dysfunction, and social problems (Table 44). In reality, however, learning problems are typically the result of a complex interaction of child-, family-, and school-related factors. For example, a subtle learning disability or mild mental retardation may result in devastating learning problems when a child also is confronted with parental divorce, poverty, or a school of inferior quality. Thus, any assessment of learning problems must include a search for "clusters" of adverse influences and consider the child's capabilities and weaknesses within the context of social and environmental circumstances.

Specific Learning/Language Disabilities

Specific learning disabilities are the most prevalent and perplexing of the many reasons for learning problems. Learning disabilities traditionally have been regarded as biologically based developmental disorders characterized by disturbances in the processes involved in understanding or using language. Learning-disabled children most commonly have problems with the language arts—reading, spelling, and written expression. However, such children may display pervasive academic delays, having difficulties also with arithmetic and handwriting skills,

**Table 44. — Conditions Commonly Associated With Problems
in Learning**

Specific learning and language disabilities

Attention deficits

Mental retardation

Sensory impairment

Emotional problems

Chronic illness

Family and social dysfunction

Ineffective schooling

or, less commonly, may have isolated problems with arithmetic. The hallmark of learning disabilities is a discrepancy between a student's potential for academic achievement as suggested by intelligence testing, and actual performance as documented by achievement tests. Although prevalence rates of 1% to more than 30% are reported in different series, best estimates suggest that approximately 3% to 5% of students are learning disabled and that such students account for about 40% of those eligible for special education services within the United States.

Because learning/language-disabled (LD) children frequently have experienced delayed or disordered language acquisition, and such children often perform poorly on a variety of oral language measures, learning disabilities have been regarded as the expression of a general linguistic disability. Recently, research also has emphasized the importance of weaknesses in higher-order cognitive functions, such as thinking and reasoning processes and memory. Difficulties in such "metacognitive" skills as being able to access acquired information when needed and apply learned skills may result in LD students being unable to focus attention on the salient features of tasks or effectively devise problem-solving strategies.

Psychoeducational evaluation is of critical importance in the diagnosis of specific learning disabilities. A variety of school personnel may participate in such evaluations, including psychologists, special educators, learning disability specialists, speech-language pathologists, and social workers. The goals of assessing a child for learning disabilities are to examine the child's academic strengths and weaknesses, determine intellectual ability, examine communicative ability, and assess social and emotional adaptation. There is no one standardized test battery appropriate for all learning-disabled children and the specific tests used depend on the preference and expertise of the examiners, the child's needs, and local resources. Typically administered tests include intelligence tests; tests of general learning abilities; academic achievement tests; diagnostic reading, math, and writing tests; tests of perceptual and motor function; measures of speech and language skills; and informal assessment techniques, including diagnostic teaching.

Developmental assessment has demonstrated that learning-disabled children typically display deficits in various areas of functioning. In addition to previously discussed speech and language difficulties and deficits in cognitive and conceptual thought, findings include motor abnormalities and clumsiness, confusion with sequences and time relationships (temporal-sequential deficits), difficulties with right-left discrimination (directional disorientation), failure to appreciate spatial relationships and visual detail (visuoperceptual difficulties), difficulties integrating auditory (eg, sounds of words) and visual (eg, visual configuration of letters) stimuli, deficits in intersensory integration, and evidence of neurological immaturity (so-called neuromaturational delay, or "soft" neurologic signs). While such *clinical correlates* should not be presumed to be actual causes of learning disabilities nor serve as a basis for diagnosis, clusters of such findings should be viewed as "red flags" indicating the need for psychoeducational evaluation.

Attention Deficits

Whether attention deficits represent a specific disorder, termed attention deficit-hyperactivity disorder in edition 3 (revised) of the *Diagnostic and Statistical Manual of Mental Disorders* of the American Psychiatric Association, or rather are the result of highly complex interactions between child-related and environmental factors is controversial. Regardless, there clearly does exist a group of children for whom difficulties with inattention, distractibility, lack of persistence, and impulsivity contribute to learning problems. Such attention deficits often coexist with other learning problems, such as specific learning disabilities. Suggested causes of attention deficits include adverse prenatal or perinatal events; delayed maturation of the central nervous system; genetic factors; metabolic abnormalities of the biogenic amines (dopamine, norepinephrine); exposure to toxins—either prenatally (eg, alcohol) or during childhood (eg, lead, artificial food additives, naturally occurring salicylates); and adverse social circumstances. Consequences of attention deficits include poor classroom work skills, low educational achievement, an increased need for special educational services, and social and emotional problems, including diminished self-esteem and difficulties with social adjustment. Recent research has emphasized the extent to which attention deficits may persist through adolescence and adulthood. Within North America, estimates of the incidence of attention deficits range from 2% to 4% of schoolchildren. While boys reportedly are affected more often than girls, with suggested ratios ranging from 5:1 to 9:1, recent research has emphasized a higher incidence among girls.

Behavioral management techniques are of major importance in the management of children with attention deficits. A well-structured, highly organized classroom is desirable. Demands on the child are clear and consistent. Special education, including academic remediation and specialized educational programs, addresses problems with academic achievement. Drug therapy, including stimulant medications (methylphenidate, dextroamphetamine, pemoline) and such alternative drugs as tricyclic antidepressants (desipramine, imipramine) and clonidine, should be reserved for use as adjunctive therapy that "sets the stage" for improved learning by enabling the child to respond more favorably to behavioral management and special education. To date, the most promising results of intervention for attention deficits has been reported for "multimodality" therapy, combining behavioral management, drug therapy, and counseling.

A variety of nonstandard therapies have been suggested for use with children with attention deficits, specific learning disabilities, and other learning problems. Neurophysiologically based treatments include patterning, optometric training, sensory integration therapy, and α-wave conditioning. Examples of therapies considered to have a biological basis include megavitamins, mineral therapy, dietary manipulation and the exclusion of food additives, and treatment of presumed hypoglycemia. In general, these approaches are not supported by controlled research studies. Neither dietary crossover studies nor specific challenge experiments support a major role for dietary therapy.

Mental Retardation

Although more severe forms of retardation are identified during early childhood, mild mental retardation is typically not identified until the child is confronted with the cognitive demands of school. Since 85% to 90% of retarded individuals are mildly retarded, the peak prevalence of discovery of mental retardation is during the school years. The academic performance of children with mild mental retardation, also termed "educable mental retardation," is characterized by a slow learning rate with the optimal acquisition of skills up to the fourth- or fifth-grade level.

No specific etiology is apparent for the majority of children with mild mental retardation. However, a limited number of conditions may result in mild retardation identified during the school years. Examples include sex chromosome abnormalities, such as the fragile X syndrome, as well as such diverse entities as neurofibromatosis, tuberous sclerosis, fetal alcohol syndrome, and fetal hydantoin effects.

Sensory Impairment

Hearing and vision are obviously the most crucial senses for academic learning. This is why no child should undergo evaluation for learning difficulties without a recent vision and hearing (audiometric) screening. Of the two, hearing loss results in the more profound educational handicap.

Although estimates vary, approximately 5% of school-age children have hearing levels below normal in at least one ear and some 10% to 20% of this group are sufficiently impaired to require some type of special educational services. The learning problems of such children typically include difficulties with reading as well as arithmetic reasoning and problem solving, with relatively better performance in arithmetic computation, spelling, and art. The learning problems of hearing-impaired children are generally regarded to be a result of impaired language acquisition and communication skills. Children with hearing impairments also have a greater frequency of difficulties with maladjustment, behavior problems, and social immaturity.

Children with vision impairment usually fare rather well within the classroom. In fact, many partially sighted and even blind children function adequately in a regular classroom program with relatively minor modifications. Those visually impaired children with major learning problems tend to have additional handicaps such as low intelligence or hearing loss. Some 50% of blind children and 40% of partially sighted children have additional handicaps.

Emotional Problems

Within different studies, 30% to 80% of students with emotional illness have learning and behavior problems in the classroom. The extent to which emotional disturbances, such as depression and conduct disorder, directly result in learning problems is unclear. While emotional illness is probably the primary cause of learning problems for a relatively small number of children, emotional factors may be far more important in the exacerbation of academic difficulties from other causes. For example, a learning-disabled child's school functioning may be even further impaired by the inevitably accompanying feelings of frustration and diminished self-esteem. From a practical standpoint, emotional difficulties should not be presumed to be the cause of a child's learning problems. Rather, evaluation must include a search for possible underlying causes, such as specific learning disabilities, attention deficits, or mild mental retardation.

Chronic Illness

A fourth to a third of children with chronic illness have learning problems. A variety of factors may adversely impact on such children's school performance, including limited alertness or stamina, chronic pain, medication side effects (eg, anticonvulsants, bronchodilators, antineoplastic drugs), excessive absenteeism, altered or inappropriate expectations of teachers or parents, psychosocial maladjustment, and the inferior quality of alternative placements, such as segregated classes or special schools.

Family and Social Dysfunction Problems

Social and environmental factors are important contributors to learning problems. Within the United States, approximately 1 in 4 children have learning, behavioral, emotional, or developmental problems as a result of family dysfunction. Learning disabilities are more common when children are raised in poverty and when parents themselves are of low educational levels. Other social problems that may contribute to a child's learning problems include parental separation or divorce, child abuse or neglect, illness or death of immediate family members, parental emotional illness, early parenthood, and substance abuse.

Ineffective Schooling

The specific school that a child attends may influence academic performance. Surprisingly, physical and administrative features of schools, such as whether the school is public or private, class size, age and spaciousness of buildings, and student-teacher ratio, appear to have a limited impact on students' learning and classroom behavior. Rather, learning is more heavily influenced by aspects of school processes, such as the school's expectations for academic attainment, amount of homework, teachers' prompt starting of lessons and more time spent discussing topics rather than disciplining the class, more group rather than individual instruction, the generous use of rewards and praise for students' achievements, and good working conditions for students. School climate and the social environment may be particularly important for children living in poverty and experiencing family dysfunction and social problems.

Evaluation of Learning Problems

Detection

Teachers form the front line of the detection process. As noted in chapters 7 and 13, the school health team can play a major role in screening frequent health office visitors and in regularly reviewing with teachers, students consistently performing in the lowest academic percentiles.

All children identified with learning problems should undergo pediatric evaluation. The responsibility for performing a pediatric evaluation will vary among school systems and depend on local resources. Ideally, such an evaluation may be performed by the child's personal pediatrician who has the advantage of observing the child over time and is able to consider findings within the context of the child's general well-being and social situation. Alternatively, such evaluations may be performed by a school physician or, via contractual arrangements, by a pediatrician with special interest and expertise in learning problems. School nurse practitioners may perform aspects of this evaluation with appropriate pediatrician consultation.

History

Information should be sought from parents, the child, and teachers. Questionnaires may facilitate information gathering. Details concerning *school functioning* should be sought, including information about the child's academic achievement, classroom behavior, school attendance, results of past psychoeducational testing, and whether any special educational services have been provided. Discrete delays in select subjects (eg, language arts) from the outset of schooling or the later emergence of select difficulties (eg, mathematics, written expression) may suggest the possibility of specific learning disabilities, while pervasive academic delays from the outset may raise concerns for mental retardation. Long-standing, pervasive problems with inattention, impulsivity, and overactivity may suggest attention deficits, while acting-out behavior, sadness, or a reluctance to participate may be the consequence of poor school performance due to specific learning disabilities. Excessive absenteeism may reflect school phobia, truancy, or a chronic illness, such as asthma. Past psychoeducational testing may document the discrepancy between a child's learning potential and actual academic achievement, which is the hallmark of a specific learning disability or a low level of intellectual and adaptive functioning diagnostic of mild mental retardation. The child's response to special educational services may suggest specific learning disabilities, while a description of special school services provided may raise concerns regarding an inappropriate or inferior classroom placement.

Aspects of the traditional medical history may yield findings with possible implications for learning problems. The *perinatal history* of children with learning disabilities and attention deficits is characterized by an increased incidence of "clusters" of adverse events, such as anoxic encephalopathy, prematurity, low birth weight, and often associated bronchopulmonary dysplasia. Maternal alcohol or drug intake may suggest possibilities such as fetal alcohol syndrome or fetal hydantoin effects, which can be associated with learning problems. Findings from the *past medical history* with implications for learning problems include chronic illness, recurrent or persistent otitis media, lead exposure, iron deficiency anemia, seizures, frequent accidents due to hyperactivity, and the use of such medications as phenobarbital, theophylline, and antihistamines. With regard to the *developmental history* of learning, disabled children may suggest delayed or disordered language acquisition and communication skills, mild delays in select milestones (eg, first words, sitting, walking), or an "uneven" pattern of skills. More global delays may suggest mild mental retardation. *Behavioral history* may suggest long-standing, pervasive problems with attention span, impulsivity, and overactivity characteristic of attention deficits or sadness indicative of depression. Acting out, antisocial behavior or shyness, and a tendency to withdraw are possible manifestations of low self-esteem accompanying long-standing school failure and chronic frustration.

Family history also may suggest clues as to the cause of learning problems. An increased incidence of learning disabilities is observed among first degree relatives of affected individuals. Parents of children with attention deficits have an increased incidence of attention deficits themselves, as well as antisocial behavior and alcoholism among fathers and hysteria among mothers. *Social history* may identify stressors known to contribute to learning problems, such as child abuse or parental divorce, and information should be sought concerning family composition, socioeconomic status, parents' educational attainment and employment status, parents' age and patterns of childbearing, and parents' aspirations for their children.

Physical Examination

Although the physical examination of most children with learning problems is normal, certain aspects deserve special emphasis. *General observation* of the child may reveal limited alertness or stamina due to a chronic disease; moodiness or sadness suggesting depression; or a short attention span, impulsivity, and overactivity suggesting possible attention deficits. Tics may be noted indicating the possibility of Tourette syndrome, which is associated with learning disabilities and attention deficits. A careful examination of *phenotypic features* may reveal an increased incidence of minor congenital anomalies (eg, fine, "electric" hair, hypertelorism, low-set ears, epicanthic folds, high-arched palate, clinodactyly, and syndactyly of the toes), which has been particularly noted among some boys with attention deficits and specific learning disabilities. Alternatively, stigmata of genetic syndromes known to be associated with learning problems may suggest such disorders as fragile X syndrome, Turner syndrome, or fetal alcohol syndrome. *Hearing and vision screening* should exclude sensory impairment. *Growth measurements* may indicate microcephaly or macrocephaly, which is noted more frequently among both learning-disabled and retarded children. Short stature is associated with an increased incidence of learning problems among boys.

Certain other aspects of the traditional examination also deserve emphasis. *Skin* examination may reveal multiple cafe au lait spots suggestive of neurofibromatosis or, less commonly, "ash leaf" spots and adenoma sebaceum of tuberous sclerosis. Examination of the *tympanic membranes* may indicate evidence of recurrent or chronic otitis. Examination of the *genitalia* may suggest evidence of sexual abuse. Also, among older boys, delayed sexual maturation is associated with an increased incidence of learning problems.

Mental Status Examination

Simple projective screening techniques may be helpful in suggesting emotional problems such as depression, poor self-esteem as a consequence of learning problems, or anxiety related to family dysfunction. Examples of such techniques include asking the child for three wishes, requesting that the child draw a family picture, and the Winnicott squiggle game, in which the child is asked to complete a picture after the examiner draws some squiggles on a page. (See Dworkin, 1992, in "Suggested Readings" at end of chapter.)

Neurodevelopmental Assessment

Performing an "extended" neurological examination to survey a child's functioning in different areas of development may be helpful in identifying factors contributing to learning problems. During neurodevelopmental assessment, the child is asked to perform age-appropriate tasks representing various areas of development, such as gross- and fine-motor skills, auditory-language function, temporal-sequential organization and memory, visuospatial orientation, and minor neurologic indicators or neuromaturational ("soft" neurologic) signs. Children with specific learning disabilities typically display an uneven developmental profile, with discrete areas of relative strength and weakness. In particular, learning-disabled children are more likely to have deficits in aspects of language functioning. In contrast, children with mild mental retardation typically have delays in all areas assessed. Behavioral observation during such an assessment may suggest the possibility of attention deficits or emotional problems.

The significance of minor neurologic indicators or "soft" neurologic signs is controversial. However, such findings as dysdiadochokinesis (difficulty with rapid alternating movements), synkinesia (mirror movements), and marked dystonic posturing of the upper extremities with heel walking are observed more frequently among boys with attention deficits and, to a lesser degree, specific learning disabilities.

Laboratory Studies

No laboratory studies are routinely indicated in the pediatric evaluation of school failure. Rather, tests should be performed when children are considered to be at increased risk for conditions known to be associated with learning problems. Screening for *iron-deficiency anemia* is indicated for children at risk because of nutritional or socioeconomic factors. *Lead screening* should routinely be considered for children because of past history, living environment, or pica. *Thyroid function studies* should be reserved for children with signs or symptoms of thyroid disease other than isolated overactivity or short attention span. *Chromosome analysis*, including a search for the fragile X site, is recommended for all retarded boys and retarded girls with a family history of retardation. Chromosome analysis is otherwise unlikely to be helpful unless suggested by phenotypic features suggesting a genetic syndrome. *Drug screening* for substance abuse may be indicated when older children or adolescents demonstrate erratic, unpredictable behavior or a precipitous decline in school performance.

Neuroanatomical and neurophysiologic studies similarly should be reserved for specific indications. An *electroencephalogram (EEG)* is indicated only when a seizure disorder is suspected. A *computed tomographic (CT) scan* or *magnetic resonance imaging (MRI)* should be reserved for children with microcephaly, macrocephaly, or hydrocephaly, or suspected central nervous system malformations. Computer-assisted neurophysiologic techniques, such as *neurometrics* and *brain electrical activity mapping (BEAM)*, should be reserved for research protocols until clinical applicability is demonstrated.

Care of the Child With Learning Problems

Educational programming is the mainstay of treatment for learning problems. Nonetheless, the school health program may participate in the management of children's learning problems through a variety of roles.

Specific Medical Treatment

Medical treatment of underlying conditions that contribute to learning problems is the most traditional of pediatric roles. Examples include the use of anticonvulsant medication for the control of seizures interfering with learning and the treatment of asthma in order to promote school attendance and minimize the side effects of drugs such as theophylline. Pharmacologic management of attention deficits should be reserved for use as one component of multimodality therapy, including also behavioral management, special education, and counseling. If pharmacologic therapy is attempted, the school health program should actively monitor the child's behavior and achievement and regularly provide this information to the prescribing physician.

Counseling

Pediatric evaluation may be helpful in clarifying a child's strengths and weaknesses and setting appropriate expectations for the child's performance. Health professionals may be particularly important for children with chronic illness or developmental disabilities for whom misunderstanding may contribute to inappropriately altered expectations and preferential or prejudicial treatment by teachers or parents. Explaining the developmental basis for certain learning problems may alleviate parental, student, or teacher guilt and anxiety. A particularly important aspect of counseling is offering scientifically based opinions about nontraditional treatment strategies lacking documented benefit, such as dietary manipulation, megavitamin therapy, optometric training, or sensory integration therapy. Depending on expertise, counseling also may include advice regarding the use of such behavioral management strategies as positive reinforcement and time-outs.

Arranging Further Investigations and Referrals

Evaluation may suggest the need for laboratory studies or referral for further investigations. A traditional pediatric role is the coordination of such studies and arrangement for further evaluations by other medical specialists (eg, neurology, ophthalmology). In general, psychoeducational evaluation preferably should be done in the school system. This may not be feasible in some cases due to limited school resources or parents' demands for an independent assessment.

Promoting Utilization of Community Services and Resources

The school health programs may facilitate communication between families and school systems by advocating for appropriate services for the student. This role may be particularly important when adversarial relationships arise between parents and school personnel. Outside of the school, families may find other resources to be helpful, such as parent groups, peer support groups, and mental health and social service agencies.

Planning Educational Strategies

Responsibility for planning educational strategies for the child with learning problems resides with the appropriate educational personnel. While the health service has neither the training nor experience to suggest specific educational interventions, participation with other professionals in the development of a child's educational program is feasible and often reassuring to parents, who often view the health personnel as the child's advocate. For children with attention deficits, the school health program should ensure that pharmacologic treatment is not relied on exclusively and that a comprehensive plan also includes behavioral management, educational services, and counseling. For children with chronic disease, educational plans should include appropriate expectations based on a clear understanding of the child's limits and potential.

School Implications

Collaboration between health and educational personnel inside and outside the school is essential in the assessment of children's learning problems. As previously discussed, assessment must consider the multiple factors that may contribute to learning problems and include a search for "clusters" of adverse influences. Furthermore, the child's capabilities and weaknesses must be considered within the context of the learning environment. Such assessment should not be performed in isolation. Rather, an interchange of ideas and communication between professionals—an interdisciplinary approach—is necessary. Multiple observations within different settings (ie, the classroom and the health office) offer an important opportunity to share information and increase the reliability of individual assessments.

The goal of pediatric assessment as performed by the school health program will vary, depending on the student's individual circumstances. When psychoeducational evaluation already has identified a reason for learning problems, such as specific learning disabilities or mild mental retardation, the goal of the evaluation is rather limited: the exclusion of medical problems as contributors to learning difficulties. The yield from such an evaluation is generally low. Alternatively, for the child with unexplained learning problems, evaluation involves the detection of medical conditions that may contribute to school difficulties (eg, seizure disorder or hearing impairment), as well as a search for clinical correlates of such causes of learning problems as specific learning disabilities, mental retardation, and attention deficits. The identification of such correlates emphasizes the need for diagnostic input from other disciplines (ie, psychoeducational evaluation).

The role of the school health program in the early identification of learning problems also will vary, depending on local resources and circumstances. When the school physician also serves as a child's personal pediatrician, an active role in early identification is feasible. Ideally, such early identification is facilitated by monitoring the child's developmental and behavioral progress from infancy. Effective developmental surveillance includes eliciting and attending to parental concerns, obtaining the opinions of other relevant professionals such as preschool teachers, inquiring about the child's acquisition of certain skills and milestones, and observing the child's development and behavior within the office setting. Such observations may be performed informally, using a collection of age-appropriate tasks, or may involve the use of a formal developmental screening test. While tools such as the Denver Developmental Screening Test (DDST) and the Pediatric Readiness Experimental Screening Scale (PRESS) are of only limited value in the early identification of learning problems, they may be useful in confirming age-appropriate tasks or in suggesting suspicions and concerns. Such screening tests should not be used in isolation, but rather as part of an overall monitoring strategy.

When the school does not have access to children prior to school entry, the role of the school health program in early identification is limited to working with educators who are in regular contact with the child in the teaching environment. Pediatric assessment should be part of the evaluation of preschool children referred to the school system because of concerns that they may be at increased risk for later learning problems or may not be ready to begin the task of academic learning. When school systems perform readiness screening prior to school entry, school health personnel should ensure that findings are interpreted in the context of the child's overall well-being and not used in isolation to plan a child's program or label the child. Alternatively, findings from the school entry pediatric examination may suggest the need for psychoeducational evaluation to identify possible learning problems. The school health program should conduct in-service training to alert teachers and other school personnel to the adverse influences of chronic diseases on school learning, so that learning problems may be promptly identified.

The school health program can assume an active role in monitoring the progress of children with identified learning problems. Frequent visits to the school health office or excessive school absenteeism may reflect school avoidance due to frustrating learning problems. Visits to the school nurse provide important opportunities to monitor children's self-esteem, observe for signs of depression, and offer encouragement and praise for progress.

As specified within Public Law 94-142 (the Education for All Handicapped Children Act), special education for learning problems must be provided within the least restrictive environment (see chapter 6). Schools will develop expanded capabilities to deal with a variety of learning problems that previously may have been addressed within a substantially separate classroom or, even, school building. Many chronically ill children are now being educated within the regular classroom. School health personnel, including the school nurse and school physician consultant, should ensure that teachers have sufficient understanding of the prognosis and educational implications of chronic disorders to maintain appropriate expectations for such children.

Suggested Readings

Dworkin PH. *Learning and Behavior Problems of School Children.* Philadelphia, PA: WB Saunders Co; 1985

Dworkin PH. School failure. *Pediatr Rev.* 1989;10:301-312

Dworkin PH. School learning problems and developmental differences. In: Hoekelman RA, ed. *Primary Pediatric Care.* 2nd ed. St. Louis, MO: Mosby Year Book; 1992

Levine MD, Satz P, eds. *Middle Childhood: Development and Dysfunction.* Baltimore, MD: University Park Press; 1984

Yule W, Rutter M. "Reading and other learning difficulties." In: Rutter M, Hersov L, eds. *Child and Adolescent Psychiatry: Modern Approaches.* 2nd ed. Oxford, England: Blackwell Scientific Publications; 1985:444-464

CHAPTER 15

BEHAVIOR AND DISCIPLINE PROBLEMS

Children's behavioral and discipline issues have concerned adults for some time. The many changes our society has undergone have led to the school setting playing an increasingly important part in recognizing and addressing both normal and pathological behavioral problems. What had traditionally been the domain of the home now is shared between home and school. Significant behavioral problems that interfere with adequate academic achievement now can be formally treated within special education as a "handicapping condition." Deciding with whom, when, how, and why to intervene falls increasingly on the classroom teacher, school nurse, psychologist, counselor, pediatrician, and principal. This chapter reviews common pitfalls, provides suggestions on how to gather needed information, and discusses methods for interpreting that information and a system for planning interventions.

Types of Problems

Because of variation in the definition used to describe school behavioral difficulties and the population characteristics of children and families, there are no precise population estimates as to the extent of behavioral concerns among schoolchildren. We know that upward of 10% of *all* children have had complaints of a stomachache during their school years. Such complaints are often a manifestation of underlying or existing behavioral and psychosocial difficulties. Surveys of various groups of parents and teachers suggest that as high as 30% to 50% of children in some schools are disruptive and overactive, and therefore can't perform as well as the others do. In a survey done 20 years ago, about 24% to 26% of parents reported having concerns regarding their child's schooling, with 25% reporting that the child had a learning problem.

Since this chapter will not go into details regarding each specific behavioral disorder, the reader is referred to competent local behavioral and mental health professionals for assistance with a specific problem. This chapter will attempt to provide a framework for the assessment and a guideline for treatment of a wide variety of behavioral concerns.

An informal survey of school psychologists in different parts of the country generated the following list of behavioral problems that each had been required to address in the course of their duties: refusal to do homework; nail biting; enuresis; schizophrenia; attention deficit disorders; stealing; making rude noises; excessive crying; school phobia; bringing weapons to class; truancy; rudeness; assaultive behavior; vandalism; masturbating; auto theft; poor hygiene; biting; disobedience; falling asleep in class; satanism; tardiness; organic brain syndrome; antisocial behavior; attention seeking; underachievement; and talkativeness. This partial list demonstrates the wide variety of problems faced by school personnel and emphasizes the need for a system with which to analyze unwanted behaviors and decide upon appropriate interventions.

Pitfalls and Important Distinctions

It is important not to draw too hasty a conclusion about the cause of an unwanted behavior. By way of example, one counselor interviewed for the survey mentioned a case in which she was asked to work with a new student who was from a disadvantaged background and who seemed depressed and unresponsive. The counselor observed the child in the classroom and was indeed concerned about the lack of eye contact, minimal attempts to socialize with peers, and general unresponsiveness. When she brought the student to her office, it took her very little time to realize the student was hard of hearing—a fact soon confirmed by the school nurse. Involvement of social services and the purchase of a hearing aid brought a dramatic change in the student's class involvement.

This anecdote illustrates that the first step in developing an effective intervention is to obtain an accurate observation of the behavior that has raised concern. While this may be obvious, time constraints, large caseloads, and increased classroom sizes have minimized the amount of time school personnel have to devote to each individual child. Consequently, a tendency to come to conclusions based solely on written questionnaires, partial observations, or a concerned party's report has become common, and often results in reaching a conclusion before the nature of the problem is understood. Another of the great pit-falls is using descriptions of a behavior and explanations for a behavior interchangeably (eg, the reason he is so active is he is hyperactive). This thinking again leads to hasty conclusions and makes it difficult to get either good information or a good solution.

Descriptions vs Explanations

Confusing these two very different but interdependent concepts is quite common. (It's much like confusing counting and measuring.) A description is a factual, observable accounting of events. It is doing what every good newspaper reporter does in trying to answer the basic questions: who, what, where, and when. "Why" falls under the domain of an explanation. "Why" explanations do not purport to represent factual data, but rather are assumptions used to explain the existence of factual data. Explanations are always dependent on the observer's assumptions, beliefs, and philosophies and may have little to do with the state of mind of the observed. More simply put, explanations can be wrong. However, it is only with an explanation (an assumption as to why a child performs a given behavior) that one can effect some sort of intervention. In the same way a "count" is either exactly right or wrong, so is a description accurate or inaccurate.

Similarly, measurements are always inexact, but denote relationships. Explanations will always be incomplete but will denote relationships between external events and internal thought processes. Using the list of issues from the national survey, nail biting, enuresis, falling asleep in class, and tardiness are observations. They are either true or false. Attention-seeking behavior, organic brain syndrome, and attention deficit disorders are all explanations. They are never complete, but can link observed behaviors to internal states of mind. They purport why a behavior exists. Accurate descriptions are always true, but alone do not provide direction for intervention. Explanations are always imprecise but provide guidance and understanding in developing strategies.

Diagnosis

A special category of "explanation" is the diagnosis. A diagnosis is a type of explanation that limits itself to specific sets of observed behavior, ie, criterion. Using a diagnosis can convey a great deal of information quickly about both the observed behavior and its causes, but there are the same inherent dangers in reaching conclusions before all the facts are in. By way of example, one of the survey participants mentioned a child he was asked to evaluate for possible learning disabilities because of apparent letter reversals. While this was somewhat of a puzzlement, as the child was already in fourth grade and had been receiving good grades and there had not been any concerns raised by previous teachers, the psychologist reasoned that as it was a new teacher reporting the problem, perhaps she was more sensitive to such problems because of more up-to-date training. When psychological testing was unable to corroborate the teacher's observations, the psychologist queried further and was given a list of spelling words with which the child was clearly having difficulty learning the rule "i before e, except after c"—a problem in reversing the letter order, but not a problem with letter reversal.

It also is imperative to be extremely cautious in using a diagnosis when discussing a problem behavior with parents. The diagnosis is often misunderstood and perceived to be a judgment or criticism of the child, rather than a defined set of observable behaviors that are explained by the diagnosis. Sticking to a discussion of the observed behavior and what makes it problematic generally elicits greater parental support. Biting, enuresis, and making rude noises are clearly descriptions of unwanted behavior that parents are likely to agree are best to stop. Attention deficit disorders, schizophrenia, and conduct disorder are diagnoses that are implicitly judgmental and likely to alienate.

Steps to Effective Observation

History Taking

Good observation begins with good history taking. The art of history taking has probably suffered more from modern time pressures than any other diagnostic tool. It is essential to gather information about the undesirable behaviors from the primary parties. This information needs to include (at the risk of being redundant): who, what, where, and when. It is important to determine if the problem is of recent onset or chronic in nature. If it is a chronic problem, what has happened to bring it to a head at this time? Has there been an exacerbation of the unwanted behavior, a change in the behavior, or has the reporting party simply had enough? Does the behavior occur in a variety of settings, or is it restricted to one or two places? If the behavior is "localized," are there any obvious antecedents, and are the same individuals always involved? As important as the antecedents to a behavior are the observed consequences. We may learn more about the "why" of a behavior from the consequences it entails than we do from what events or circumstances led up to the behavior.

One school nurse related a story of one of her young students who seemed particularly accident prone. Numerous trips to the doctor's office were unsuccessful in establishing a medical explanation for the numerous accidents. Observations of the student on the playground and in physical education class revealed nothing out of the ordinary, nor did the accidents happen at any particular time of the day. They did happen almost exclusively at school. It was only after one of the teachers mentioned the child was doing poorly in school and that her accidents often occurred on the day of a major test that the "cause" of the accidents was suggested. Psychoeducational testing and placement in a resource specialist program has brought an end to the "accidents."

Direct Observation

Once an adequate history is gathered (hopefully from more than one source and including the family), direct observation is the next step. All too often, a single report is used as both the history and direct observation. The same questions, issues, and conditions explored during the history taking should now be directly observed. Who is involved? How does it start? Does the behavior always occur, or is it more intermittent?

Analysis of Observations

When all of the observational data is in, analysis needs to follow along several dimensions.

Pathological vs Normal: Not all undesirable behaviors are abnormal. Indeed the vast majority of problems faced in the school setting are reassuringly "normal" problems. Abnormal or pathological problems are abnormal either by kind or by degree. By kind it is meant that the behavior is so out of the ordinary, maladaptive, and destructive that there is no social, developmental, or biological explanation of the behavior that would alleviate concerns about the individual's well-being without some significant intervention. The child who actively hallucinates, demonstrates echolalia, or is self- mutilating presents with a pathology of kind. Behavior that is not strikingly bizarre, aberrant, or unusual but either by its frequency, absence, duration, or persistence has crossed the line from normal to abnormal represents a pathology of degree. The 7 year-old child who sucks his thumb in class and arouses his classmates' ridicule, the 12 year old without any friends, or the 10 year old who is unable to attend or concentrate well enough to profit from his/her classwork are examples of pathology of degree.

Cultural Context: It is fundamental to any analysis of an individual's behavior to recognize that cultural context may determine if the behavior is, first of all, a problem, and, second, if the behavior is abnormal or normal. In addition, cultural sensitivity in all phases of evaluation and treatment is mandatory. Many children in traditional rural settings are brought up with firearms as a normal part of the everyday setting. Unfortunately, many children in highly urban settings are now also brought up with guns as a part of everyday life, but the context of the individual setting clearly alters how one would view a 13 year old owning a gun. In some cultures, direct eye contact is a sign of respect and implies the individual is "listening." In other cultures, direct eye contact is a sign of disrespect and reflects escalating anger. One school counselor working in a rural district in the southwest related a story of her first misadventures with her Native American students. She had been raised and educated in a large eastern city and was attracted to the "adventure" of the southwest. Initially impressed with the friendliness of the small rural community, she was ill prepared for the children's unwillingness to give her their "real" names during casual conversation. Alarmed, she approached her principal, a Native American as well, who informed her that in some native beliefs, a person who knows your name can have power over you. Therefore, an alias was often used with non-tribal acquaintances.

Active vs Passive: Behaviors that are problematic by their presence arc different than behaviors that are problematic by their absence. The child who talks out of turn or hits other children is different from the child who doesn't turn in homework or does not interact with others.

Organic vs "Functional": If the undesired behavior is primarily due to organic, medical, or biological factors, interventions necessarily must be different than if the primary cause is functional in nature (by functional, it is meant that the misbehavior has a function or purpose and is not biologically determined). Attention deficit disorders, Tourette syndrome, mental retardation, "drug exposed infants," and organic brain syndrome are all medical conditions that, to varying degrees, have direct bearing on behavior. Not as obviously, asthma (particularly the side effects of some of the medications), allergy, arthritis, sleep disorders, and chronic ear infections also may have an indirect effect on classroom behavior.

Whenever an organic, biological, or medical condition is suspected, a referral to the pediatrician is warranted. If an organic cause is established, close communication with the physician and any other "specialist" knowledgeable about the condition is imperative. Interventions generally will require specialized personnel and may well include medications, behavioral management programs, and placement in special education classes.

Motivation: Assuming the behavior is found to be functional in nature, the next step in analysis is to determine what the "function" of that behavior is. Here is where the "why," or the explanation of a behavior, comes into play. There are a number of personality theories outlining motivation, drives, needs, and developmental courses, but most of these are too cumbersome and impractical for use in the classroom. One theory, that of Adler, argues that humans are inherently social beings, most behavior has a goal, and behavioral problems are created either from inappropriate expectations or by some failure to meet one of three basic social needs: to be loved, to belong, and to be productive. Failure to meet any or all of these social needs will

produce misbehavior with one of the four "functions" or purposes
in mind: to seek revenge, to seek attention, to engage in a power
struggle, and to assume a disability. Revenge seeking is just as
it sounds; there is an attempt to retaliate for wrongs believed
to have been caused by others. Attention seeking also is relatively straightforward, and usually involves a child who is un-
sure of his belonging or place within a group. Power struggles
are attempts to exert influence. Assumed disabilities are an
attempt to avoid an unpleasant task or responsibility.

Any of these motives for misbehavior can arise from any combination of unmet social needs. However, observing the outcome
of the misbehavior, including your own reaction to the behavior,
will provide insight into resolving the problem.

Determining the Goals of Misbehavior: As stated above,
one's own reaction to misbehavior can often prove diagnostic.
If the child's behavior draws one's attention in an annoying
fashion, it is likely the child is asking for attention. If the behavior is provocative and threatening, an attempt to establish
personal power is the likely goal. Behavior that produces a sense
of frustration and a desire to "quit" is likely to have an assumed
disability as its object, while behavior that is hurtful is likely
aimed at seeking revenge. Combinations of goals not only are
possible, but are usually the case. Observing the reactions of
others and the general outcome of an event can be quite useful
in developing the multiple goals.

A child in music class would hum a specific tune whenever
her music teacher would begin a lesson. Ignoring the problem
and direct confrontation both proved ineffective in eliminating
the humming. It was noticed that one of the outcomes of her
humming was the stopping of the lesson and the embarrassment of the teacher. Review of the history of the problem
revealed that the student had not made the choir taught by
the same teacher, and the misbehavior was aimed directly at
seeking revenge and demonstrating the student's power. After
lengthy discussion, it was decided the girl would function as
a helper for the music teacher with the choir, and there
were no more disruptions from her in the class. This anecdote
directs us well into the "what do you do about it" part of this
chapter.

Intervention

Once observations are complete, the problem analyzed, and it is determined if it is an "organic," "pathological," or "functional" problem, appropriate interventions need to be developed. With both organic and/or pathological problems, the child needs to be referred, first to his or her pediatrician and then to experts in that particular field, if indicated. Functional or purposeful misbehavior usually can be addressed within the school setting. A system for matching types of interventions to types of problems is imperative. The following methods can be usefully employed.

Logical vs Natural Consequences

In order to evaluate the outcomes of an intervention or treatment, one must distinguish between logical and natural consequences. A logical consequence is one that is imposed, whereas a natural consequence is one that will happen without intervention. The child who goes outside during inclement weather without proper clothing and becomes uncomfortable suffers the natural consequences of his/her actions. As guardians of children, we all are sometimes guilty of protecting children from the natural consequences of their misbehavior. We do need to provide for their safety, but the child who is too "bossy" with friends and is consequently snubbed will soon learn to modify his/her behavior if there is no adult intervention. More often, however, there is a need to develop logical consequences. This may include ignoring the child who is attention seeking, giving a "special job" to the youngster who seeks revenge, avoiding direct challenges and liberally using humor for the power-seeking child, and providing attention to the child who is trying to avoid responsibilities through assumed disabilities; these are all examples of logical consequences. Repair of the damaged or unmet social needs to be loved, to belong, and to be productive also must be addressed.

Redirection

The child who is occupied with one task will not have time to misbehave at another. The child who helps clean the chalkboard is unlikely to act the class clown during transitions in the classroom.

Modeling

There are occasions when an unwanted behavior occurs out of lack of knowledge. Assuming that this is the case, teaching or modeling a wanted behavior to replace the unwanted behavior will prove effective.

Reframing

There are occasions, particularly when the goal of a misbehavior is revenge or power seeking, when reframing an incident can be very effective. One school psychologist recounted her interaction with an inner city gang member who was increasingly belligerent. This took the form of meeting teachers in the parking lot and taunting them about the many dangers of the neighborhood. The psychologist turned these taunts around by thanking the student for the warnings and acknowledging his superior knowledge about the neighborhood. He then asked the young teenager for suggestions on improving safety. Although the student put on a good face-saving show, he did indeed come back later to offer a number of useful suggestions that were then put in place.

Appropriate Expectation

Children who display avoidance behaviors or assumed disabilities are usually children who believe themselves unable to meet the expectations of their environment. This is particularly true of the slow or learning-disabled student, and careful consideration to making sure that goals and expectations are both appropriate and challenging is necessary.

Overall Approach

Sharing groups, "magic circles," and "feeling groups" are all excellent methods for understanding why an unwanted behavior exists and methods for intervening. Judicious use of peer pressure and, in general, developing a positive approach to classroom activities will mitigate many problems. Parental involvement is a *must*; in that regard, if parents can't come to you, find a way to go to them. Above all, take the time to see the individual strengths and weaknesses of each child, and do your best to help each develop the skills needed for more productive functioning. Children will recognize that you have their best interests at heart, though they are very unlikely to show it.

Armed with these approaches, and with the support of school and community health and mental health professionals, the school health team can play an important part in the assessment and treatment of behavioral problems presented in the school setting.

Suggested Readings

Dreikurs R, Grunwald BB, Pepper FC. *Maintaining Sanity in the Classroom: Illustrated Teaching Techniques*. New York, NY: Harper & Row; 1971

Levine MD, Carey WB, Crocker AC. *Developmental-Behavioral Pediatrics*. 2nd ed. Philadelphia, PA: WB Saunders Co; 1992

CHAPTER 16

CHILDREN WITH CHRONIC ILLNESS

Having a chronic illness may affect a child's school participation and educational capabilities. At least 10% to 20% of children have some chronic health condition. The large majority of these conditions are mild, and have little impact on the child's ability to attend or participate in educational activities. Severe chronic illnesses that commonly interfere with school participation affect 2% to 4% of children.[1]

Children face a large number of different severe chronic illnesses; yet, with few exceptions, each individual condition is quite rare. The more common conditions include asthma, spina bifida, arthritis, seizure disorders, cystic fibrosis, sickle cell anemia, congenital heart disease, diabetes mellitus, and leukemia. Of these, only asthma occurs with a frequency much greater than 1 in 1,000 school-age children, and most conditions occur much less frequently. These figures mean that a school with 1,000 students will rarely have more than one or two children with any specific severe chronic illness other than asthma. However, the total number of children in that school with different severe chronic illnesses will be 20 to 40.

The current mortality rates for children with severe long-term illnesses indicate that at least 80% to 90% survive to age 20 years; therefore, schools can plan for the eventual graduation of most children with severe health impairments, rather than expect their early death. These rates are distinctly different from those of two or three decades ago, when many children with severe illnesses died younger than the age of graduation, and their educational planning often followed these expectations. The current low mortality rates suggest that the numbers of children with severe long-term illnesses are relatively stable throughout the childhood years. If major technological advances lead to the prevention of many chronic illnesses, the size of the population will decrease. New populations that may increase the numbers with severe long-term illnesses include children surviving with acquired immunodeficiency syndrome (AIDS), children experiencing the long-term effects of maternal sub-

Table 45. — Classification of Childhood Long-term Health Conditions

Conditions that *may* affect cognition directly

Complex craniofacial anomalies
Spina bifida
Epilepsy

Conditions that *may* affect cognition through side-effects of treatment

Leukemia
Asthma

Conditions with little or no cognitive impact

Arthritis
Cystic fibrosis
Hemophilia
Diabetes mellitus

stance abuse, and children who leave neonatal intensive care units with major pulmonary or neurologic sequelae.

Impact of Childhood Chronic Illness on Education

Illness can affect a child's education both by impairing cognitive abilities and by placing physical limitations on school participation.[2,3] Although most severe chronic illnesses have no associated cognitive impairments, some directly affect brain function, and treatment of others may have impact on cognitive abilities (Table 45). Some cases of spina bifida or seizure disorder, for example, affect a child's cognitive abilities directly. Here, careful collaboration among health providers (both generalists and specialists) and educational staff will clarify the direct impact of the health condition on the child's ability to learn and lead to optimal school placement.

Most chronic illnesses, such as arthritis or cystic fibrosis, have no apparent direct effect on cognitive functioning and thereby should not interfere with the child's ability to learn. Children with these conditions can participate well in regular education classes. Even here, there remain important controversies, such as whether conditions such as diabetes (with its periods of significant hyperglycemia) affect cognitive abilities. Such children in regular education settings may require other special health services, such as transportation or specialized therapies, to participate in school.

Other conditions can affect cognitive functioning indirectly, through the effects of medication. Some asthma medications affect cognition, many anticonvulsants affect brain function, and children with leukemia may have cognitive impairments following central nervous system irradiation. Careful testing can help identify these illness-related cognitive impairments.

In addition to affecting cognitive abilities, some conditions cause mobility problems for children. (See chapter 6, "Special Education," and chapter 17, "Technology Supported Students," for a discussion of laws related to access for the disabled.) Lack of elevators or ramps may decrease access to school buildings or to specific classes for some children. Some conditions require barrier-free schools and special transportation services for the child. Other health conditions create enough fatigue to curtail the child's participation and require special remedial efforts. Illnesses and their treatments frequently lead to greater-than-usual school absence and may, in that way, also hinder educational progress.

Health Services in Schools

Medications and Emergencies

Many school systems provide school health services with full-time personnel; however, the majority of schools lack full-time personnel, and many school districts provide very limited health services. Children with chronic illnesses may need specialized programs to ensure access to medications and planning for potential health emergencies. Restricting these children to schools that have in-building health services markedly limits access to regular education services. School policies should include a medication policy, even in situations in which the school lacks full-time health personnel.[4] Medication policies for children with chronic illnesses should be integrated with policies for all the children in the school. Each school should have a designated person who is responsible for overseeing medication distribution. Where school-based nursing is unavailable on a full-time basis, it should be clear who the designated person is and what backup arrangements exist in that person's absence. That designated person could be a specific teacher or administrative person in the principal's office. The person should have specific training and in-service monitoring provided by a licensed health professional, such as a registered professional school nurse. The medication plan should define storage and labeling for medicines at school. Policies should allow capable students to take their own medications when appropriate (such as use of inhalers for children with asthma). Medication should be provided only with the parents' written permission and with written authorization of a physician or other health provider who is legally able to prescribe medications. Where self-medication occurs, methods should be available to monitor students' proper use of equipment and medication and their adherence to prescribed medication regimens.

Many children with long-term illnesses experience medical emergencies in the school setting, such as seizures, acute episodes of asthma, or serious bleeding episodes. Each school should have policies and procedures for handling emergency situations.[5] Schools should establish an ongoing relationship with local health facilities to expedite a student's transfer when necessary.

Each child with a chronic illness should have an individualized plan with respect to medications and emergencies, conforming to the school's basic medication policy and developed with the child's physician and the family. The individualized plan also should address special modifications of the school program, such as for physical education. One state's guidelines and procedures for meeting the specialized physical health care needs of pupils are available (write to the Department of Education, State of California, Sacramento, CA, 95814). If you have any questions, contact your own state's department of education.

Other Special Services

Public Law 94-142 (see chapter 6) guarantees to children with developmental disabilities and many with chronic illnesses an education in the least restrictive environment. This law has greatly improved the availability of many health services in schools, which assist children to participate in regular school activities. Many school districts, however, limit access to needed health-related services to children who are enrolled in a special education program and attend a special education classroom. As noted previously, however, most children with long-term illnesses do not require special education classes. Means should be developed to provide these related health services without requiring placement of the student in a special education category. If this is not possible, one may want to use the special education category of "other health impaired" to provide these services.

Home Tutoring and Absence Policies

Many chronically ill children require tutoring at home at certain times in their illness.[3] Yet, policies regarding teaching at home often do not meet well the needs of children with chronic illnesses. Many school districts require a certain number of *consecutive* days of absence from school (2 to 4 weeks) before a child becomes eligible for home tutoring. Many children with chronic illnesses, such as arthritis or asthma, miss only a few days at a time, although the aggregate number of days of absence may well exceed 2 to 4 weeks. Even where a child is eligible, home tutoring is generally limited to less than 10 hours/week and consists of a generalist teacher providing instruction in all of the different subjects the child is studying. Home tutoring programs face further problems in ensuring the quality and monitoring of services provided.

Several school districts have implemented special programs for home tutoring for chronically ill children by developing registries of children whose chronic conditions are likely to lead to frequent absences.[6,7] These children then become eligible for home tutoring without the usual waiting period. These flexible policies allow more timely response to the needs of such children, and help them to stay on course with their classmates. Home tutoring, nevertheless, is a poor substitute for the socialization and schoolmate contact that comes from direct participation in school activities. Thus, it is important that the child with chronic illness return to the classroom as soon as possible. Encouraging classmates to bring schoolwork to the child with chronic illness who is at home for several days or more helps to decrease the social isolation accompanying home tutoring.[8]

Absence policies in some school districts interfere with the child's educational progress. Some districts require a minimum number of days present for graduation or promotion, regardless of the child's performance of academic tasks. Yet, some children face lengthy periods of school absence due to their illness (for example, leukemia or cystic fibrosis), even though the child's educational progress may be excellent and otherwise support promotion to the next grade level. Absence policies should be flexible enough to allow the proper grade progress for the child with a chronic illness.

Physician Collaboration With Schools

Beyond their ongoing counseling with families whose children have long-term illnesses, physicians can play an important role in working with the schools regarding children with chronic illnesses. First, physicians can share information about the health care issues of specific children that may affect school planning, including health treatments needed in school, the management of emergencies, special restrictions on the child's classroom activity or participation, and planning for physical education. The physician can help especially in sharing information about the impact of the illness or its treatments on the child's ability to learn. Information that is shared with the school should always be done with the full consent of the parents, and when appropriate, the child as well.

Second, physicians can serve as a resource for teachers and other school personnel regarding specific illnesses by providing information in understandable terms about the illness, its consequences, and its long-term expectations.

Third, physicians can help improve health curricula to include general information about chronic illness and health disability, so that children can learn more about these issues and be more accepting of individuals with long-term illnesses. In a similar fashion, the manner in which a teacher accepts a child with chronic illness can serve as a model for how a child is accepted by peers. Physicians and parents working together can help teachers with these tasks.

Future Issues

Many schools are increasing their ability to provide in-school direct-health services and comprehensive school health programs. Where these programs develop, they can help to coordinate multidisciplinary care for children with chronic illness and take an active role in school and patient education about illness. As much as possible, children should be attending school, and enhancement of school-based services will diminish the time that children need to be out of the school receiving treatment in more distant places. Teaching self-care in developmentally appropriate ways is a central part of the management of long-term illness in children. The school, collaborating with other health providers, can be a central resource in helping to teach self-care skills and education about chronic illness in general to children with long-term illness. Schools also can monitor progress and recommend adjustments as needed in the child's education about the particular health condition.

Many families whose children have severe long-term illnesses participate in some form of care coordination or case management. Most families coordinate their own care, but in other circumstances care coordination may be provided by physicians, social workers, or nurses, among others. An advantage of care coordination and case management efforts has been more careful attention to developing goals for educational activities along with more traditional health care planning. Insofar as schools are the major workplace for children, coordination of services for chronically ill children could be effectively carried out by school-based personnel, especially nurses. Coordination at this level will likely maximize the amount of time a child is in school and diminish the impact of illness on education.

References

1. Hobbs N, Perrin JM, Ireys HT. *Chronically Ill Children and Their Families.* San Francisco, CA: Jossey-Bass; 1985

2. Walker DK, Jacobs FH. Public school programs for chronically ill children. In: Hobbs N, Perrin JM, eds. *Issues in the Care of Children With Chronic Illness.* San Francisco, CA: Jossey-Bass; 1985: 615-655

3. American Academy of Pediatrics, Committee on Children With Disabilities and Committee on School Health. Children with health impairments in schools. *Pediatrics*. 1990;86:636-638

4. American Academy of Pediatrics, Committee on School Health. Guidelines for the administration of medication in school. *Pediatrics*. In press

5. American Academy of Pediatrics, Committee on School Health. Guidelines for urgent care in school. *Pediatrics*. 1990;86:999-1000

6. Case J, Matthews S. CHIP: the chronic health impaired program of the Baltimore city public school system. *Child Health Care*. 1983;12(2):97-99

7. Ushkow M. Some children have occasional obstacles to learning (SCHOOL). *Pediatrics*. 1980;66:333

8. Weitzman M. School and peer relations. *Pediatr Clin North Am*. 1984;31:59-69

CHAPTER 17

TECHNOLOGY-SUPPORTED STUDENTS

Some children, because of a medical condition, have been denied not only an education, but the chance to associate and integrate with their peers. Each year there is an increasing number of educators, parents, and physicians who realize that with a minimum of modifications of educational programs and school structure, these students, even though they have a disability, may attend regular school programs. The passage of the Education for All Handicapped Act, Public Law (PL) 94-142 and PL 99-457, mandates education of such children, and schools must adapt programs and facilities in ways that exclude no one. More attention is being put on the positive attributes possessed by these children, rather than on their disabilities.

To call further attention to each child's individuality, the educational plan is referred to as the Individual Educational Plan (IEP). For purposes of discussion and program development it is necessary to create artificial groupings. These groupings have boundaries that are constantly shifting as our knowledge expands. Youngsters who at one time were kept in hospitals and institutions are now cared for at home. Those who were once confined to home care now attend school. Children who were sheltered in schools are now in the workplace. Change is occurring rapidly as society learns to adapt.

As early as 1978, Healy et al[1] proposed the following grouping for school children with impairments.

The first level of disability might be illustrated by what is categorized as a chronic disease (for example, asthma, diabetes, cystic fibrosis, epilepsy, hemophilia, leukemia, congenital heart disease, and renal problems). Those with level 1 disabilities will benefit most by placement in a regular classroom (Table 46).[2,3] The more severe forms of impairments may be placed in level 2. It is important to note that no change in program planning is necessary by school officials for this level of integration, but schools need to be prepared for unusual occurrences.

The next level of functioning, level 3, contains students with diseases that present frequent crises or interfere with the ability to learn. For these students, school activities will have to be

Table 46. — Level of Functioning and Program Modifications Associated With Severity of Impairment*

	Level 1: Mild	Level 2: Mild To Moderate	Level 3: Moderate	Level 4: Severe
Is the child disabled?	No	Possibly	Yes	Yes
How does it affect the child's functioning?	Health impairment does not interfere with day-to-day functioning and learning.	Health impairment does not interfere with learning, but there is a possibility of unusual episodes or crises.	Health impairment either presents frequent crises, or so limits the child's opportunity to participate in activities that it interferes with learning.	Health impairment is so severe that special medical attention is regularly needed. The child's opportunity for activity is so limited that regular classroom participation may not be possible.
Must the program be modified?	No	No change in program planning is necessary. Be aware of the potential for unusual occurrences. Report them to the parents or doctor. Know any first aid procedures that might be required.	Activities will have to be modified to allow a health-impaired child to participate. Staff must know proper first aid procedures and be prepared to deal with children's questions about crises.	Extensive staff and program alterations are necessary to accept child into program. Home- or hospital-based programs may be more appropriate. Classroom support from medical services will be necessary if child is in classroom.

*Adapted from Symposium on Chronic Disease in Children. *Pediatr Clin North Am.* 1984;31(1):224. Reprinted with permission.

modified. Another category or definition is, "conditions that interfere with daily functioning for greater than 3 months in a year, cause hospitalization of more than 1 month in a year, or (at the time of diagnosis) are likely to do so."[4] Chronic renal disease, heart disease, malignancies (including leukemia), hemophilia, sickle cell disease, and cystic fibrosis in their most severe forms are illustrations of the types of chronic illness requiring both hospital and community-based care. Youngsters in this category have been referred to as being at risk, but not necessarily requiring specialized technology or care in the school setting.

The most severe level of impairment (level 4) as defined by the Office of Technology Assessment states that a technology-dependent child is "one from birth through 21 years of age having a chronic disability, who needs *both a medical device* to compensate for the loss of a vital body function and substantial *and ongoing nursing care* to avert death or further disability."[5] Rather than use the words "technology-dependent," an increasing number of authors are preferring the more positive expression, *technology-supported*. This terminology will be continued in the chapter. This group includes children who are ventilator supported, require prolonged use of intravenous medications or nutrition, have a gastrostomy, nasogastric tube, or tracheostomy, or require oxygen support, cardiorespiratory monitors, and substantial nursing care.

Incidence and Scope

It is difficult to give the exact number of technology-supported children. We know that approximately 10% of the children in this country are eligible for placement in special education programs because of a disabling condition.[6] The smallest group consists of those with physical and sensory disabilities (2% to 5%), as contrasted with those who have learning disabilities, speech impairment, emotional disorders, and mental retardation. The number of children who need technology support is extremely small. Small as this number may be, it will rise. Children with severe disabilities are slowly gaining entrance to our schools. Youngsters who were hospitalized, kept in institutions, or stayed at home in the past are now attending school. Newer technology is constantly being developed, especially in the fields of communication, that allows children with severe disabilities to attend school. Caretakers are being trained with greater frequency to provide medical care and support. We constantly are learning that more and more can be done in a less restrictive environment. For these reasons, these children will become more visible to the population. Newer technology will support children with disabilities who previously would have died at an earlier age.

History and Progress Toward Normalization

In prior years, the skills and technology to maintain a severely disabled child had not been developed; the child's life was short due to the inability to combat severe infection, the absence of mechanical apparatus able to support vital life functions, or poor nutrition.

Neonatal intensive care units and hospital intensive care units are becoming more proficient in prolonging life. Patients who were able to survive remained in hospitals and state institutions. As we progressed, these children began to be cared for at home. Now they have entered the community via the schools and workplace. Not only is survival a prime goal, but also quality of life is being improved.

The earlier a person in need receives help, the greater is the progress toward normalization. Lack of intervention often resulted in persons failing to reach their maximum potential; their condition was "maintained." Little thought was given to the quality of life, only survival mattered. Public Law 94-142 gave support to the school-age child with a disability; PL 99-457 now is supporting early intervention for the preschool child (see chapter 6). Together, these laws were renewed as PL 102-119.

Specific Legal Case Examples Related to Provision of School Services

At present, specified school health services are provided to schoolchildren as part of related services mandated under PL 94-142. The law does not require that schools provide medical services except for evaluation and diagnostic purposes. The entire category of "technology-supported" is new and is constantly in flux. Just a short time ago Amber Tatro, a child with spina bifida, desired to attend school. She required intermittent bladder catheterization. The case was presented to the Supreme Court, which ruled that intermittent bladder catheterization was not a medical service but a nursing service, which could be provided in a school setting. Now it is common for students with spina bifida to receive intermittent bladder catheterization in school.

In Auburn, NY, a student named Melissa Detzel was supported by a ventilator and required the constant services of a nurse to monitor and assist her. The Supreme Court ruled that this was a related nursing service. Another wrinkle in this case recently has been ironed out, in that Medicaid was willing to pay for a nurse if the child remained at home, but not if she attended school. The courts have decided that Medicaid is obligated to pay when the child is in school.

The law does not clearly define related services. The community (including the medical community) did not fully realize or understand how far we have progressed in assisting the person with a disability to approach normalization. Today it is commonplace for children who require bladder catheterization to receive it in school. Ventilator-supported children are now coming to schools in increasing numbers.

Attitudes Concerning the Child in School

For general education, success is often measured by group norms, and the objective is to do the best for the most children. Special educators are trained with a focus on attention to personal/individual needs; they measure success by individual progress relative to each student's starting point, and they depend on the support and cooperation of physicians, nurses, therapists, psychologists, and paraprofessionals.[7]

Studies have shown that teachers were more accepting of individuals with physical disabilities such as amputations, harelip, and epilepsy, than of individuals who were mentally retarded, had cerebral palsy, or were emotionally disturbed.[8] Teachers especially were concerned about how to deal with medical emergencies in the classroom and about the repercussions for other children. On the whole, their knowledge of the causes and treatments involved was rudimentary.[9] Educating teachers to understand individual problems is progressing. In an epidemiological study in Hamilton, Ontario, the authors[10] confirmed the importance of friendship and contact with persons with disabilities as determinants of more accepting attitudes.

Physicians should play a large role in helping the children they care for, their families, and schools, in providing special education programs. In one survey,[11] 70% of the physicians interviewed professed no knowledge of a patient's current special education program. Some physicians of very involved patients do familiarize themselves with their patients' day-to-day school lives; many other physicians are poorly informed about the school activities and functional status of their young patients with disabilities.

Where Does the Medical Responsibility for the Child Rest?

The ultimate responsibility for a child lies with the parents. Parents should be made part of all decisions concerning their child with a disability. Very often, a team of professionals needs to be assembled to advise and support the parents. In a severely disabled child, the first advisors usually are tertiary care specialists in a medical center. As soon as possible, the physician who will be providing a medical home for the child should be included. In most situations, it will be necessary to network with community resources. This may take the form of special transportation, financial support, the development of coping skills, or respite care.

It is most important with the special education model that early intervention be started. This is a shared responsibility among the parents, those who provide the medical care, and those who provide the educational care. A team usually is formed and all efforts coordinated by a "case manager." Parents, if they so desire, can be supported to be effective "case managers."

There will be many changes in the problem; new problems will arise. What is more important is that better problem-solving techniques and support systems also will be developing.

Health Care Services Required in School

Very early, it becomes necessary to transport a severely disabled child from place to place. There are various types of car seats built especially for children with disabilities. Specific recommendations have been made in statements by the AAP Committee on Injury and Poison Prevention.[12,13] The National Association of State Directors of Special Education also has developed a manual addressing the issue.[14]

Some children who have gastrostomies will require special diets. In school districts that have large school food service departments, the dietitian should have no problem in providing nutritious meals and snacks. In smaller districts, cooperative programs with parents and schools will be required to meet the child's specific nutritional needs.

Schools are required to deliver nursing, not medical, care. Classroom teachers and aides also are quite capable of supplying care for children with disabilities. Parents (lay persons) have been taught many nursing skills in order to provide for their children. They are quite capable of administering medication, doing bladder catheterization, suctioning tracheostomies, performing tube feeding, and running a nebulizer. These skills can be taught to teachers and aides. Specific guidelines and procedures are available (see chapter 16). Advanced skills requiring more evaluation, interpretation, and medical decision making should be done by a nurse. There are differences of opinion as to what a teacher and what a nurse can and should do. This may present a dilemma when teachers' unions, nurses' unions, and legal counsel have varying views. All should be guided to perform in a way that best serves the interest of the child. Each case should be evaluated individually.

Case Managers for Health Care and Education

We previously presented the concept of team management, including a case manager. The parents, the medical and nursing caretakers, the educator, and others, depending on the problem, make up the team. Quite often, the one person left out is the child. The child should be included in the decision-making process to a level commensurate with the ability and willingness of the child to participate. Other team members may include a psychologist, speech therapist, physical therapist, occupational therapist, social worker, transporter, or financial advisor.

It cannot be stressed too strongly that the more severe the disability, the greater the number of people who will have to become involved. A committed case manager, the parents, and the child are the primary members. Each member of the team can provide support and coping mechanisms for the other members. In this way, the problem of "burnout" in any one person can be diminished or promptly addressed. Because of many medical/legal issues that may arise in some cases, it might be a good idea to have a member of the legal profession participate as a team member.

Ethical Issues

As the number of technology-supported students increases, so will the ethical issues. The challenge of medicolegal issues has been discussed previously. The question already has been asked, "What about the child with multiple severe disabilities who has a 'do not resuscitate' order"? What responsibility and liability may a school district incur? Should schools be required to have oxygen, suction, stimulant medications, and a defibrillator on site? Who will make the decisions? Who will carry them out? There is a very small number of children who might be subject to this anticipated dilemma. The vast majority of children never would be in such a situation, and should not be penalized by the words, "It could happen." There is a risk inherent with everything we do. Risks are controlled and minimized, yet continue to exist. The child with a severe disability deserves the same dignity for risk taking that is part of everyone's daily life.

Costs and Financing

The costs for leading or maintaining a technology-supported student in a normal life-style and of providing an education can be most expensive. In most cases, a level of expense is reached that cannot be supported by the family. Careful fiscal guidance will call on the third-party payors, such as Medicaid and private insurers. There are many philanthropies that support research and help students afflicted with certain disorders. Government is recognizing the needs of those with severe disabilities by mandating other tax-supported agencies to provide certain services. More and more dollars are being required as children with various types of disabilities are beginning to benefit from the extensive developments in the field of electronic and microcomputer technology. Currently, many devices exist to assist children with physical or communication disabilities.[15]

Costs and ethics will become linked at some time. We may be able to justify expense as long as the student continues to progress toward normalcy. However, are we ready to justify expenses for a child with severe disabilities who has reached a plateau and is no longer progressing?

We prefer not to use phrases such as "priority for care" or "rationing of care." The demand created by those needing services and the continued technical advancements will increase. Can finances available for this purpose keep up?

What Does the Future Hold?

It cannot be denied that within the past 10 years students who are technology-supported have progressed toward normalcy. This has required the efforts of many pediatricians, nurses, health care workers, scientists, and teachers. Vast sums of money have been required. The greatest changes taking place have been in attitudes toward those with disabilities. No longer are they to be hidden away. Structural changes in conveyances (ie, buses, wheelchair cabs) and in buildings (ie, ramps, specially designed rest rooms) are now commonplace. Students with disabilities have become more visible and accepted at home, in school, and in the workplace.

Situations once thought insoluble have been solved. This progress should be continued. Realistically, for some individuals, we may reach a state in which progress will be slower and, in some cases, come to a halt. We do not know what this level is, and for that reason we must continue.

References

1. Healy A, McAreavey P, von Hippel CS, et al: Mainstreaming preschoolers: children with health impairments. In: *Symposium on Chronic Diseases in Children. Pediatr Clin North Am.* 1984; 31(1):224

2. Walker DK. Care of chronically ill children in school. *Pediatr Clin North Am.* 1984;31(1):221-233

3. Gearheart BR, Weishahn MW. *The Handicapped Child in the Regular Classroom.* St Louis, MO: CV Mosby; 1976

4. Hobbs N, Perrin JM. *The Constant Shadow: Childhood Chronic Illness in America.* San Francisco, CA: Jossey-Bass; 1985

5. US Congress, Office of Technology Assessment. *Technology – Dependent Children: Hospital v. Home Care – A Technical Memorandum*. Washington, DC: US Government Printing Office; May 1987; OTA-TM-H-38

6. *Sixth Annual Report to Congress on the Implementation of Public Law 94-142: The Education for all Handicapped Children Act*. Washington, DC: US Office of Special Education and Rehabilitative Services; 1984

7. Haas TJ. A Convergence of Two Cultures in the Implementation of PL 94-142. Presented at the Annual Meeting of the American Educational Research Association; 1982; New York, NY

8. Tripp A. Comparison of attitudes of regular and adapted physical educators toward disabled individuals. *Percept Mot Skills*. 1988;66(2):425-426

9. Eiser C, Town C. Teacher's concerns about chronically sick children: implications for pediatricians. *Dev Med Child Neurol*. 1987;29(1):56-63

10. King SM, Rosenbaum P, Armstrong RW, Milner R. An epidemiological study of children's attitudes toward disability. *Dev Med Child Neurol*. 1989;31(2):237-245

11. Palfrey JS, Sarro LJ, Singer JD, Wenger M. Physician familiarity with the educational programs of their special needs patients. *J Dev Behav Pediatr*. 1987;8(4):198-202

12. American Academy of Pediatrics, Committee on Accident and Poison Prevention and Committee on Fetus and Newborn. Safe transportation of premature infants. *Pediatrics*. 1991;87(1):120-122

13. American Academy of Pediatrics, Committee on Injury and Accident Prevention. Safe transportation of newborns discharged from the hospital. *Pediatrics*. 1990;86(3):486-487

14. Bluth LF. *Transporting Handicapped Students: A Resource Manual and Recommended Guidelines for School Transportation and Special Education Personnel*. Washington, DC: National Association of State Directors of Special Education Inc; 1985

15. Desch LW. High technology for handicapped children: a pediatrician's viewpoint. *Pediatrics*. 1986;77(1):71-87

CHAPTER 18

A SCHOOL-BASED RESPONSE TO TRAUMATIC STUDENT DEATH

Suicide and homicide are, respectively, the second and third leading causes of death among American adolescents.[1] Accidents are also a common cause of death; accordingly, many adolescents will experience the traumatic death of a schoolmate. The literature suggests that exposure to any of these types of traumatic death may be detrimental to adolescents and that community-based interactions may attenuate these harmful effects.[2-4]

Deleterious Effects of Exposure to Traumatic Death

Suicide

Publicity about suicide can be followed by an increase in the rate of suicide and suicide attempts, particularly among adolescents. This has been documented by studies of media publicity about suicide. The increase in the rate appears to be proportional to the amount of publicity.[5-7] Adolescent suicide clusters have been described anecdotally[8-12] and by rigorous statistical definition.[13] Suicide victims are more likely to have been exposed to suicidal behavior than matched controls.[14] Exposure to suicide confers about a threefold increase in psychiatric disorders among friends and acquaintances, as compared with unexposed controls.[15] The disorders that are most common are the depressive disorders, along with an exacerbation of preexisting difficulties of conduct and substance abuse.[15] Those who witnessed the suicide or discovered the body of the victim were particularly likely to have symptoms of post-traumatic stress disorder (PTSD).[15,16] Depression or PTSD symptoms are more likely to occur in the friends and acquaintances of suicide victims than is imitative suicidal behavior.[15]

A psychopathological reaction to exposure to suicide, including depression, PTSD, and perhaps imitative suicidal behavior, may be more likely to occur if the exposed young person witnessed the suicide or discovered the body, was a friend of the victim, had previous psychiatric disorder, has a family history of the same, and had endured other interpersonal losses.[9,10,15-17] Friends of suicide victims tend to have high rates of emotional disorders, suggesting that these friends themselves have extensive psychological vulnerability even antedating their friend's suicide.

Homicide

School-age children's responses to a peer's homicide have been studied primarily in the context of children witnessing a sniper attack on a schoolmate.[18] Only symptoms referent to PTSD were assessed, but the variables influencing the individual child's response were carefully documented. Children were more symptomatic if they were in close proximity to the victim (ie, experienced a threat to life themselves), had a close relationship with the victim, felt unable to help the victim, and had experienced other trauma before the exposure. A group of adolescents on a school bus witnessed a suicide and accidental shooting of a fellow student. Incident PTSD and anxiety disorders were quite common and were associated with a past history of psychiatric disorder, family history of emotional disorder, and previous interpersonal losses.[16] Other studies in adults of the correlates of PTSD indicate that preexisting psychopathology (particularly anxiety or affective disorder), family history, anxiety disorder, and the degree of life threat experienced by the individual during the exposure are the best predictors of PTSD symptoms.[19-21]

Disasters

Community-wide disasters with deaths are a third type of traumatic death that may affect students. The extent of the psychopathological reaction to a disaster is predicated on the directness of the exposure to a given individual. The likelihood of a psychopathological reaction increases the closer an individual is to the "epicenter" of a disaster, the greater the life threat experienced, and the extent to which injury to self and family, physical dislocation, and overall degree of disruption of community life have occurred.[4] The most common reactions are affective and anxiety disorders.[4,22]

Time Course of Sequelae

Studies of exposure to all three types of traumatic experiences indicate both immediate effects of exposure that take the form of dysphoria, grief, symptoms of PTSD, and perhaps imitative suicide.[15,16,18] More enduring effects, lasting at least 6 or 12 months, are the effects of depression, PTSD, and prolonged grief.[4,15,16,23]

School-Based Interventions

The goals of school-based intervention *after* a traumatic death are to:
1. Inform students and staff about the death, so as to dispel rumor and innuendo.
2. Allow students to grieve appropriately.
3. Provide a means for identifying and referring for mental health treatment those students who are experiencing difficulty in response to the death.
4. Provide a secure and stable environment that acknowledges the death and student responses, yet allows for a return to a normal school routine as soon as possible. By structuring the school environment appropriately, the risks of "contagion" in the case of suicide or PTSD in the case of homicide are lessened.

Preparation for a Crisis

Policy decisions about how schools should respond to the traumatic death of a student should be formulated during a calm period, rather than in the midst of a crisis.[3,24] Policy decisions must be approved by the school board and superintendent and should be documented in writing, so as to avoid policy disputes that may erupt during the pressure of responding to a crisis. The steps involved in preparing for such a crisis include: (1) formulation of a crisis team; (2) staff training; and (3) development of an action plan.

Administrative Structure and the Crisis Team

One person within the hierarchy, usually the superintendent, assistant superintendent, or director of pupil services, should be designated as the person who will initiate and take ultimate administrative responsibility for the response to traumatic death, including consulting with and updating the school board about actions taken after the event. The building principal should be responsible for the day-to-day administrative issues of the crisis team's interventions, such as convening a staff meeting, coordinating mailings to parents, holding parent meetings, and assessing building security and space needs.

Designating crisis team members is the first responsibility of the administrator mentioned above. Small school districts of 10 schools or fewer may find one crisis team of six to eight persons to be sufficient, while large districts will require several such teams, perhaps assigned to particular regions of the district.

The crisis team may consist of school psychologists, guidance counselors, nurses, and social workers who are regular full-time employees of the school district. Membership on a crisis team should be voluntary, as individuals who do not wish to serve in a crisis situation usually are not effective. Specialized training is not a prerequisite for membership on a team, but the team should consist of the most clinically skilled staff available in the district. We have found it helpful to have crisis team members who also can provide crucial, nonclinical services (eg, escorting students to offices, maintaining records on students who are referred and screened by the team). A calm, reliable paraprofessional or secretary, for example, can be an invaluable asset to a team. Particularly in smaller schools, mental health professionals from a local community mental health center or hospital should be part of the crisis team, participate in joint training, and share in policy decisions and planning. The minimum effective size for a crisis team is about six members, based on our own experience and that of others.[3] Within the crisis team, one person should be designated as the crisis team leader (sometimes referred to in the suicide literature as the "postvention" [post event intervention] coordinator).[3] The crisis team leader will be responsible for coordinating the efforts of the team, monitoring overall school climate, and serving as a liaison between the crisis team, school administration, school staff, parents, funeral director, the coroner, community mental health agencies, school security, and media representatives. An additional person may be designated as the clinical coordinator, whose responsibility it is to review and supervise the screening and referral process, to facilitate referrals to appropriate mental health services, and to review with school guidance counselors the extent to which referral recommendations have been followed by children and their parents.

Training

In order for a school or school district to respond successfully to a crisis, a comprehensive district training program is necessary. Certain aspects of the training should be mandatory for all educational professionals, whereas more intensive training should target those members of the crisis team. Each school building staff needs to meet and develop its own crisis plan. This straightforward document might consist of a listing of the faculty administrative and office staff with room assignments and telephone numbers. We have found it very helpful to have a school also submit a floor plan of the building, indicating spaces that could be redeployed for individual and small group meetings in the event of a crisis.[25] Finally, each crisis plan should provide a detailed map for crisis team members coming from other schools and agencies.

Once the school's plan is developed, it may be reviewed in a 1-hour in-service program that also includes the following topics: review of the district's policy, review of warning signals for suicide and depression, and an overview of the goals for postvention. All employees in the building should attend this meeting, which may be led by a member of the administrative or pupil service staff.

For all pupil services and administrative staff, more in-depth training will be required. This training should include the following: risk factors for suicide in the school setting, usual and pathological responses of students to a peer's death, identification of those individuals who are experiencing difficulty subsequent to the death, mechanisms for referral of at-risk students, and an overview of the rationale and plan for postvention.

Certain selected individuals who will constitute the crisis team, as well as the building principal, should receive additional training on how to organize and carry out a *"post event intervention"* hereafter referred to as *"postvention"* including identifying at-risk students, short-term group and individual bereavement counseling, and facilitation of mental health referrals, triage, and if necessary, the involuntary commitment process. Those mental health agency professionals who are designated members of the crisis team should undergo training simultaneously with school staff, thereby increasing the likelihood that professionals from two different agencies can work together in an intervention with a minimum of tension and a maximum of efficiency.

Central office staff, superintendents, and school board members may receive copies of the individual school crisis plans and a brief overview of the planned activities in the event of a traumatic student death. School security staff and public information and/or public relations officers also need this information so they can respond quickly and efficiently during a crisis.

The final aspect of training is often overlooked: stress management strategies and support activities for the crisis team members. While the team may not initially identify the need for this additional support, their stress will become evident after repeated postvention or crisis situations.

Procedure

In this section, the sequence of events followed by the school and the crisis team are outlined. Naturally, such a sequence is somewhat artificial, insofar as certain actions may proceed simultaneously or be delayed because of logistical reasons (such as a weekend or holiday). This sequence is outlined in Table 47. Each step will be described below in greater detail, including the goals and rationale for each action.

Contact With the Coroner or Medical Examiner

Before proceeding with a plan, it is vital to have contacted the coroner to have precise knowledge about the circumstances and cause of death. Rumors and innuendos about the death will circulate throughout school, and it is vital that the crisis team be aware of the facts as they are known. For example, it is common for students to deny a suicide, claiming it was an accident or even a homicide or, alternatively, to lay the blame for the suicide on a person or group of persons. The coroner also can provide information about whether anyone witnessed the death or discovered the body, since these individuals are likely to be at higher risk for a psychopathological reaction to the death.[15,16,26] Occasionally, based on suicide notes or interviews with witnesses, it may be possible to uncover a suicide pact.

Contact With the Mental Health Center

A post event plan may be run by a member of the mental health agency or the school, depending on previous training and arrangements. Regardless of whether the crisis team leader is

Table 47. — Sequential Steps Following a Traumatic Student Death

1. Prepare for a crisis before the crisis occurs.
2. Pass board policy.
3. Designate spokesperson to deal with reporters.
4. Crisis team leader (CTL) formulates a plan with superintendent and building principal(s).
5. Contact other schools where death might have an impact.
6. CTL contacts coroner or medical examiner.
7. CTL contacts community mental health center to enlist help for the crisis team, and a clinical coordinator is designated.
8. CTL contacts appropriate other outside referral agencies (eg, hospital emergency rooms, hospitals, other community mental health programs), alerts them to potential referrals.
9. CTL contacts parents of suicide victim.
10. Contact clergy and funeral director.
11. Conduct staff meeting with school staff in which plan is discussed.
12. Make appropriate security arrangements and implement rumor control switchboard.
13. Inform parents by mail and through a parent meeting.
14. Identify available rooms for screening and counseling.
15. Inform students of death and orient them to signs of grief and when to seek help for themselves or their friends.
16. Provide ongoing monitoring and support for selected students.
17. Screen students as necessary, inform parents of outcome of screening, and make referrals as needed.
18. Follow up to ensure that all vulnerable adolescents were screened and that these referrals were completed.
19. Evaluate efficacy of services, revise crisis plan, and identify additional training needs.

a member of the catchment area community mental health center (CMHC), it is vital to involve staff from the CMHC. Mental health professionals can help make announcements to the students, run support groups, screen students, and make referrals. The CMHC should designate an "on-call" clinical coordinator who works closely with the crisis team leader, supervises the screening of students, and facilitates referrals, particularly emergency evaluations and admissions to psychiatric inpatient units. The clinical coordinator should have the authority at the CMHC to authorize emergency evaluations and transfers to a facility equipped to handle psychiatric emergencies. Reassignment of staff to outpatient assessment duties may protect a CMHC from being overwhelmed with a sudden increase in demand for appointments. Extending clinic hours is another way to respond to the likely increase in referrals.

Contact With Other Agencies

If there are other agencies, such as private psychiatric facilities or hospital emergency rooms, to whom the school is likely to make referrals, the clinical coordinator should identify a contact person at each of the agencies and alert the contact about possible emergency referrals. It has been our experience that emergency referrals increase dramatically during the first week of postvention, as a function of increased "case-finding" and self-referrals prompted by the crisis.

Crises affect adults as well as students, so it is helpful to call on the employee assistance program (EAP) for the school district. The EAP might assign a staff member to be at the school on the first day of the intervention to talk with staff members and to recommend follow-up counseling.

Contact With Parents of the Victim

The crisis team coordinator should contact the parents of the suicide victim to convey condolences from the school. The coordinator may determine how the parents and siblings of the victim are doing and provide information about support groups and other services for the family. Informing the parents about the intervention plan procedure is courteous and may prevent parents from making requests that increase the likelihood of contagion (in the case of suicide). For example, they may want a memorial assembly at school or some other type of publicity with regard to their child. Such publicity may make their child appear to be a hero, unduly publicizing and glamorizing the suicide. If this is explained to the parents in advance, the likelihood of misunderstanding on the part of parents and interested friends is minimized. The coordinator or principal also makes arrangements for the safe return of all personal belongings the victim might have left at school. Families have reported to us their appreciation for the schoolwork papers, school photographs, and other reminders of the children's lives as students.

The parents and siblings may answer questions about the circumstances of death, especially with regard to the precipitants and possible predisposing psychiatric conditions. To identify those potentially vulnerable to the impact of exposure to the death, the parents should indicate with whom the victim last spent time, who were the closest friends of the victim, if there was anyone who may have witnessed the death or found the body, and others that the family expects will have difficulty coping with the death. Discussing these issues with bereaved family members requires a great clinical sensitivity on the part of the interviewer. This list of friends, who were either recently involved with the victim or who may have been exposed to the death or death scene, constitutes a beginning list of those considered to be at risk subsequent to exposure. The parents need to know that they may be contacted by the reporters and may refer any direct calls to the crisis team leader or designated spokesperson (often the school district's public information officer).

Contact With the Clergy and Funeral Director

The funeral director is contacted in order to understand the funeral arrangements, to communicate to the director the postvention strategy, and to encourage the director to make any referrals or call for consultation if it becomes apparent that a particular student is having difficulty. The signs of depression, suicidality, and other emotional disturbance may be reviewed with the clergy who are involved with friends of the victim to aid in identification of adolescents at risk.

Contact With Other Schools

Usually, other schools are affected by the student's death, as may be revealed by conversations with the teachers, administrators, friends, and parents of the victim. The most likely circumstances in which this may be the case are when the student: (1) had attended other schools; (2) had friends in another school; (3) had siblings in another school; or (4) was killed by a student in another school. While a full-scale intervention in the other school may not be required, it may be necessary to screen some of those students most likely to be affected.

Staff Meeting

Meeting with all teachers is a critical early step. Teachers may be misinformed about a death, and they must know the facts if they are to help their students. Faculty members closely involved with the victim may require individual or small group support. The school staff need to know the overall plan and the criteria for identifying students at risk.

Make Appropriate Security Arrangements

In the case in which the death occurs on school grounds or on a school bus, students should be evacuated from the scene as quickly as possible to prevent personal injury and to diminish secondary exposure. Following a traumatic event, several other potentially disruptive activities may occur. Representatives of the media often try to gain access to the school; students may try to create a publicly visible memorial for the deceased student (such as a mural); or unsupervised students may gather. Reporters should be banned from the school premises or any parent meetings. The creation of any memorial on school property should be stopped. In the case of suicide, memorials tend to glorify the victim and this form of death. Generally, students can be persuaded to find another equally fulfilling way to memorialize the victim, such as donating to a general memorial fund, planting a tree, or creating a "time capsule" to be buried. Finally, students may gather together almost as a form of counterculture protest. ("You adults don't understand us. We kids need to talk with each other.") The crisis team leader should be alerted to disband any such groups, to encourage the students to meet with responsible adults, and to encourage such youth not to take the responsibility of a friend's life on their own young shoulders. If students refuse to meet with adults at school, it may be helpful to introduce a "neutral," but trusted, third party—a member of the clergy or a community youth leader.

Dealing With the Media

A designated spokesperson from the school district or the crisis team leader should deal with the media. Neither this person nor any other school or mental health professional should comment on the method or circumstances of the student's death or the status of any other student. It is best to try to be proactive with the media by trying to explain how publicity can be harmful and how it can be helpful. For example, publicity about the manner of the suicide victim's death is not likely to be helpful, and may enhance contagion. Videotape footage showing the death (whether by suicide or homicide) may be traumatizing. On the other hand, it is helpful to publicize the intervention effort, the signs of grief, and typical and worrisome responses to the death of a friend; when to get help; and how to obtain help.

Informing Parents of Students

A vital step early in postvention is to inform all parents about the student's death and the action to be taken by the school. This should be done by sending a letter home, ideally the afternoon before the screening of students actually begins. However, for logistical reasons, such as if a suicide occurred on a Friday evening, it may be necessary to begin screening on Monday and simply inform parents after the fact. The letter should let the parent know about the death, the postvention procedure, who to call in case of any questions, and the time of a parents' meeting. Figure 3 shows a sample parent letter used for an elementary school postvention. Figure 4 shows a sample parent/ student letter more appropriate for adolescents.

Parents have reported their relief in having a list of signs of stress in children and adolescents, as they may not have connected their children's different behavior with the crisis at school. It is important to keep the letter focused on helping strategies, with few details about the death. (Media representatives may get copies of the parent letter and quote from it.) Parents or school staff may request a parent meeting. If one is held, it should be scheduled soon if the intervention has begun in order to explain in further detail the procedures and to educate parents about the mental health effects of exposure to traumatic death, how to identify if their child is having difficulty, and what steps to take in order to get help. Media representatives may try to attend and take notes. To ensure parents' privacy as they ask questions, insist that "outsiders" leave this meeting. The other points of contact with the parent will be during the screening interview with the child. The parent is called to corroborate or enhance the information received and is informed about the outcome of the screening, including any recommendations for further follow-up or treatment.

Date

Dear Parent/Guardian:

Our school is very sad to learn of the death of our student *(name)* who died on *(date)*. If you would like to make a memorial contribution, you may send it to the school. We will be sure the family receives all contributions.

We are concerned about your child's feelings after this tragedy, as sad events often bring out strong feelings in children. To help our students, we have called in a team of counselors from *(agency or school district)*. Today, counselors met with students during their classes to give them an opportunity to talk about the tragedy. Counselors from the school district will be available for several days to help children cope.

Here are some things you may notice in your child as he or she adjusts to this news. First, your child may feel sad and may cry. Your child might not feel like eating or may eat too much. Nightmares and bad dreams may be a problem. Also, you may notice that your child is absent-minded, forgetful, or having trouble paying attention to you. Your child may complain of a headache or stomachache. Anger is another feeling that children sometimes have. Finally, your child may be afraid that something will happen to him or her. Please take time to talk with your child about what has happened, as talking with a parent can be very helpful to children coping with a tragedy.

Your child should begin to feel better within 2 weeks. If your child is still having a difficult time 2 weeks from now, please call the school so that we can help.

We appreciate your support during this tragedy and hope you will call us if you have any questions. Our number is *(school telephone number)*.

Sincerely,

School Principal

Fig 3. Sample letter for the parents of elementary schoolchildren (use school letterhead).

Date

Dear *(School Name)* Student and Parent/Guardian:

Our school is very sad to learn of the death/accident of our student, *(name)*, who died/was injured on *(day, date)*. (Insert here one factual statement about the manner of death.)

We are concerned about your feelings after this tragedy, as sad events often bring out strong feelings in everyone. In order to help our students, we have called in counselors and social workers from the *(school district)*. They have met with students in their classes, individually, and in small groups to give them an opportunity to talk about the tragedy. Counselors and social workers from the school district will be available for several days to help students cope with their feelings.

People react in different ways to sudden death/accident. You may feel shock, fear, anger, grief, confusion, sadness, or numbness. Or you may have a different reaction. Whatever your response to this tragedy, it is understandable.

Because of these strong feelings, you may experience a change in eating or sleeping habits. You may have difficulty concentrating, experience mood swings, or have headaches or stomachaches. You may have concerns about your own safety.

We are encouraging family members to discuss what has happened and their feelings about this tragedy.

Gradually you should begin to feel better. If you are still having a difficult time 2 weeks from now, please call the school so that we can help.

We appreciate your support during this time and hope you will call us if you have any questions or concerns. Our number is *(telephone number)*.

Sincerely,

School Principal

Fig 4. Sample letter for high school students and their parents (use school letterhead).

Informing Students of Death

Students should be told about the death, including the cause of death, during the earliest available time. Use only the cause of death *as reported by the coroner*! If the cause of death has not been definitively determined, this should also be stated. Tell students about the death in small groups. Never use a school-wide announcement on the public address (PA) system or a school-wide assembly. The individual reactions of the students can be monitored in small groups, while the PA announcement or large assembly could have the additional disadvantages of contagion insofar as it further dramatizes the event. After this announcement, students are encouraged to ask questions, with the primary aim being to dispel rumors about the death. The presenter (a member of the crisis team or the teacher) will describe typical reactions to death, indicate "warning signs," and indicate how the student can receive additional help, either through a support group at school and/or an individual screening interview. Also, the letter to parents may be given to students to take home. Students are encouraged to self-refer and also to go to a responsible adult if they are concerned about a friend.

Support Group

The support group is for those who were close to the victim, witnessed the death, or were noted to be psychiatrically vulnerable. It should be stressed that attendance is voluntary. Each group should be no longer than 50 minutes and no larger than a membership of 20. The group can be run after school in order to interfere least with the day-to-day functioning of the school. The goals of the group should be clear: to allow students to share feelings, express concerns, correct misconceptions about the death and their own sense of responsibility, and to facilitate normal, healthy grief. A secondary role of such groups is to identify those who would benefit from a screening interview, individual support, and/or referral for further treatment. Students who should be excluded from such groups would include those with serious current psychopathology who are not that closely connected to the victim, an individual who might be victimized by other group members because of his or her relationship to the victim (eg, ex-girlfriend of suicide victim who was "implicated" in the suicide or those students who want to run an adultless support group). The latter should not be tolerated on school grounds, insofar as adolescents should not have such responsibility or authority over their peers.

The group is best led by two facilitators from the crisis team skilled in group process. Students should identify themselves and give their names and phone numbers to be recorded on a sign-up sheet for use by the adult. Each student should describe the following: (1) relationship with the deceased; (2) how the student learned of the death; (3) whether the student witnessed the death or was at the death scene; (4) the student's reaction to the death, including any thoughts of self-blame; (5) how the student is coping; and (6) the student's plans to visit the funeral home and/or attend the funeral. The facilitators should use these individual reports as a basis for discussion about typical reactions to death and ways of coping. The students also should be oriented to possible danger signs, in themselves and their friends, of suicide, depression, and PTSD. Distributing student help cards with the telephone numbers of 24-hour hotlines and other available mental health sources enhances this process. At this point in the discussion, the facilitator can discuss with the group members how to obtain help and distribute the appropriate handouts.

If students plan to attend the funeral, it is useful to review what they might anticipate. Youths should be encouraged to attend the funeral and visit the funeral home *only* with responsible adults; this message should be conveyed to parents as well. The students can be encouraged to consider ways in which they can be supportive of each other and the family after the service.

Additional meetings may be needed. It is recommended that two additional meetings be scheduled at weekly intervals from the first but—like the first meeting—it should be stressed that attendance is entirely voluntary. After the initial days of the intervention, the pupil services staff of the school building may be able to resume full responsibility for the follow-up of the students. If this plan is not adequate, one or two members of the school district's crisis team may be reassigned to the crisis site for a few hours a week until students are able to relinquish the extra support.

Screening of Students

Certain students may be considered at higher risk for a pathological reaction to a traumatic death. As noted earlier, this would include those who were close friends of the victim, who have had previous psychiatric problems, who were exposed to the scene of death or actually witnessed the death, and those self-identified or noted by teachers to be having difficulty coping with the death. Such students should be referred to a crisis team member with a clinical background for a psychiatric screening interview, which covers the following: (1) relationship to the deceased; (2) type of exposure to death; (3) current and past symptomatology of depression, suicidality, conduct disorder, and substance abuse; (4) family history of psychiatric problems; and (5) current stressors. The parent then is called to review and verify these findings, after which point a disposition is formulated.

Three outcomes are possible. First, students may display a normal, circumscribed grief reaction and not require further referral for mental health evaluation and treatment. These students should be monitored with regard to school attendance, performance, and behavior. Second, students may have had prior psychiatric difficulties, have witnessed the death, or have been a very close friend; these students are more likely to be symptomatic.[15,16,18] If such students are showing evidence of an exacerbation or recurrence in a preexisting psychiatric disorder, or evidence of PTSD, they should be referred for further treatment after these findings are discussed with their parents. Third, such psychiatrically vulnerable students may evidence significant suicidality,[12] which will require making a no-suicide contract with the evaluator. The no-suicide contract is a written agreement between the student and the evaluator that the student will refrain from suicidal behavior, and that, if the student feels suicidal, the student will call the evaluator, go to another responsible adult (to be specified), or call an emergency room telephone number (to be specified), in order to obtain help.[12] The evaluator should review with the student plans to cope with specific stressors associated with this suicidality and rehearse the use of the no-suicide contract.[27] Parents should definitely be notified about suicidality in their children, and the need to remove any available firearms should be stressed.[28,29] If the adolescent cannot make a no-suicide contract or manifests other significant risk factors for suicide, this is an indication for immediate emergency evaluation and possible admission to an inpatient psychiatric unit.[12]

The students who are referred for more specialized mental health treatment should sign a two-way release of information to make it possible to share the results of the in-school screen with the referral agency. The release also enables the evaluator to follow up and learn whether the referral recommendation was followed. All such students should be monitored as to attendance, performance, and behavior, to track their progress and need for further interventions. The crisis plan should designate who will maintain evaluation and screening forms.

Evaluation of the Efficacy of Services

A follow-up staff meeting with the faculty and crisis team should be held to review how the intervention proceeded from an administrative and process point of view. Ambiguous policies or procedures should be addressed by the crisis team leader with the principal and superintendent. If any of the interventions seemed to have an untoward effect, this should be discussed and a modification in procedure and board policy should be considered. For example, students attending support groups may claim that such groups were prolonging or exacerbating their grief. Therefore, the voluntary nature of attendance at support groups should be emphasized in subsequent intervention.

Emergency facilities and mental health agencies can be monitored to assess if compliance with recommendations was achieved. Also, the attendance, performance, and behavior of targeted individuals can be monitored. Overall, the goal of postvention is to return the school climate to normal as soon as possible. If this has not been achieved within 3 weeks, further discussion is merited.

Finally, the members of the crisis team should be debriefed, as participation in such an intervention can be highly stressful. Provision of adequate support to these professionals is necessary to their long-term viability in this role.

Special Circumstances

Sudden Death or Suicide of a Teacher

Similar procedures may need to be followed in the case of a teacher suicide or accidental death. Vulnerable students and those with whom the teacher had a relationship (eg, teacher, advisor) should be screened. Students may experience very strong reactions to a teacher's sudden death, so it is best to have a complete crisis team "on call" for this situation. Young children often exhibit separation fears and increased anxiety; the selection of the substitute or replacement teacher is critical, and the transition must be handled with great sensitivity. The EAP can be very helpful in the event of an adult death, as the impact is felt by colleagues.

Death of Student Not Attending School

If the victim was well known but graduated or dropped out of school, an announcement, letter, and parent meeting may not be necessary. A meeting with staff members who knew the student should elicit names of other students who should be notified and possibly screened. Unless the death was by suicide, students may be encouraged to organize some kind of memorial.

Disasters

The guidelines for postventions outlined related primarily to traumatic death. In the case of a community-wide disaster, the school still may be an important focal point, and many of the same principles remain. However, close coordination with governmental agencies and medical relief agencies will be required, such as in the case of an earthquake or flood.[4,24] As disasters attract widespread public attention, it will be even more important to protect students from upsetting interactions with media representatives.

Other Types of Death

The traumatic types of death that have been emphasized have been suicide and homicide, where more is known about the risk factors for depression, suicidality, and PTSD subsequent to exposure, thereby informing the postvention procedure. Our recommendation is to follow similar procedures for sudden accidental death, particularly if the student was well known in the school or if more than one student was hurt in the accident.

There is less empirical information about the usual and pathological responses to accidental death, but it may be safe to assume that the risk factors for depression and PTSD are similar for exposure to all types of traumatic death. In the case of the natural death of a student, we recommend a more focused postvention aimed at informing students about the cause of death, offering support and screening to those closest to the student, and alerting the school nurse about possible increases in health-related concerns and somatic symptoms among students. However, as in the case of accidental death, we know less about students' usual modal and pathological responses to a peer's natural death.

Role of the Pediatrician

After a traumatic death, a member of the crisis team should alert emergency rooms and community physicians about a possible increase in referrals related to the exposure to the death. Pediatricians in the office, emergency room setting, and particularly those involved in supervising school nurses should be aware of covert agendas of those coming to the nurse and alert to somatic manifestations of grief, injuries that may relate to increased risk-taking behavior, and more overt concerns of depression and anxiety subsequent to exposure. After a natural death of a student, a pediatrician's input to the school and student can be helpful in explaining the cause of death and putting it in perspective with respect to the overall low rate of mortality in this age group.

Summary

Traumatic death is a common cause of mortality among adolescents. Therefore, it is highly likely that many high school students will experience the death of at least one of their peers due to suicide, homicide, or an accident. Because of the evidence that exposure to suicide or homicide has significant mental health effects, screening and counseling of vulnerable youth in the school setting is recommended. The most important aspect is *prevention*, that is, having a policy and detailed plan of action, a well-trained faculty and crisis team, and good relations among schools and with medical and mental health agencies. While the proposed model closely follows that recommended by the American Association of Suicidology[3] and the Centers for Disease Control,[2] it has not been subjected to rigorous evaluation as to its efficacy in attenuating the short- and long-term morbidity due to exposure to traumatic death.

References

1. Centers for Disease Control. *Youth Suicide Surveillance 1970-1980.* Atlanta, GA: US Department of Health and Human Services, Public Health Service, Violent Epidemiology Branch, Center for Health Promotion and Education; 1986

2. Centers for Disease Control, Center for Environmental Health and Injury Control, Division of Injury Epidemiology and Control. CDC recommendations for a community plan for the prevention and containment of suicidal clusters. *MMWR.* 1988;37(suppl)

3. American Association of Suicidology, School Suicide Prevention Programs Committee. *Postvention Guidelines.* Denver, CO: American Association of Suicidology; 1989

4. Pynoos RS, Nader K. Prevention of psychiatric morbidity in children after disaster. In: Shaffer D, Philips I, Enzer NB, eds. *OSAP Prevention Monograph-2. Prevention of Mental Disorders, Alcohol, and Other Drug Use in Children and Adolescents.* Rockville, MD: US Department of Health and Human Services, Public Health Service, Alcohol, Drug Abuse, and Mental Health Administration; 1989:chap 7. DHHS Publication No. (ADM) 89-1646

5. Gould MS, Shaffer D. The impact of suicide in television movies. Evidence of imitation. *N Engl J Med.* 1986;315:690-694

6. Phillips DP, Carstensen LL. Clustering of teenage suicides after television news stories about suicide. *N Engl J Med.* 1986;315:685-689

7. Schmidtke A, Hafner H. The Werther effect after television films: new evidence for an old hypothesis. *Psychol Med.* 1988;18:665-676

8. Dizmang LH, Watson J, May PA, Bopp J. Adolescent suicide at an Indian reserve. *Am J Orthopsychiatry.* 1974;44:43-49

9. Ward JA, Fox J. A suicide epidemic on an Indian reserve. *Can Psychiatr Assoc J.* 1977;22:423-426

10. Robbins D, Conroy RC. A cluster of adolescent suicide attempts: is suicide contagious? *J Adolesc Health Care.* 1983;3:253-255

11. Coleman L. *Suicide Clusters.* Boston, MA: Faber & Faber; 1987

12. Brent DA, Kerr MM, Goldstein C, Bozigar J, Wartella U, Allan MJ. An outbreak of suicide and suicidal behavior in a high school. *J Am Acad Child Adolesc Psychiatry.* 1989;28:918-924

13. Gould MS, Wallenstein S, Kleinman MH, O'Carroll P, Mercy J. Suicide clusters: an examination of age-specific effects. *Am J Public Health*. 1990;80:211-212

14. Shafii M, Carrigan S, Whittinghill JR, et al. Psychological autopsy of completed suicide in children and adolescents. *Am J Psychiatry*. 1985;142:1061-1064

15. Brent DA, Perper JA, Moritz GM, et al. Psychiatric effects of exposure to suicide among the friends and acquaintances of adolescent suicide victims. *J Am Acad Child Adolesc Psychiatry*. 1992;31:629-640

16. Brent DA, Perper JA, Moritz GM, et al. *Adolescent witness to a peer suicide*. Paper submitted for presentation at the 38th Annual Meeting of the American Academy of Child and Adolescent Psychiatry, San Francisco, CA, October 1991

17. Brent DA. Suicide and suicidal behavior in children and adolescents. *Pediatr Rev*. 1989;10:269-275

18. Pynoos RS, Frederick C, Nader K, et al. Life threat and posttraumatic stress in school-age children. *Arch Gen Psychiatry*. 1987;44:1057-1063

19. Helzer JE, Robins LN, McEvoy L. Posttraumatic stress disorder in the general population. Findings of the epidemiologic catchment area survey. *N Engl J Med*. 1987;317:1630-1634

20. Goldberg JL, True WR, Eisen SA, Henderson WG. A twin study of the effects of the Vietnam War on posttraumatic stress disorder. *JAMA*. 1990;263:1227-1232

21. Breslau N, Davis GC, Andreski P, Peterson E. Traumatic events and posttraumatic stress disorder in an urban population of young adults. *Arch Gen Psychiatry*. 1991;48:216-222

22. Shore JH, Tatum EL, Vollmer WM. Psychiatric reactions to disaster: the Mount St. Helens experience. *Am J Psychiatry*. 1986;143:590-595

23. Pynoos RS, Nader K, Frederick C, Gonda L, Stuber M. Grief reactions in school-age children following a sniper attack at school. *Isr J Psychiatry Relat Sci*. 1987;24:53-63

24. Klingman A. School community in disaster: planning for intervention. *J Community Psychol*. 1988;16:205-216

25. Kerr MM. *Crisis Team Handbook*. Pittsburgh, PA: Pittsburgh Board of Public Education.

26. Rudestam KE. Physical and psychological responses to suicide in the family. *J Consult Clin Psychol*. 1977;45:162-170

27. Rotheram MJ. Evaluation of imminent danger for suicide among youth. *Am J Orthopsychiatry*. 1987;57:102-110

28. Brent DA, Perper J, Allman CJ. Alcohol, firearms, and suicide among youth. Temporal trends in Allegheny County, PA 1960-1983. *JAMA*. 1987;257:3369-3372

29. Brent DA, Perper JA, Goldstein CE, et al. Risk factors for adolescent suicide. a comparison of adolescent suicide victims with suicidal inpatients. *Arch Gen Psychiatry*. 1988;45:581-588

CHAPTER 19

COMMUNICABLE DISEASES

Communicable diseases are easily transmitted in schools since children are brought together in groups of various sizes. This has long been a cause for concern for parents as well as for schoolteachers and administrative personnel. The control of these diseases in the school setting is multifaceted and requires the close collaboration of parents, school personnel, and health care professionals to institute a rational commonsense approach. In general terms, control may involve antimicrobial therapy or prophylaxis, exclusion, or cohorting. Closing of an educational facility for the purposes of communicable disease control is almost never required.

General Principles of Inclusion and Exclusion

Mild illnesses are very common during the school years. However, there are very few illnesses that mandate exclusion from participation in school. Children with minor illnesses should not be excluded from school unless:

1. The illness prevents the child from participating in school activities.
2. The child requires more care than the school staff can provide.
3. Fever, lethargy, irritability, persistent crying, difficulty breathing, or other signs suggesting severe illness are present.
4. There are mouth sores associated with inability to control saliva, unless medical authority states that the child's condition is noninfectious.
5. There is rash with fever or behavior changes (until illness is determined by a physician not to be communicable).
6. As indicated in the discussion of specific diseases in the following section.

There is no evidence that the incidence of acute common respiratory diseases such as the common cold, croup, bronchitis, or pneumonia can be reduced by exclusion; thus, exclusion is not recommended for these diseases.

Detection and School Management of Specific Diseases

The following diseases are spread primarily by the respiratory route.

1. Erythema infectiosum
   a. Description of clinical disease: Erythema infectiosum (fifth disease) is a mild infectious disease with fever in only 15% to 30% of cases. It is characterized by a distinctive rash that begins with red cheeks and progresses in 1 to 4 days to a lacy maculopapular rash on the arms that spreads centripetally to involve the trunk. The rash recurs and fluctuates in intensity over a 1- to 3-week period.
   b. Age group most commonly affected: School-age children.
   c. Seasonal incidence: Highest incidence is in the winter and spring.
   d. Incubation period: Most commonly 4 to 14 days to development of rash, but can be as long as 20 days.
   e. Period of communicability: Not well delineated, but greatest just before onset of rash and probably not thereafter.
   f. Exclusion: Children are most infectious before the onset of illness and unlikely to be infectious after the onset of rash and other associated symptoms.

2. Measles
   a. Description of clinical disease: Measles is a very contagious disease, with a 1- to 2-day prodrome of malaise and fever followed by the onset of coryza, conjunctivitis, a dry cough, and the appearance of a maculopapular rash. Characteristically, the rash starts on the head and neck, spreads over the rest of the body, and disappears 5 to 7 days after onset.
   b. Age group most commonly affected: Most cases occur in preschool children. However, currently more than 40% of cases occur in those older than 10 years.
   c. Seasonal incidence: The peak incidence of infection is during the winter and spring.
   d. Incubation period: 8 to 12 days from exposure to onset of symptoms with an average interval of 14 days to appearance of rash.

e. Period of communicability: 1 to 2 days before the onset of symptoms, or 3 to 5 days before the appearance of rash until 4 days after rash appearance.

f. Exclusion: Children should be excluded from school at least 4 days after the onset of rash.

3. Mumps

a. Description of clinical disease: Mumps is an acute contagious disease, with onset of low-grade fever, headache, anorexia, and malaise followed in 24 to 48 hours by swollen, painful, tender salivary glands, primarily the parotid. In about 25% of cases the swelling is unilateral. The salivary gland involvement lasts 7 to 10 days and the lack of a prodrome is not unusual. Approximately one third of cases of mumps infection are not characterized by glandular swelling.

b. Age group most commonly affected: Infection occurs throughout childhood with infection in the older patient being more likely to result in severe disease.

c. Seasonal incidence: Mumps is more common during late winter and spring.

d. Incubation period: 16 to 18 days, but cases may occur as early as 12 or as late as 25 days after exposure.

e. Period of communicability: Usually 1 to 2 days. However, the period may be as long as 7 days before onset of parotid swelling and occasionally as long as 9 days after onset.

f. Exclusion: Children should be excluded from school until 9 days after the onset of parotitis.

4. Pertussis

a. Description of clinical disease: Pertussis (whooping cough) is a contagious disease that begins with mild upper respiratory tract symptoms and proceeds to severe cough paroxysms with the characteristic inspiratory "whoop," often followed by vomiting. Fever is not a prominent feature, and the total course of the disease is usually 6 to 10 weeks.

b. Age group most commonly affected: Approximately 30% of cases occur in infants younger than 6 months, and 75% of cases occur in children younger than 5 years. Recently, pertussis in adolescents varying from a mild illness to the full-blown syndrome has been increasingly frequent.

c. Seasonal incidence: There is little seasonal variation in the occurrence of pertussis.

d. Incubation period: 6 to 20 days, but usually 7 to 10 days and rarely longer than 2 weeks.

e. Period of communicability: Most common during the early catarrhal stage before paroxysms, and extending until 3 weeks after this onset of paroxysms of coughing. When treated with erythromycin, the period of infectiousness is usually limited to the 5 days after onset of therapy.

f. Exclusion: Cases should be excluded from school until 3 weeks after onset of the paroxysmal stage or until on erythromycin therapy for 5 days.

5. Rubella

a. Description of clinical disease: Rubella is usually a mild illness with a minimal fever and a maculopapular rash that usually starts on the face or upper trunk and extends over the rest of the body. The rash usually lasts about 3 days and is often accompanied by postauricular and suboccipital lymphadenopathy. As many as half of rubella infections do not manifest a rash.

b. Age group most commonly affected: In the prevaccine era, rubella was primarily a disease of childhood. Today, infections in adolescents have become important.

c. Seasonal incidence: Rubella is more common during late winter and early spring.

d. Incubation period: 16 to 18 days, with outside limits of 14 to 21 days.

e. Period of communicability: One week before until 5 to 7 days after onset of rash.

f. Exclusion: Children should be excluded from school for 7 days after onset of rash.

6. Streptococcal pharyngitis

a. Description of clinical disease: Streptococcal pharyngitis is a contagious disease usually characterized by fever, sore throat, exudative tonsillitis, and tender anterior cervical lymph nodes. However, symptoms may be minimal.

b. Age group most commonly affected: The 3- to 15-year age group is most commonly affected.

c. Seasonal incidence: The highest incidence is during late fall, winter, and spring.

d. Incubation period: The incubation period is short, usually 2 to 5 days, occasionally longer.

e. Period of communicability: The period of communicability is 10 to 21 days in untreated cases. Transmissibility usually ceases 24 to 28 hours after institution of adequate therapy. Untreated persons may carry the organisms in their throats for weeks to months, most commonly in decreasing numbers. The contagiousness of these carriers is markedly reduced after 2 to 3 weeks.

f. Exclusion: Children should be excluded from school until they are afebrile and at least until 24 hours after the institution of appropriate antimicrobial therapy.

7. Tuberculosis

a. Description of clinical disease: Primary tuberculosis is almost always a disease of the lungs. Most children are asymptomatic when first infected and early clinical manifestations, which may include hilar lymphadenitis, involvement of a lung segment, atelectasis, or pleural effusion, may not be apparent for 1 to 6 months. Fatigue, fever, and weight loss may occur early while cough, chest pain, hemoptysis, and hoarseness may follow.

b. Age group most commonly affected: All ages are susceptible, but infants and pubertal children are at higher risk.

c. Seasonal incidence: No increased seasonal incidence has been identified.

d. Incubation period: The incubation period from infection to development of a positive skin test is 2 to 10 weeks. After infection, the maximum risk of disease is during the first year. Months to years may elapse between infection and development of disease. Usually infection does not progress to clinical disease.

e. Period of communicability: In adults on therapy, the period of infectivity is a few days to a few weeks. In contrast, if cavitary disease is not present, children are generally not infectious.

    f. Exclusion: Until the child's physician or local health department authority states that the child is noninfectious. Children with primary tuberculosis may attend school if they are on chemotherapy.

8. Varicella-zoster

    a. Description of clinical disease: Primary varicella (chickenpox) is an acute, very contagious disease having an onset with low-grade fever and malaise and accompanied by a generalized vesicular rash, which usually starts on the scalp or upper trunk. Characteristically, the lesions are in different stages of evolution and there is very little subclinical disease. A latent infection may occur following primary infection. Reactivation of the latter results in herpes zoster (shingles) with its characteristic dermatomal distribution.

    b. Age groups most commonly affected: Most cases of chickenpox occur in children between 5 and 10 years of age. Disease in the older patient tends to be more severe.

    c. Seasonal incidence: Chickenpox is more common during late winter and early spring.

    d. Incubation period: 14 to 16 days, with outside limits of 11 to 20 days.

    e. Period of communicability: 1 to 2 days before and shortly after onset of rash, but contagiousness may persist as long as 5 days after the appearance of lesions.

    f. Exclusion: Children should be excluded from school until the sixth day after onset of rash, but may return sooner if lesions are dry or crusted. Children with zoster may return to school when the lesions have crusted.

The following diseases are spread primarily by the fecal-oral route.

1. Acute gastroenteritis

    a. Description of clinical disease: Gastroenteritis is primarily a disease of infants and young children characterized by fever and vomiting, followed by watery diarrhea that occasionally may be severe. Symptoms last 2 to 5 days.

    b. Age group most commonly affected: Disease most commonly occurs in infants and young children.

c. Seasonal incidence: Cases occur at all times of the year, but rotavirus infections, the most common cause of diarrhea in children, occur more commonly in the colder months.

d. Incubation period: 24 to 72 hours.

e. Period of communicability: During the acute stage of the illness and for a short time thereafter while the infectious agent is still being excreted.

f. Exclusion: Vomiting two or more times in the previous 24 hours should result in exclusion from school unless disease is determined to be noncommunicable and the child is not in danger of dehydration. Children in whom stool cannot be contained by toilet use also should be excluded. Handwashing after toileting and before eating is essential.

2. Hepatitis A

a. Description of clinical disease: Hepatitis A usually has an abrupt onset with malaise, fever, anorexia, and nausea, followed by the onset of jaundice in a few days. The illness ranges from very mild to very severe and disabling. Many infections in children are asymptomatic or mild.

b. Age group most commonly affected: The disease is most common among older schoolchildren and young adults.

c. Seasonal incidence: There is no appreciable seasonal variation in the incidence of disease.

d. Incubation period: 15 to 50 days, with an average of 25 to 30 days.

e. Period of communicability: Period of contagiousness is about 1 to 3 weeks, with the highest titers of virus being present in stools 2 weeks before the onset of illness. The infectivity risk then diminishes and is minimal 1 week after the onset of jaundice.

f. Exclusion: Children should be excluded from school for 1 week after the onset of the illness and until jaundice, if present, has disappeared or until passive immunoprophylaxis has been administered to appropriate children and staff as directed by the health officials.

The following diseases are spread primarily by direct contact.
1. Conjunctivitis
   a. Acute bacterial conjunctivitis
      (1) Description of clinical disease: Infection begins with hyperemia and increased lacrimation, followed by swollen eyelids and mucopurulent discharge. The infection may last from 2 days to 2 to 3 weeks.
      (2) Age group most commonly affected: Children younger than 5 years are most susceptible and the incidence decreases as children grow older.
      (3) Seasonal incidence: There may be some seasonal predilection depending upon the organism, but, in general, occurrence is increased in warmer climates.
      (4) Incubation period: Approximately 24 to 72 hours.
      (5) Period of communicability: Children are infectious during the course of active infection.
      (6) Exclusion: Children should be excluded from school during the acute stage.
   b. Viral hemorrhagic conjunctivitis
      (1) Description of clinical disease: Onset of disease usually is sudden with redness, swelling, and pain. Subconjunctival hemorrhages are frequently present and lymphoid follicles may develop. The disease lasts from 4 to 15 days.
      (2) Age group most commonly affected: Infections occur at all ages and reinfections and/or relapses can occur.
      (3) Seasonal incidence: Adenovirus infections have an increased incidence in late winter, spring, and early summer; enteroviruses peak in summer and fall.
      (4) Incubation period: Adenovirus infection, 2 to 14 days, with a mean of 8 days; enteroviruses, 12 hours to 5 days.
      (5) Period of communicability: Adenovirus infections may be transmittable for 14 days after onset, while enteroviruses are communicable for at least 4 days after onset.
      (6) Exclusion: Children should not attend school while disease is active. Some experts do not feel exclusion is necessary if there is clear, watery discharge without fever, eye pain, or eyelid redness.

2. Impetigo
   a. Description of clinical disease: A superficial skin infection that commonly proceeds through vesicular, pustular, and encrusted stages.
   b. Age group most commonly affected: Incidence of impetigo is highest in young children.
   c. Seasonal incidence: Disease is most common in late summer and fall.
   d. Incubation period: Usually 7 to 10 days.
   e. Period of communicability: Disease is transmissible when lesions are active by draining or until 24 hours after institution of therapy.
   f. Exclusion: Children should not attend school until at least 24 hours after institution of therapy, and they are afebrile.
3. Pediculosis (head lice)
   a. Description of clinical disease: Pediculosis is an infestation of the head or body with lice, larvae, and nits, resulting in severe itching and excoriation. When secondary infection occurs, regional lymphadenitis may result.
   b. Age group most commonly affected: Infestations are most common in child care and school-age children.
   c. Seasonal incidence: There is no appreciable seasonal variation.
   d. Incubation period: Unknown.
   e. Period of communicability: Disease transmission may occur as long as lice or eggs are viable on the infested person or clothing.
   f. Exclusion: Children should be excluded from school until the morning after the first treatment.
4. Scabies
   a. Description of clinical disease: Scabies is caused by mites whose skin penetration is characterized by papules, vesicles, or linear burrows, commonly containing the mites and their eggs. Frequently involved areas include finger webs, wrists, elbows, anterior axillary folds, beltline, thighs, and buttocks. Pruritus is prominent, particularly at night. Lesions may become secondarily infected secondary to scratching.

b. Age group most commonly affected: All age groups are affected.

c. Seasonal incidence: There is no significant seasonal variation in disease.

d. Incubation period: In persons without previous exposure, 4 to 6 weeks before onset of itching; in reexposure, 1 to 4 days.

e. Period of communicability: Communicable until eggs and mites are destroyed by therapy.

f. Exclusion: Infected individuals should be excluded from school until the day after therapy is completed.

5. Tinea capitis (ringworm of the scalp)

a. Description of clinical disease: Ringworm of the scalp begins as a small papule and spreads radially, resulting in scaly patches of baldness. Infected hairs become very brittle and have a tendency to break off. Boggy suppurative lesions known as *kerions* may develop.

b. Age group most commonly affected: All ages are susceptible, but particularly children between the ages of 2 and 10 years.

c. Seasonal incidence: No particular seasonal predilection has been noted.

d. Incubation period: 10 to 14 days.

e. Period of communicability: Communicable as long as fungi can be cultured from the infected area or demonstrated by fluorescence.

f. Exclusion: Children should be excluded from school until 24 hours after initial treatment.

The following diseases are spread primarily by body fluids such as saliva, urine, blood, and semen.

1. Acquired immunodeficiency syndrome (AIDS) (see chapter 20)

a. Description of clinical disease: AIDS is a severe, life-threatening disease that progressively damages the immune system. The onset of clinical illness is usually insidious and characterized by nonspecific symptoms such as malaise, anorexia, fatigue, diarrhea, weight loss, lymphadenopathy, and fever. Eventually the patient is afflicted with serious infections, frequently opportunistic.

b. Age group most commonly affected: Young adults.

c. Seasonal incidence: There is no evidence of seasonal predilection.

d. Incubation period: Variable. Antibodies are usually detectable 1 to 3 months after infection. Period from infection to detection of disease ranges from 2 months to 10 years or longer.

e. Period of communicability: Unknown, but presumed to extend from shortly after infection through life.

f. Exclusion: Since human immunodeficiency virus (HIV) infection or AIDS is not acquired by casual contact, children and adolescents infected with HIV should be allowed to attend school without restriction unless they manifest severe aggressive behavior, such as biting, or have weeping skin sores that cannot be covered.

2. Cytomegalovirus

a. Description of clinical disease: Congenital infection is usually asymptomatic, but unusually can result in mild or severe mental retardation or even death. Acquired infection is usually asymptomatic but may unusually cause a disease similar to Epstein-Barr virus—induced mononucleosis in young adults. Immunodeficient or immunosuppressed patients may develop severe disseminated infection.

b. Age group most commonly affected: In highly developed countries, serum antibody prevalence in young adults approximates 40%, while in developing countries it is almost 100%. Acquisition of antibody is inversely related to socioeconomic group.

c. Seasonal incidence: There is no seasonal predilection.

d. Incubation period: Incubation period for acquired disease varies from 3 to 12 weeks.

e. Period of communicability: Months to years as virus is excreted in urine and saliva for prolonged periods.

f. Exclusion: Exclusion from school is not indicated.

3. Hepatitis B

a. Description of clinical disease: Hepatitis B usually has an insidious onset with anorexia, vague abdominal pain, nausea and vomiting, and, occasionally, joint pain and rash. Jaundice is often present, but fever may be absent or mild. Clinical presentation ranges from inapparent to fulminant. The disease is milder and often anicteric in children.

b. Age group most commonly affected: In North America, infection is most common in young adults.

c. Seasonal incidence: Very little seasonal variation.

d. Incubation period: Incubation period is 45 to 160 days, with an average of 120 days.

e. Period of communicability: Blood from infected persons is infectious many weeks before onset of symptoms through the clinical course of the acute disease and during the chronic carrier state, if such ensues.

f. Exclusion: There is no reason to exclude from school unless there is unusually aggressive behavior, such as biting.

4. Hepatitis C

a. Description of clinical disease: Hepatitis C, like hepatitis B, is characterized by an insidious onset of malaise, anorexia, nausea, vomiting, and abdominal pain. Jaundice is less likely than with hepatitis B, and severity ranges from inapparent infection to fulminant disease.

b. Age group most commonly affected: Disease is most frequently recognized in adults, and reported cases in children younger than 15 years are uncommon.

c. Seasonal incidence: There is no seasonal predilection.

d. Incubation period: 7 to 9 weeks, with a range of 2 to 12 weeks.

e. Period of communicability: From 1 or more weeks before onset of symptoms through the acute disease and into the carrier state, if such ensues.

f. Exclusion: There is no reason to exclude from school unless very aggressive behavior, such as biting, is present.

5. Herpes simplex, oral

a. Description of clinical disease: Herpes simplex is a viral infection characterized by localized vesicular lesions with a tendency to latency and recurrence (fever blisters or cold sores). The primary illness may be mild or inapparent, or may manifest with extensive lesions accompanied by fever and malaise lasting a week or more.

b. Age group most commonly affected: Initial infection usually occurs before age 5 years, with recurrent disease covering many subsequent years.
c. Seasonal incidence: No seasonal variation has been noted.
d. Incubation period: 2 to 14 days.
e. Period of communicability: As long as 7 weeks after recovery from disease.
f. Exclusion: Exclusion of children from school is not indicated.

Suggested Reading

American Academy of Pediatrics, Committee on Infectious Diseases. *Report of the Committee on Infectious Diseases (Red Book)*. 22nd edition. Elk Grove Village, IL: American Academy of Pediatrics; 1991

CHAPTER 20

HIV — STUDENTS AND SCHOOL PERSONNEL

The human immunodeficiency virus (HIV) epidemic has been with us since cases of HIV infection first were reported in 1980. Treatment regimens are available, but treatment is not yet fully effective. Because the HIV virus is transmitted almost exclusively by sexual behavior that adolescents and adults can alter, educational programs could be effective in the prevention of the spread of HIV infection. Children with HIV infection most likely have acquired it at birth or from a transfusion of contaminated blood products.

Children with HIV infection can participate in all activities in school to the extent that their health permits. They should not be excluded from school, nor should they be isolated within the school setting.

Epidemiology

Acquired immunodeficiency syndrome (AIDS) is a major leading cause of death among children 1 to 4 years of age and in young people between the ages of 15 and 24. As of July 1992, there were 222,419 cases of reported AIDS in the United States. Of these cases, 3,694 were infants and children under the age of 13, and 854 were adolescents through age 19 (630 males and 224 females). For every child who actually has AIDS, it is estimated that 2 to 10 children are infected with the HIV virus. By 1995, 5.7 million people will be infected with HIV in the United States. A total of $10 billion will be expended for treatment of people infected by HIV. That figure will jump to $15 billion annually in the mid-1990s. New York state has the highest incidence of AIDS in patients under the age of 13, with 1,043 cases of which 940 were in New York City. This is followed by Florida (588), New Jersey (378), California (241), and Puerto Rico (200).

Although HIV has been found in blood; saliva; urine; cervical secretion; cerebral, spinal, and pleural fluid; and human milk, transmission of the virus has only occurred through blood, semen, cervical secretions, and, sometimes, through breast milk. Transmission from an infected person to an uninfected person has occurred by only three major routes: sexual intercourse, inoculation of blood (ie, drug users who share syringes and need-les for injections), and blood transfusion from an infected source. Congenital or perinatal transmission from a woman to her fetus or newborn accounts for the majority of infants and children with HIV infections. Due in part to the unusually long latency period between the onset of HIV infection and the appearance of symp-toms, HIV infection among adolescents may be much greater than the apparent low incidence of AIDS cases in adolescents. There is every indication that HIV infection can spread, and is spreading, to all segments of our society.

The HIV infection has a devastating impact on children and their families, schools, and communities. Handicaps resulting from the disease can cause social and psychological problems. Myths circulate that the disease can be transmitted by casual contact. This causes fear and anxiety and results in discrimina-tion. Increasing costs for AIDS patients threaten to absorb a disproportionate amount of health care funds, thus placing other valuable social welfare resources and needs in competition with HIV-related services. A collaborative approach will be needed.

Children with HIV infection can be admitted freely to all schools to the extent to which their health will permit. This places a great burden on special services, however, and confidentiality problems ensue involving the patient's right-to-privacy versus the school's right-to-know. Related services may need to be util-ized without the school knowing the true diagnosis.

Children with HIV infections show evidence of increasing cog-nitive dysfunction resulting in a higher incidence of learning disabilities and school problems. These children may progress to a need for home instruction as well as occupational and physi-cal therapy similar to that needed to treat cerebral palsy. Be-havioral problems also occur involving depression, anxiety, family disruption, and hostility, resulting in the need for in-creasing mental health services.

Prevention offers the chief means of decreasing the incidence of HIV infection. Thorough screening methods have practically eliminated infected blood transfusions as a source of HIV. Use of condoms together with virucidal vaginal gels can prevent HIV infection during intercourse. Sterile needle exchange programs for drug abusers combined with treatment programs have been proposed to reduce this particular source of HIV infection. Many authorities believe that these are the most effective ways to prevent HIV infections. Voluntary neonatal screening programs together with counseling will help us to track and treat newborn HIV infections. The most effective and universally accepted method of HIV prevention is education done in an organized, comprehensive, well-developed manner by a coalition of schools and the community. The pediatrician can play a pivotal role in implementing these efforts and acting as a case manager when required.

AIDS Education as a Major Prevention of Transmission

Educational programs can be effective in the prevention of the spread of HIV infection. In October 1986, Surgeon General C. Everett Koop, MD, issued a report on AIDS in which he stated: "AIDS education should start in early elementary school and in the home so the children could grow up knowing the behavior to avoid in order to protect themselves." The Office of School Health and Education Projects at the Centers for Disease Control (CDC) in 1986 convened a special task force in order to write guidelines for effective school health education to prevent the spread of AIDS.

These guidelines state that:

1. Education about AIDS would be most appropriate and effective when carried out within a comprehensive school health program; that State Departments of Education and Health should work together in order to establish this; that community involvement was essential; and that programs should be developed also to address the developmental needs of students in school and out-of-school youth and minorities.
2. Programs should be taught by qualified teachers.
3. Young people should abstain from sexual intercourse until ready to establish a mutually monogamous relationship.
4. Students should refrain from using illicit drugs and avoid sharing needles.
5. If abstinence cannot be practiced, then a latex condom should be used with a virucidal spermicide.
6. Students should seek counseling and testing when HIV infection is suspected.

These guidelines also contain specific suggestions as to the content of AIDS education. In early elementary school, AIDS education should be designed to allay excessive fears of the epidemic and discuss the difference between sickness and health. In late elementary school, the concept of viral infection and the nature of AIDS can be discussed. In junior and senior high school, the specifics of the sexual transmission of AIDS and prevention, discrimination, civil rights issues, and other social aspects should be discussed. The report also suggests that sufficient curriculum time and resources be allotted at each grade level to ensure that the student acquire essential knowledge and that the criteria for program assessment be provided. The report was delayed for over a year due to governmental concerns about its content, but it finally was released and published in *Morbidity Mortality Weekly Report* in January 1988.

In September 1987, the CDC had awarded funds totalling $6 million for underwriting a number of model education programs. Funds for training and developmental grants were awarded to national educational organizations and groups serving minorities and out-of-school youth, to the state and local educational agencies in areas with a high incidence of AIDS, and to private curriculum development organizations. As a result of these efforts, a number of organizations established effective AIDS education programs. Included among these were the American School Health Association, the National Education Association, and the American Association of Superintendents and Administrators. These organizations sought consultation with the American Academy of Pediatrics in order to help develop their programs. The CDC also established a combined health information data base in order to provide information about AIDS education programs to organizations wishing to develop programs. Organizations or individuals can contact the data base and obtain information regarding programs registered with the CDC. Further information about these programs can be obtained by written request from the Division of Adolescent and School Health.* Additional information about AIDS education programs is also provided in this chapter.

---

*Division of Adolescent and School Health, Mail Stop K-31, 4770 Buford Highway NE, Atlanta, GA 30341-3724.

Policies

Hysteria and fear were encountered when efforts were made to admit children with HIV infections to public schools. In many states and school systems, children were put in special self-contained classrooms or educated at home. The CDC and the American Academy of Pediatrics have issued statements stating that children with HIV infection can attend school. Both the CDC and the American Academy of Pediatrics now believe that children with HIV infection can attend school in an unrestricted manner and do not need to be isolated within the classroom, either for the protection of other children or for their own protection. School district policies should reflect these official policies.

Confidentiality

Confidentiality is the keystone to ensuring the education of the child with HIV. The school's request for information needed to educate the child must be balanced by the need to safeguard the rights of the patient. The primary role of the pediatrician is to represent the patient and the family. Although the school environment has improved in the past 6 years, disclosure of the child's HIV status to anyone in the school might result in possible fear and hysteria and possibly prejudice the child's education. This should therefore be done only with the informed consent of the parents and age-appropriate consent of the child. Should special education services be required, these usually can be done without revealing the diagnosis. A successful AIDS education program should reassure teachers about the nature of the disease and improve the environment so that the school staff can feel comfortable with educating an HIV-positive child should the diagnosis become known.

There are now treatments available for HIV infection, such as orally administered zidovudine (AZT), which may need to be administered during the school day. These treatments should be given in the manner developed for all children who require medication while in school. Since the nature of the medication may identify a child as HIV infected, only those intimately involved with the administration of the medication in school need to be informed. In these cases, this would be only the school medical advisor and the school nurse. The decision for this limited disclosure should be made by the parents and the physician.

Reaction to the disclosure of HIV status may result in discrimination for children with HIV infection in school. Teachers should take the lead in discouraging this by educating students about tolerance of children with chronic illnesses. The pediatrician can play a role in educating parents and the community and discouraging discrimination by utilizing the assistance of public health authorities, American Academy of Pediatrics statements, and the help of religious leaders and others in the community.

Employees

Staff members infected with HIV generally should be allowed to stay at school or on the job as their state of health permits. They should seek the advice of their physicians as to attending work/school. The school policies covering the employment of HIV-infected personnel should prohibit discrimination.

Pupil Needs

A child with HIV symptomatic infection should be regarded as a chronically health-impaired child. School personnel need to be oriented toward the needs of this child. Health services should be available in the school. Special education should be provided as needed under Public Act 94-142 and, for children from birth to age 3, under 99-457. The physician should participate actively as a member of the team. Due to intercurrent illnesses, children with HIV infection may be absent from school frequently and may require occasional home instruction. This should be provided as quickly as possible upon authorization of the team. The child's physician, together with school nurse, should facilitate the transition between school and home instruction.

Health-Related Therapy

Children with symptomatic HIV infection may demonstrate visual, spacial, and perceptual dysfunction. Neurologic findings, including poor fine-motor coordination, clumsy rapid alternating movements, or abnormal gait, have been demonstrated in many such children. These children also may need occupational therapy, physical therapy, and/or speech or language help under appropriate medical supervision.

Behavioral Aspects

Children with HIV infection may present behavioral problems such as anxiety, depression, anger, and withdrawal. These may be due to the neurologic effects of the disease or to the problems associated with family disruption and the resulting parental isolation, guilt, and alienation. Physical changes, such as weight loss and declining cognitive function, may lead to additional emotional problems during the middle school years. The family should be given support by school mental health personnel, and the pediatrician should work with the school and the family in order to provide behavioral counseling and support.

Universal Precautions

Because all infected children will not necessarily be known to the school and officials, policies and procedures should be developed in advance to handle incidences of bleeding because blood is a possible source of contagion. Washing exposed skin with soap and water is the most important preventive measure in this setting. Lacerations and other bleeding lesions in school should be managed in a manner that minimizes direct contact of the caregiver with blood. Under no circumstances should the urgent care of a bleeding child be delayed because gloves are not immediately available. Since many infectious agents may be transmitted by other body fluids such as urine, stools, vomitus, tears, and nasal or oral secretions, hand washing is recommended.

Health Education

The American Academy of Pediatrics believes that AIDS education should be part of a comprehensive school health education program. This should be taught from kindergarten until 12th grade with a planned, sequential health curriculum. During the early elementary grades, a regular, trained teacher is sufficient; however, at the middle and high school level, a qualified health educator should be appointed to supervise AIDS education. Programs might be started during the high school years but then expanded downward to the elementary grades and kindergarten. Finally, parental involvement should be actively encouraged. Parents can obtain AIDS education themselves from schools, community resources, local public health departments, and their own pediatrician.

The Role of the Pediatrician and/or Family Physician

Physicians have an important part to play in AIDS education because of their role as a case manager for children with chronic illnesses, their opportunity to communicate with parents, their knowledge about family structure, and their participation in community affairs. The role of physicians in AIDS education is to begin educating themselves about AIDS. In Connecticut, it was found that the best way of training office physicians in private practice was to train physicians and their office staff together. This was done in six regional areas and took place during a single 3-hour course given in the early evening for physicians, nurses, and all members of their office staffs. Once trained, physicians and their staffs can be effective in promoting school-based AIDS educational programs as well.

The AIDS education programs in schools should be advocated for and supervised by a school health advisory committee or similar school-related organization in each community. This committee may consist of a school medical advisor, community pediatrician and/or public health physician, school nurse, health educator, mental health professional, school administrator, faculty member, parent, and community representatives.

The school medical advisor should be instrumental in educating physicians and nurses in the community. Once trained, they would then: (1) conduct education programs for teachers, parent groups, and other personnel; (2) assist schools and organizations in developing educational programs; (3) review, adapt, and develop education materials; and (4) participate in media events and in discussions between administrators, faculty, and parents.

Physicians can review videocassettes for content and developmentally appropriate levels. They also can participate in review of curriculum materials to make sure they are medically correct and timely. Broadcast media, radio and TV, also are appropriate media for discussing the nature of HIV disease. Physicians may participate in hotlines about the topic or do television interviews. Printed media also may be appropriate vehicles to discuss the subject with parents. Networking is an important aspect of AIDS education. Organizations such as Parents of Children With Chronic Diseases, AIDS support groups, and health education coalitions are appropriate organizations to involve.

Legislation to outlaw discrimination toward HIV patients, both at a local and national level, should be supported. Mandatory testing should be discouraged and voluntary testing supported. Financial support should be provided for the many difficulties faced by parents with HIV infection.

Conclusion

The pediatrician must network effectively with parents and public health authorities in order to ensure the educability of HIV-infected children in school and the education of other children about this disease.

Resources

Pediatricians frequently seek information about AIDS education for use as school medical advisors, for networking purposes, or for their own information and use in their offices. There are now several excellent sources to access. These include the CDC National AIDS Clearinghouse, the CDC National AIDS Information and Education Program (NAIEP), the National Pediatric HIV Resource Center at the Children's Hospital of New Jersey, the National School Boards Association, the Council of Chief State School Officers Comprehensive Health Education Network (CHEN), and the National Association of State Boards of Education.

The CDC National AIDS Clearinghouse

This clearinghouse is a comprehensive information center for people working in HIV and AIDS, including public health professionals. The center operates information services, distributes materials, facilitates networking, and operates NAC ONLINE. One can call the clearinghouse toll free at 1/800/458-5231. Specialists will answer inquiries and make referrals and help locate publications. They can access the following computer data bases in order to put the caller in touch with organizations providing materials:

The Resource Data Base contains a description of more than 16,000 organizations providing HIV-related services and resources.

The Educational Materials Data Base provides a collection of information on more than 9,000 hard-to-find HIV-related educational materials.

The AIDS School Health Education Data Base is produced by the CDC Center for Chronic Disease Prevention and Health Promotion, Division of Adolescent and School Health. This was developed in 1987 to help organize the various educational resources available to teach children and youth about AIDS and HIV infection. In order to access this combined health information data base, one should call 1/800/289-4277. Use one's own computer terminal and obtain a subscription to BRS, a communications soft package and a modem. (AIDS School Health Information Data Base Maxwell On-line BRS Information Technology Division, 1200 Route 7, Latham, NY 12110.) The data base publishes a manual with a list of references in alphabetical order (audiovisuals, books, brochures, journal articles, etc). The manual also contains a description of the 1989 Cooperative Agreements giving the addresses and phone numbers of national, state, and local programs in AIDS education and national training programs. If you need more information about the School Health Education Data Base or wish to submit materials or information related to AIDS Education, contact the CDC at the Centers for Disease Control and Prevention, Center for Disease Prevention and Health Promotion, Division of Adolescent and School Health, Mail Stop 814, ATTN: AIDS School Health Education Data Base, Atlanta, GA 30333.

The Funding Data Base describes funding activities for community-related HIV and AIDS service organizations. It includes information about application processes, deadlines, and eligibility requirements.

One can obtain materials from the Clearinghouse such as selected reprints from the CDC's *MMWR* and the *HIV/AIDS Surveillance Reports.*

The Clearinghouse also works with national, state, and local organizations and with a number of minority, adolescent, and women's organizations in order to provide exchange about HIV- and AIDS-related services.

Finally, the Clearinghouse operates NAC ONLINE, which is a computerized information network facilitating information exchange among AIDS service providers.

National AIDS Information and Education Program (NAIEP)

This program is responsible for informing the American people about the HIV virus and AIDS. This includes a media communication effort and national information hotline and clearinghouse for the public. The public information aspect creates and promotes "America's response to AIDS" information materials. This is the largest federally sponsored health campaign in history. The CDC National AIDS Hotline operates around the clock, providing anonymous, confidential information in English (1/800/342-AIDS); information also available in Spanish and for the deaf. Trained specialists answer questions about HIV and AIDS. They also work with the National Partnership Development activity that works with private sector organizations to encourage their participation.

National Pediatric HIV Resource Center

This is located in the Children's Hospital of New Jersey, 15 S 9th St, Newark, NJ 07107; telephone number 1/800/362-0071. The center provides consultation and technical assistance to programs serving children with HIV infection, promotes development and distribution of educational materials for patients and family, provides technical assistance on legal issues facing providers, as well as educational opportunities for professionals including an HIV core curriculum. This is an in-depth theory and clinical curriculum for pediatric HIV professionals, including physicians, nurses, and social workers. Mini-fellowships at the Children's Hospital are designed to enhance providers' clinical skills. Workshops are given on ethical and cultural issues as well as "train the trainer" workshops for pediatric professionals to utilize within their own communities.

Interested pediatricians should contact Carolyn Burr, the coordinator, or Dr Samuel Grubman, who is a coordinator of medical education and arranges the clinical training experiences (Telephone: 201/268-8251).

National School Boards Association

This educational organization maintains an HIV and AIDS resource data base that enables policy makers and educators to make informed decisions about HIV and AIDS policy in educational issues. These provide information about AIDS-related issues important to school officials. Pediatricians may want to utilize this source to help discover worthwhile AIDS education curricula to utilize in schools. The data base contains more than 600 entries including resources such as sample policies, curricula, court decisions, books, journals, and videotapes. School officials are encouraged to submit policies and other relevant materials for inclusion and request data base searches to aid in decision making involving HIV and AIDS education policies. The data base may be accessed by calling the National School Board Association, 1680 Duke St, Alexandria, VA 22314 (703/838-6754).

Comprehensive Health Education Network (CHEN)

The Council of Chief State School Officers is funded by the CDC to create a computer network, entitled "The Comprehensive Health Education Network" (CHEN), which enables state education agencies, local education agencies, and national organizations funded by the CDC to share information about HIV/AIDS education and other related issues. Users can also exchange private messages and post information. Users of this data base are able to share and request information about a number of topics, including source materials, curriculum assessment, and policy issues in education. One can also reach select groups of health educators. Those requesting further information may contact Martha Bush, (202/336-7031). Council of Chief State School Health Officers, 1 Massachusetts Ave, NW, Suite 700, Washington, DC 20001-1431.

National Association of State Boards of Education (NASBE)

A useful policymaker's guide to help in planning effective state programs about AIDS education has been published by this association. Entitled *Effective AIDS Education*, the guide can be obtained from the National Association of State Boards of Education, 1012 Cameron St, Alexandria, VA 22314. The National Association of State Boards of Education also has published an *HIV/AIDS Education Survey*, which profiles state actions in each individual state. These publications contain materials, highlights of state policies and programs, and state health education requirements in each of the 50 states.

AAP Provisional Committee on Pediatric AIDS

In 1986, the Academy issued a statement entitled "School Attendance of Children and Adolescents With Human-T Lymphotrophic Virus 3, Lymphadenopathy Associated Virus Infection," which was the first statement on HIV infection in school children and complemented a CDC statement issued earlier. The statement stated that children could attend school on a case-by-case basis and that routine screening for children with HIV infection was not indicated. This paper now is retired and has been replaced by a newer policy statement that includes recommendations listed below. It was of value primarily in that it served to reassure the nation and provide impetus for successful AIDS education programs.

In the course of the need to develop policy and better educate pediatricians about HIV infections, the Academy appointed a Task Force on Pediatric AIDS in the summer of 1987. The Task Force—now a Provisional Committee—meets three times a year and consists of pediatricians with experience in infectious disease, HIV infections, adolescents, perinatal AIDS, foster care, psychosocial issues, disability issues, and school health.

In 1988, the AAP Committee on School Health issued a policy statement entitled, "AIDS Education in Schools," which was reviewed by the Provisional Committee. Recommendations are similar to those described by the CDC and have been described earlier in this chapter. The statement was in agreement with the CDC position that all schools should develop a comprehensive AIDS education program to include children from kindergarten through 12th grade. It recommended that all physicians, especially pediatricians, provide leadership by encouraging development of local AIDS education programs.

In November 1988, the Provisional Committee on Pediatric AIDS published a statement entitled "Pediatric Guidelines for Infection Control of HIV Virus in Hospitals, Medical Offices, Schools, and Other Settings." This report attempted to differentiate high-prevalence areas from low-prevalence areas and provided further reassurance to the public concerning HIV infection control. The paper stated that:

1. Children with HIV who are old enough to attend school could be admitted freely to all activities, to the extent that their health permits.

2. Because all infected children would not necessarily be known to school officials in high-prevalence areas, and because blood was a potential source of contagion, policies and procedures should be developed in advance to handle instances of bleeding. Because of minimal risk, the only mandatory precaution should be washing exposed skin with soap and water. In schools in high-prevalence areas, access to gloves should be provided for those individuals wishing to further reduce the risk; especially if they will be involved in handling of body fluids.
3. Even in high-prevalence areas there is no need for separate examining rooms or visiting rooms for HIV-infected patients, unless the patient is sufficiently immunosuppressed to require reverse isolation.
4. Needles should be placed uncapped in closed puncture-proof containers, which then should be disposed of as infectious waste.
5. All children could be admitted to school and to day care if their health, neurologic development, behavior, and immune status were appropriate.

This paper served as a foundation for subsequent statements on HIV infection and freed physicians from their concern about contagion.

A list of current statements developed by the AAP Provisional Committee on Pediatric AIDS is included below. Also listed are AIDS-related statements developed by other AAP committees. The reader is referred to the Academy for updated information.

AAP Policy Statements

Guidelines for Human Immunodeficiency Virus (HIV)-Infected Children and Their Foster Families

Perinatal Human Immunodeficiency Virus (HIV) Testing

Education of Children With Human Immunodeficiency Virus Infection

Pediatric Guidelines for Infection Control of HIV (AIDS Virus) in Hospitals, Medical Offices, Schools, and Other Settings

Perinatal HIV Infection (AIDS)

Acquired Immunodeficiency Syndrome Education in Schools

Human Immunodeficiency Virus (AIDS Virus) in the Athletic Setting

Suggested Readings

American Academy of Pediatrics, Committee on Children With Disabilities, Committee on School Health. Children with health impairments in schools. *Pediatrics*. 1990;86:636-638

American Academy of Pediatrics, Committee on School Health. Administration of medication in schools. *Pediatrics*. 1984;74:433

American Academy of Pediatrics, Committee on School Health. Concepts of school health programs. *AAP News*. December 1985

American Academy of Pediatrics, Committee on School Health. Guidelines for urgent care in school. *Pediatrics*. 1990;6:999-1000

American Academy of Pediatrics, Committee on School Health. Medically indicated home, hospital, and other non-school based instruction. *AAP News*. February 1992

American Academy of Pediatrics. *Proceedings From a National Conference on Public Law 99-457; Physician Participation in the Implementation of the Law*. Elk Grove Village, IL: American Academy of Pediatrics; 1988

Belman AL, Diamond G, Dickson D, et al. Pediatric AIDS neurologic syndrome. *Am J Dis Child*. 1988;142:29-35

Burger JE, ed. *Responding to HIV and AIDS*. Washington, DC: National Education Association, Health Information Network; 1992

Centers for Disease Control. Education and foster care of children infected with HTLV III/LAV infection. *MMWR*. 1985;34:517-521

Epstein LG, Sharer LR, Oleske JM, et al. Neurologic manifestations of human immunodeficiency virus infection in children. *Pediatrics*. 1986;78:678-687

Majer LS. HIV-infected students in school: who really does "need to know"? *J Sch Health*. 1992;62:243-245

Sklaire MW. Role of the pediatrician in school health. *Pediatr Rev*. 1990;12:69-70. Commentary

Ultmann MH, Belman AL, Ruff HA, et al. Developmental abnormalities in infants and children with acquired immune deficiency syndrome (AIDS) and AIDS-related complex. *Dev Med Child Neurol*. 1985;27: 563-571

Zlotnik JL. AIDS: helping families cope. Recommendations for meeting the psychosocial needs for persons with AIDS and their families. *Rep Nat Inst Ment Health*. 1987

CHAPTER 21

ABUSE*

Nature and Significance of the Problem

While the physical and sexual abuse of children has been occurring for centuries,[1] it is only within the past three decades that significant public and professional concern has been paid to the problem, marked by many with the coining of the phrase "battered child syndrome" in 1962 by Kempe.[2] This landmark paper led to the rapid growth and development of the multidisciplinary field of child abuse and neglect, which now includes more than the recognition and care of battered children. Included in modern definitions of abuse are:

1. Physical abuse: The nonaccidental injuring of a child or adolescent by a caretaker or (usually) older individual.
2. Sexual abuse: The engaging of a child in sexual activities the child does not understand, to which the child cannot give informed consent, which are developmentally inappropriate and/or which violate the laws or taboos of society.

Other forms of child maltreatment include emotional abuse and neglect,[3] physical neglect,[4] medical care neglect,[5] and Munchausen syndrome by proxy.[6] The reader is referred to cited reviews for information on these issues.

Physical and sexual abuse of children can occur in intrafamilial and extrafamilial settings. The widespread nature of the problem, and its significant sequelae should make the recognition, treatment, and above all, prevention, of all forms of abuse and neglect of children a national priority.

Extent of the Problem

By estimates, there were 302 hospitalized cases of battered children in 1962.[1] Between 1965 and 1968 states passed legis-

---

* This chapter is reprinted with permission. From Krugman RD. Abuse. In: Wallace HM, Patrick K, Parcel GS, Igoe JB. *Principles and Practices of Student Health*. Oakland, CA: Third Party Publishing Company; 1992;1:chap 10

lation requiring that professionals report suspected abuse and in 1974 with the passage of PL 93-247 and subsequent amendments, federal funds were tied to expanded definitions that included mental injury, neglect, and sexual abuse. By 1979, a reported 669,000 cases of abuse and neglect were received by county and state child protective services agencies.[7] By 1986 (the last year official data were collected) that figure had tripled to 2.1 million reports.[8] There have been substantial problems in the collection of accurate, reliable data on the incidence of abuse. Definitions vary, as do the criteria used in different states to substantiate reports. Inexplicably the federal government has historically contracted this task of measuring and monitoring incidence to nongovernmental entities. The most recent studies, however, suggest that approximately 1.6% to 2.5% of children are abused and neglected annually in the US[9]—a figure dramatically higher than most other health problems affecting school-age children. Approximately 40% of the over 2.1 million reports are substantiated on a national basis although wide variation exists from state to state. Approximately 25% of cases are physical abuse, 20% sexual abuse, and 55% are neglect.[9]

Factors Known to Promote the Problem

The physical and sexual abuse of children should be viewed in an ecological perspective.[10] There are individual,[11] social,[12] and cultural[13] factors that contribute to the problem. Although nearly all abusers of children were inadequately parented in their childhood and were often abused as they abuse children,[11] this does not mean that all abused children will grow up to be abusive adults. Most do not repeat the cycle, although their risk is higher than nonabused children.[14] Reduced socioeconomic status, family violence, unemployment, substance abuse, and adolescent parenting have been associated with physical abuse; substance abuse, family violence, concomitant physical abuse, pornography, and cult or satanic behavior have been associated with sexual abuse, but none of these are particularly helpful associations to the practitioner dealing with an individual case.

Recognition

The recognition of abuse as a problem is dependent on the willingness of the practitioner to entertain the possibility that the condition exists.[15] There is much societal and professional denial of the existence of child abuse, especially sexual abuse, which has been called a "hidden pediatric problem."[16]

Physical abuse may be recognized when one obtains a discrepant history—that is, the history of what the caretaker said happened to the child does not fit with medical findings.[17] The discrepancy may not be obvious to the practitioner without other information generally available only to those making a site visit, such as a child protective services (CPS) worker, public health nurse, or law enforcement officer. For example, we may believe the history that a child's bruises resulted from a fall down a flight of stairs, but if we know there is no flight of stairs at the house, we might suspect abuse. Kempe often said that no child ever died of a social work evaluation; many have died because we didn't get one. Other features found in the multidisciplinary evaluation of physical abuse are listed in Table 48.[18] There are also visual clues to the diagnosis, bruises and burns being most common. Certain bruises are more suspicious—such as those resembling belts, cords, pinch marks, slap marks, cigarette burns, or scald-immersion burns.

In addition, spiral fractures of the long bones in nonambulatory children, and intracranial hemorrhage, duodenal intramural hematomas, or pancreatic injury in any child in the absence of a history of major trauma is suspicious for abuse.[17]

Sexual abuse has a variety of presentations, most of which are nonspecific (Table 49).[19] The most specific symptom of all these relatively nonspecific findings is sexual acting-out behavior. The diagnosis of sexual abuse is generally made on the history. Physical findings are usually not helpful except in the acute sexual assault, although certain hymenal changes in pre-pubertal children have been associated with a history of sexual abuse.[20-22] Certain sexually transmitted diseases can be presenting signs of sexual abuse. Gonorrhea and syphilis in prepubertal children are diagnostic of sexual abuse; chlamydia, trichomonas, herpes 2, and condyloma acuminata are suspicious for sexual abuse.[23]

When any behavior, discrepant history, or physical finding makes the practitioner suspicious of any form of abuse, it must be reported to the agency mandated to accept reports. Many worry about "being wrong" in the report. As long as it is done in good faith, there is immunity from successful suit. Failure to

Table 48. — Features Differentiating Accidental and Nonaccidental Trauma

1. Discrepant history
2. Delay in seeking care
3. Crisis in abuser's life
4. Triggering behavior by child
5. Prior history of abuse in childhood of abuser
6. Social isolation
7. Unrealistic expectations for the child
8. Pattern of increased severity of injury over time
9. Use of multiple hospitals or providers

report is a misdemeanor and may also lead to a malpractice action. In a time when so many children are cared for by caretakers other than their parents, it is critical that practitioners remember that the person who brings the child for care may not be the abuser. Thus, whenever it is suspected, an approach could be: "There are a number of potential causes for this finding, including abuse. Is that a possibility?" A report can follow, with the practitioner being available for follow-up.

Sequelae of Abuse

There are both survivors and casualties—physically and emotionally—of child abuse. As previously noted, not all abused children repeat the cycle as adults, but certainly the risks are significantly higher for this group compared to the general population.[14] It is less the physical injury (except for the sequelae of brain injury) or the sexual acts that are harmful to children as it is the emotional context of the injury or sexual relationship being perpetrated by a family member or someone in a position of trust.

The degree of "survivability" is dependent on a number of factors. In general, the longer the abuse persists, the younger the child at the age of onset, the closer the relationship of the abuser to the child, and the more severe (physical) or intrusive (sexual) the abuse, the worse the prognosis. The sequelae of physical abuse have been suggested by retrospective analyses of high-risk or pathologic populations. They include in children and adoles-

Table 49. — Presentations of Sexual Abuse

Early warnings

General statements
  Sexualized play

Direct statements

Behavioral changes
  Sleep disturbances (eg, nightmare, night terrors)
  Appetite disturbance (eg, anorexia, bulimia)
  Neurotic or conduct disorders
  Phobias; avoidance behavior
  Withdrawal, depression
  Guilt
  Temper tantrums, aggressive behavior
  Excessive masturbation
  Runaway behavior
  Suicidal behavior
  Hysterical or conversion reactions

Medical conditions
  Genital or urethral trauma
  Genital infection
  Sexually transmitted diseases
  Recurrent urinary tract infections
  Abdominal pain
  Enuresis
  Encopresis

Pregnancy

School problems

Promiscuity or prostitution

Substance abuse

Perpetration to others

cents: aggressive to violent behavior, juvenile delinquency, suicide, homicide, and runaway behaviors, in addition to a risk of physical abuse to other children.[24] The sequelae of sexual abuse include all those listed below "Behavioral Changes" in Table 49; and in older adolescents and adults: depression, difficulty with relationships, drug or alcohol addiction, adolescent pregnancy, multiple divorces, sexual dysfunction, and a higher risk of abusing or neglecting (eg, a baby with nonorganic failure to thrive) one's own children have been described.

While child abusers are increasingly recognized by primary care providers for children, those caring for adolescents and young adults may not consider the late sequelae in their differential diagnosis. Such behaviors should trigger a referral to a competent mental health provider.

Types of Effective Approaches

Treatment

Any child who is a victim of abuse should be evaluated for the need for treatment. Combinations of individual and group, professional and self-help groups may be useful. Whether the child is abused within or outside the family, siblings and parents may also benefit from therapy.[25] In extrafamilial abuse the young child may recover more quickly than the parents, especially if the parents have a history of abuse in their childhood that has never been addressed. In intrafamilial cases, court-ordered treatment may be more effective than voluntary approaches.[26] The coexistence of substance abuse, sociopathy, or psychosis makes outcomes less likely to be positive.

Regrettably, the child protective services system is episodic and case-oriented, as is the mental health system. There are, therefore, no prospective longitudinal outcome data to guide in treatment. It is the health system that has the tradition of continuity of care, and therefore practitioners are urged to maintain follow-up and surveillance on their patients who have been abused, since adolescents who were abused in childhood have a much higher incidence of health-risk behaviors than nonabused peers.[24] There may be multiple times during the life cycle in which waves of symptoms may well up in prior abuse victims; eg, adolescence with the onset of sexual activity, marriage, childbearing, divorce, or even the watching of a television show on abuse.

Prevention

The prevention of physical abuse is possible. Studies have shown clearly that it is possible to predict with reasonable accuracy who is at high risk for physical abuse and, by providing either a lay[27] or public health nurse[28] home visitor, prevent the physical abuse of children. Other modalities such as parenting classes, hotlines, and crisis nurseries have had some success as well.[29]

The prevention of sexual abuse is more difficult. Most strategies depend on the development of resistance by the child and "telling someone." Few programs of this nature for children have been evaluated, and none are fully effective (they seem to be better at identifying existing cases than preventing new ones).[30] More attention needs to be paid to the adult components of abusive behavior and what leads to the motivation to abuse children sexually.[31]

Commentary

The last three decades have seen dramatic growth in the public and professional awareness of abuse and neglect. The past decade, however, has been marked by a steady erosion of our ability to protect abused children. Child welfare services have become less supportive of families and more investigative in nature as the number of reported cases has risen to over two million nationally. The mental health system has been flooded with the chronically deinstitutionalized mentally ill and has been unable to absorb many of the hundreds of thousands of abused children and families who need services. Further, what used to be supportive public health nursing agencies to young mothers and infants have evolved into home health care agencies that are caring primarily for children with diseased organs and, preferably, insurance. We may be the only civilized nation in the world that has no idea where all its children between 2 days and 6 years of age are.

School and college health practitioners have four main roles when it comes to abuse and neglect. Recognition and reporting of cases is the first and has been discussed. Schools can be sites of prevention activities as well, often in elementary and secondary schools, with the cooperation of parent teacher organizations. The third role is less appreciated, but for many abused children, schools are their only safe place. Many adult survivors have remarked that teachers were their best role models. Schools should be sure that children who are abuse victims get the best, most nurturing teachers. Too often there is a tendency to put these children into the classes of harsh disciplinarians so they can "shape up" these children. There is no evidence that this is helpful.

Finally, teachers in schools and colleges need to avoid their contribution to the problem. A small percentage of these (and all) professionals abuse their students—physically, sexually, or emotionally.[32] It is up to each profession to monitor the behavior of its own professionals.

In an age when there are more cases than can be handled by the overburdened child protective services system, it is critical for the health system—and especially the school and college health systems, which provide continuity of care—to get involved with these children and adolescents. Physical and sexual abuse are major etiologic agents in the new morbidity facing our youth. It is incumbent on all professionals to get involved on behalf of children.

References

1. Radbill SX. Children in a world of violence: a history of child abuse. In: Helfer RE, Kempe RS, eds. *The Battered Child*. 4th ed. Chicago, IL: University of Chicago Press; 1987:3-22

2. Kempe CH, Silverman FN, Steele BF, Droegemueller W, Silver HK. The battered-child syndrome. *JAMA*. 1962;181:17-24

3. Garbarino J, Guttman E, Seeley JW. *The Psychologically Battered Child*. San Francisco, CA: Jossey-Bass; 1986

4. Helfer RE. The litany of the smoldering neglect of children. In: Helfer RE, Kempe RS, eds. *The Battered Child*. 4th ed. Chicago, IL: University of Chicago Press; 1987:301-311

5. Bross DC. Medical care neglect. *Child Abuse Negl*. 1982;6:375-381

6. Rosenberg DA. Web of deceit: a literature review of Munchausen syndrome by proxy. *Child Abuse Negl*. 1987;11:547-563

7. American Humane Association. *Highlights of Official Child Neglect and Abuse Reporting*. Denver, CO: American Humane Association; 1979

8. American Humane Association. *Highlights of Official Child Neglect and Abuse Reporting*. Denver, CO: American Humane Association; 1986

9. US Department of Health and Human Services. *Study Findings: Study of National Incidence and Prevalence of Child Abuse and Neglect: 1988*. Washington, DC: US Government Printing Office; 1988

10. Garbarino J. A preliminary study of some ecological correlates of child abuse: the impact of socioeconomic stress on mothers. *Child Dev*. 1976;47:178-185

11. Steele B. Psychodynamic factors in child abuse. In: Helfer RE, Kempe RS, eds. *The Battered Child*. 4th ed. Chicago, IL: University of Chicago Press; 1987:81-114

12. Straus MA, Kantor GK. Stress and child abuse. In: Helfer RE, Kempe RS, eds. *The Battered Child*. 4th ed. Chicago, IL: University of Chicago Press; 1987:42-59

13. Korbin JE. Child abuse and neglect: the cultural context. In: Helfer RE, Kempe RS, eds. *The Battered Child*. 4th ed. Chicago, IL: University of Chicago Press; 1987:23-41

14. Widom CS. The cycle of violence. *Science*. 1989;244:160-166

15. Sgroi SM, Porter FS, Blick LC. Validation of child sexual abuse. In: Sgroi SM, ed. *Handbook of Clinical Intervention in Child Sexual Abuse*. Lexington, MA: D. C. Heath and Company; 1982:39-79

16. Kempe CH. Sexual abuse: another hidden pediatric problem. The 1977 C. Anderson Aldrich Lecture. *Pediatrics*. 1978;62:382-389

17. Schmitt BD, American Academy of Pediatrics. The Visual Diagnosis of Non-accidental Trauma and Failure to Thrive [slide series]. Denver, CO: University of Colorado Medical Center; 1979

18. Krugman R. The assessment process of a child protection team. In: Helfer RE, Kempe RS, eds. *The Battered Child*. 4th ed. Chicago, IL: University of Chicago Press; 1987:127-136

19. Krugman RD. Recognition of sexual abuse in children. *Pediatr Rev*. 1986;8:25-30

20. Cantwell HB. Vaginal inspection as it relates to child sexual abuse in girls under thirteen. *Child Abuse Negl*. 1983;7:171-176

21. White ST, Ingram DL, Lyna PR. Vaginal introital diameter in the evaluation of sexual abuse. *Child Abuse Negl*. 1989;13:217-224

22. Paradise JE. Predictive accuracy and the diagnosis of sexual abuse: a big issue about a little tissue. *Child Abuse Negl*. 1989;13:169-176

23. American Academy of Pediatrics, Committee on Child Abuse and Neglect. Guidelines for the evaluation of sexual abuse of children. *Pediatrics*. 1991;87:254-260

24. Riggs S, Alario AJ, McHorney C. Health risk behaviors and attempted suicide in adolescents who report prior maltreatment. *J Pediatr*. 1990;116:815-821

25. Jones DPH, Alexander H. Treating the abusive family within the family care system. In: Helfer RE, Kempe RS, eds. *The Battered Child*. 4th ed. Chicago, IL: University of Chicago Press; 1987:339-359

26. Wolfe DA, Aragona J, Kaufman K, Sandler J. The importance of adjudication in the treatment of child-abusers: some preliminary findings. *Child Abuse Negl.* 1980;4:127-135

27. Gray JD, Cutler CA, Dean JG, Kempe CH. Prediction and prevention of child-abuse and neglect. *J Soc Issues.* 1979;35:127-139

28. Olds DL, Henderson CR Jr, Chamberlin R, Tatelbaum R. Preventing child abuse and neglect: a randomized trial of nurse home visitation. *Pediatrics.* 1986;78:65-78

29. Cohn AH. Our national priorities for prevention. In: Helfer RE, Kempe RS, eds. *The Battered Child.* 4th ed. Chicago, IL: University of Chicago Press; 1987:444-455

30. Fryer GE Jr, Kraizer SK, Miyoshi T. Measuring actual reduction of risk to child abuse: a new approach. *Child Abuse Negl.* 1987;11:173-179

31. Finkelhor D, Williams LM, Burns N. *Nursery Crimes; Sexual Abuse in Day Care.* Newbury Park, CA: Sage Publications; 1988

32. Krugman RD, Krugman MK. Emotional abuse in the classroom: the pediatrician's role in diagnosis and treatment. *Am J Dis Child.* 1984;138:284-286

CHAPTER 22

USE AND ABUSE OF DRUGS

Scope of the Problem

During the last two decades, society has become increasingly concerned about the effects of alcohol and drug abuse on young people. Pediatricians, educators, mental health professionals, and chemical dependency experts, as well as law enforcement officials and the courts, all have been involved in the development of programs to prevent and manage substance abuse in teens. This chapter explores the phenomenon of drug, tobacco, and alcohol use in schools, looking particularly at ways in which medical and education personnel can work together to address the problem.

While evidence suggests that substance abuse has declined since the late 1970s and early 1980s, its effects are still to be felt in our schools. A survey of 1,237 high school student leaders in 1991 indicated that alcohol is a major problem in their schools. Nearly half identified it as the number one problem, and nearly three quarters ranked it in the top three (*USA Today*, June 25, 1991). The Monitoring the Future Survey (1991) questioned 15,500 seniors from 136 public and private school graduating classes and found that nearly one fifth of high school seniors were daily smokers and 78% had used alcohol in the previous year. Furthermore, a third reported having had heavy intake of alcohol (defined as consuming at least five drinks at one time) on at least one occasion within the past month. Use on at least one occasion of the most common illegal drug, marijuana, was reported by some 27% of graduating seniors.[1] It must be noted that this classic, ongoing study conducted on behalf of the National Institute on Drug Abuse (NIDA) by the University of Michigan tends to underestimate drug use in teenagers, as it specifically does not survey many of those who are at greatest risk, namely school dropouts. Perhaps more worrisome is the fact that students from as early as the 8th grade not only report peer pressure to drink, but studies suggest that as many as 42% of them have already done so. Data from the survey in 1991 indicated that 25% of 8th graders and 43% of 10th graders had used alcohol within the previous month. Furthermore, 13% of 8th graders and 23% of 10th graders admitted to having had an episode of heavy drinking, as defined previously.

From the health standpoint, drug and alcohol abuse affects virtually the entire body, including the cardiovascular, respiratory, immune, and central nervous systems. While some of these effects may not appear until after many years of use, even episodic and occasional use of substances such as inhalants and cocaine may result in fatality or severe long-term health effects. In addition, drugs and alcohol are implicated in fully 50% of the most common causes of death among adolescents, namely accidents, suicides, and homicides.

A major aspect of the drug and alcohol abuse problem is the effect they have on our children and their schools. Use of drugs and alcohol affects performance in dramatic and documented ways. Significant use may be associated with a falloff in attendance, resulting in truancy and trouble-filled idle time. Cognitive ability may be affected on a temporary, long-term, or permanent basis. Buying and selling of drugs, coupled with the common practice of bringing weapons to school and school functions (see chapter 30), creates a climate of potential violence. Athletes involved in illegal drug use risk damaging their bodies in critical ways . Furthermore, when school is a place where drugs can be obtained in a de facto marketplace, the safety of students and faculty, as well as the issue of liability, become major concerns.

The US Department of Health and Human Services in 1991 published the monograph entitled, "Healthy People 2000: National Health Promotion and Disease Prevention Objectives." This publication set the following goals: (1) the decrease in preventable death and disability; (2) an increase in the quality of life for all Americans; and (3) a decrease in the disparity in health status among various populations. It identified drug and alcohol abuse in schools as a major problem and offered the following description of what a school health program should provide:

> A quality school health program should provide factual information about the harmful effects of drugs, support and strengthen students' resistance to using drugs, carry out collaborative drug-abuse prevention efforts with parents and other community members, and be supported by strong school policies as well as services for confidential identification, assessment, referral to treatment and support groups (often provided through a student assistance program) for drug users.[2]

Common Drugs of Abuse and Their Effects on School Performance

While a detailed discussion of all the drugs used by adolescents is beyond the scope of this chapter, a brief review of some of the common substances and their effects—especially as they relate to school—is in order. Schuckit has written an excellent reference, with detailed discussion of drugs and their effects.[3]

Tobacco

Tobacco is one of the so-called gateway drugs—those that are legal and frequently associated with progression to illicit drugs. While the sale of tobacco to minors is illegal in most states, its ready availability makes enforcement of such laws difficult. Its effects on health are well-known, including lung and cardiovascular disease. A third of all deaths from lung cancer are linked to smoking, and smokers are especially prone to heart attacks and chronic lung conditions. Forms of smokeless tobacco (snuff and chewing tobacco) are increasingly popular among young people and have been associated with forms of mouth cancer. Passive smoking (inhaling the exhaled smoke of other smokers, especially indoors) also has been identified as a major health threat.

Acutely, nicotine acts as a stimulant. It may cause increased heart rate and respirations. Chronic smoking is associated with persistent cough, postnasal drip, bad breath, and sore throat. In addition, the nicotine in tobacco is an addicting drug, and dependent students may find it very difficult to go through the school day without a cigarette.

Alcohol

Alcohol use is epidemic among children and adolescents. As a legal substance, its availability is wide, and few children have difficulty obtaining it on demand, despite the fact that it is illegal to sell alcohol to minors in the United States. It has profound effects on behavior. In even moderate doses it may affect judgment, speech, balance, memory, learning ability, and concentration. In higher doses it may cause unconsciousness and death. Withdrawal in the long-term alcoholic results in the constellation of symptoms, frequently called "delirium tremens," which can include convulsions, delirium, hallucinations, and anxiety. Long-term use is associated particularly with gastrointestinal and central nervous system disease.

The intoxicated student may appear stuporous, agitated, lethargic, belligerent, and inattentive. Its effects on the ability to think and function in class are obvious.

Marijuana

Marijuana is by far the most commonly used illegal drug and its users are increasingly young. As many as one out of every six seventh graders reports marijuana use on at least one occasion. Its physiologic effects include increased heart rate, bloodshot eyes, and dry mouth. Because of the manner in which it is smoked (by inhaling it deeply and allowing it to stay in the lungs), it may be more harmful to lung tissue than traditional cigarette smoke. The active ingredient in marijuana, cannabis, has severe effects on learning, memory, and concentration. The so-called "amotivational syndrome" is a frequently reported problem in which the student simply cannot focus on, absorb, and process information—and feels no need or pressure to do so.

The acutely affected student may appear "spaced out" and have bloodshot eyes. Typically, heavy marijuana users pay little attention to personal hygiene, and their lethargy can be dramatic.

Inhalants

Volatile chemicals are inhaled ("sniffed" or "huffed") frequently, especially by young urban adolescents. While users report a pleasurable sensation from inhaling the concentrated vapors of these substances, they also may report unpleasant feelings such as nausea, coughing, and sneezing. These are particularly toxic substances, which when inhaled in a concentrated form (as in a plastic bag) may result in disorientation, violent behavior, unconsciousness, and death. Readily available as spray paint propellants, solvents, correction fluid, and glues, they are hard to curtail. Short-term use of inhalants clearly impairs learning ability. Long-term use may be associated with permanent damage to brain, liver, heart, and lungs.

The student acutely under the influence of an inhalant may be lethargic and show poor motor control and light-headedness.

Hallucinogens

Psychedelic drugs, so popular in the 1960s, are unfortunately staging a comeback. Lysergic acid diethylamide (LSD) is again becoming available on college campuses, as is phencyclidine

(PCP). These drugs have profound effects on the central nervous system and may result in convulsions, coma, and death, at apparently small doses. Many users report unpleasant "flashbacks."

Common effects of PCP and LSD include pupillary dilation, delirium, mood disorders, loss of muscular coordination, slurring of speech, and a vague sense of isolation and loss of perspective.

Cocaine

Cocaine is an extremely potent stimulant that produces an overpowering euphoria. Users report that it is so intense that one can be swept into compulsive use after one or two episodes. It is extremely addicting in both its standard form (which can be injected or inhaled through the nose) and its free-base derivative "crack" (commonly smoked or injected). Cocaine has been associated occasionally with sudden cardiac death, sometimes in first-time users.

Acutely, cocaine causes agitation with increased heart rate and respirations. The euphoric phase lasts briefly and is associated with hyperactivity and restlessness. This is followed by a period of lethargy and somnolence, and a craving to use again.

Stimulants

Medications such as amphetamines and their congeners ("uppers," "speed") cause effects similar to cocaine's, though they are less intense. Most users report euphoria and sensations of enhanced physical strength and competence. For this reason they appeal to many athletes, and their ability to suppress appetite may be especially appealing to gymnasts and wrestlers. Furthermore, adolescent females frequently abuse both prescription and over-the-counter stimulants for purposes of weight loss. Their usage by girls with anorexia nervosa is well documented.

These drugs have toxic effects on the cardiovascular and central nervous system, and the acutely intoxicated student may be agitated, anxious, and restless.

Sedatives and Tranquilizers

Barbiturates ("barbs"), Quaaludes ("ludes"), and other "downers" are among the most commonly abused prescription drugs.

They tend to be readily available on the street, and long-term use may create physical and psychological dependence. Severe overdosage may be lethal.

Acutely, tranquilizers create an overpowering sense of drowsiness and confusion, along with motor incoordination.

Narcotics

Use of narcotics such as opium and heroin declined in the early 1970s, and these "end-stage" drugs are less commonly used in schools today. Nonetheless, they remain extremely potent sedatives and pain relievers, and those who begin with alcohol and marijuana may progress to harder drugs and to heroin. Used intravenously, the drugs are very potent, creating an intense "rush" and a physical feeling that has been described as resembling orgasm. More recently, intensely potent uncut forms of heroin that can be inhaled through the nose have become available. Margin of safety is very narrow, and acute overdosage may be associated with coma and death.

Acute usage of narcotics is marked by constricted pupils and sometimes profound degrees of lethargy. Telltale signs such as needle tracks also may be present.

Anabolic Steroids

Usage of these compounds—derivatives of the male sex hormone testosterone—is epidemic among students today. These drugs are perceived as having the effect of increasing strength and endurance, especially when used in a training program by bodybuilders, wrestlers, and football players. They also may improve muscle definition and physical attractiveness. Unfortunately, they also have severe effects on the body as a whole, causing testicular atrophy and impotence in males and increased body hair and breast atrophy in females. Long-term use is associated with liver and heart damage.

The use of anabolic steroids (as distinct from the cortisol derivatives, which have many legitimate medical uses) is associated with particularly quick weight and muscle gain if used with a weight training program. Acne is frequently exacerbated, and purple and red spots may sometimes appear on the body. Frequently there are behavior changes, most notably increased aggressiveness.

The Stages of Drug Use in Children and Adolescents

Substance abuse develops in fairly predictable fashion in most young people. The landmark studies of Kandel, Logan, and Yamaguchi[4-6] identified alcohol and tobacco as "gateway" drugs that lead to marijuana use in many young people. This, in turn, may make the progression to other illicit drugs more likely.

Furthermore, there is a definable progression in the degree to which most young persons use drugs and alcohol. Macdonald has divided this into four stages[7]:

Stage I - Learning the Mood Swing: Early use begins at home and may mimic parental role modeling. Studies show that even at the time of first use, most children realize that drugs and alcohol are potentially harmful to their health, yet embark on usage nonetheless. During the earliest phases of drug use, society and its media messages are an important factor, as is usage by friends and peers. Initial "pleasurable experimentation" may lead to so-called "recreational use," in which social events are planned around drinking. It is during this initial phase that adolescents learn how good it feels and how easy it may be to get "high."

Stage II - Seeking the Mood Swing: Having experienced the pleasures of being high, progressive users no longer are content to "see what happens." They may actively seek drugs and begin to use on a more frequent basis. This is the stage when young people may begin to abandon old friends who do not use in favor of the peer group that does. As the teenager attempts to maintain school grades and keep parents in the dark, home life becomes chaotic as the young person becomes more isolated and communication deteriorates. Interest in school activities declines, and lack of motivation may become dramatic.

Stage III - Preoccupation With the Mood Swing: At this point, life is planned around drug and alcohol use. Psychological as well as physical dependency may develop. The behavior changes seen in stage II become more pronounced, and attitude as well as physical appearance may provide more obvious clues to drug usage. Truancy is common, school grades almost invariably drop, and there may be brushes with the law as the expense of maintaining a habit increases. Physical effects may begin to be noticed as the adolescent spends more time under the influence of drugs, and the emotional changes become dramatic. The adolescent may begin to recognize this deterioration but frequently is unwilling or unable to give up using.

Stage IV - Doing Drugs to Feel Okay: At this stage, dangerous physical and psychological dependence has developed, and the teenager may require drugs and alcohol simply to avoid withdrawal symptoms and to function. The excitement and joy of the mood swing generally are gone, and finding one's next dose becomes a full-time job. All sense of responsibility to family, friends, school, and society is gone. Most adolescents in this stage are drifting and are vulnerable to a major run-in with the law or an intoxication requiring hospital emergency room care. Untreated, these youngsters often will end up permanently disabled or dead.

Sadly, this progression may occur with alarming rapidity depending on the youngster and the social situation. It is not uncommon to see an adolescent's entire life at home and in school unravel in a 6-month period. And while not every adolescent will proceed inexorably through these stages, early detection and diagnosis is crucial to interrupt the process.

Role of the Professional in Recognizing Alcohol and Drug Abuse

Educators and physicians have a special responsibility in detecting and discouraging drug and alcohol abuse in young people. School boards of education and administration set policy that classroom personnel carry out. Athletic coaches and extracurricular activity supervisors work with their students and come to know them perhaps better than anyone else. The very special relationship that develops between a bandleader and a clarinetist or between a swimmer and a coach may be among the most honest in a teenager's world. School counselors become involved with every student at one time or another and have access to personal information that may be of great value. School nurses and health aides are responsible for the administration of school health policies and may be the first to recognize patterns of somatic complaints as they develop. Pediatricians are sources of information and advice and are usually the ones contacted when parents are concerned about their youngster's health or behavior. All involved must give careful attention to issues raised by any one of the adults involved in a student's life. While recognizing educational problems may be the province of professionals in the schools and detecting health problems that of medical professionals, the diagnosis and management of substance abuse must be everyone's concern.

There are a number of factors that predispose a young person to alcohol and drug abuse. Family history is a strong predictive factor, and careful attention must be paid to the fact that one of every eight children grows up with an alcoholic parent. The family models behavior for young children, and parental use of drugs and alcohol makes such use seem more normative to impressionable young people. Interestingly, recent studies support the concept that rigid opposition to alcohol usage actually may predispose a child to later use, perhaps because of the curiosity factor. Family disruption and divorce may create an environment in which drug and alcohol use go undetected. The environment in which the family lives is also important. Drug use is more prevalent in communities where obtaining drugs may be easier.

The role of the media has received significant attention in recent years, as the public comes to recognize how important marketing forces are in selling alcohol and tobacco to youth. Beer companies adopting animal mascots and cigarette companies using cartoons to sell their products are but two noteworthy examples. The success of these techniques is unfortunate, as two such companies have seen their market share among child users increase dramatically.

Patterns of behavior in the individual should be cause for concern. Unfortunately, many of the behaviors so typical of drug- and alcohol-using adolescents are to some degree typical of the age group as a whole. Many adolescents use drugs and alcohol to "self-medicate" depression, anxiety, or sleep problems. Yet, significant changes in behavior must not go undetected, as these may be the first signs that an adolescent is experimenting with drugs or alcohol. Mood swings, depression, angry outbursts, and increased isolation may be part of the highs and lows of drug use. Changes in appearance or dress may signify a teenager's adoption of a new life-style and a desire to fit in with drug-using peers. The argument may be made that one cannot "judge a book by its cover," but the teenager who suddenly adopts a new and more rebellious dress code, who loses pride in personal hygiene and hair care, or who self-tattoos or carves on his or her body is communicating an image to peers and adults that deserves notice.

A young person involved in drugs may come to the attention of the school nurse or physician for somatic complaints. Common concerns include cough, lethargy, decreased appetite and/or weight loss, abdominal pain, sleeping difficulties, headache, depression, irritability, dizziness, and menstrual problems. The alert health care provider, while looking for organic causes for such symptoms, will consider the possibility that drug or alcohol usage may be playing a role.

Changes in school attendance patterns, such as tardiness or truancy, may be associated with substance abuse, as the adolescent skips class to use drugs or is late because of a "hangover." Decline in school performance may be a further sign of increasing drug and alcohol involvement. Behavioral changes within the confines of the school, such as fighting, belligerence, and other inappropriate behavior, should alert school officials to a possible problem.

Causes of Adolescent Substance Abuse

An understanding of the theories of why teenagers become involved in drugs and alcohol may lead to the formation of a reasonable approach toward its prevention and treatment. Many theories have been proposed, and they fall into five categories.

1. *Problem behavior theory* suggests that drug and alcohol use are just part of a general pattern of problem behavior. Where relatively low value is placed on adherence to societal expectations, more deviant behavior is accepted. Thus, poor school performance, lack of motivation for future economic independence, failure to fit into social groups, and refusal to live up to community values are all behavior patterns that may come to include alcohol and drug use. Classic research by Jessor and Jessor[8] suggests further that when peers and parents are ambivalent about drug use, such use flourishes.

2. *Social learning theory* proposes that adolescent behavior is determined by a process in which the adolescent learns

what works and what does not. That is to say, behaviors that bring positive feedback are pursued. Thus, the risk of problem behavior is minimized if positive behavior patterns are reinforced, and opportunities to interact positively are provided. Relationships with society that are rewarding (success in school, activities, peers, members of the opposite sex, for example) might minimize the likelihood of drug use.

3. *Stage theory* as espoused by Kandel and Logan[4] states simply that readily available gateway drugs (tobacco and alcohol) are used almost universally, at least on an experimental basis. Regular use of alcohol may follow and lead to trying illegal drugs (marijuana). Further involvement almost invariably implies more frequent use and use of more potent illicit substances.

4. *Biopsychosocial theory* is based on teenagers turning to drugs to self-medicate and deal with stress. It emphasizes the fact that skills used to cope with daily stress may be different from those used to resist temptations, which may explain why some youth with poor social skills may be more easily seduced into drug use.

5. *Social stress theory* emphasizes the fact that drug use is usually the outcome of poor relationships with social systems. Thus, this model would emphasize the importance of good attachments (to family and society), the development of coping skills, good role models in the community, and the promise of community support in the form of jobs and social services.

Programs for Prevention of Adolescent Alcohol and Drug Abuse

Given the fact that young people spend the majority of their waking hours in school, the school is the logical promoter of drug abuse education programs. Properly designed and executed school-based programs can make major inroads into the problem.[9]

To be effective, school-based programs must avoid a number of pitfalls. Many begin too late, long after use has started. Programs that are brought into schools for a single presentation usually provide information but have little lasting impact. Long-term prevention activities may become routine and boring, and may not address the issues that are specific for a certain school in a certain community. Finally, those who teach the program may lack credibility, whether they are outsiders or members of the school community.

Historically, school-based drug and alcohol abuse prevention programs have fallen into five basic categories:

1. Factual, based on dispensing factual knowledge about drugs and alcohol, with the assumption that if young people know the harm that can come to them from substance abuse, they will not embark upon it. Unfortunately, there is fairly universal agreement that such programs do not decrease drug use, for while knowledge is necessary for prevention, it is not sufficient.

2. Affective, based on the theory that if a child is "immunized" against drugs and alcohol (by improving self-esteem and decision-making abilities, and providing values clarification), the child will be less likely to use these substances. Programs that focus on attitude change also have been, for the most part, ineffective. Even combining attitude and educational programs appears to be of little use.

3. Peer-based/skill training, which is perhaps the most effective of all program types. This training helps promote resistance, communication, and decision-making skills and are frequently led and developed by peers.

4. Alternative highs, predicated on the hope that if teenagers are involved in programs that provide positive recognition (activities, sports, etc) and in nondrug leisure activities, they will not feel the need to partake of mood-altering drugs. These programs can be very effective when such activities are made available to the entire school population.

5. Parental and community based, founded on the assumption that a comprehensive network of drug-free parent-supported and community-run programs can minimize the interest in drug experimentation. Combined with peer and school programs, community involvement can effect significant changes.

Drug Prevention, the Pediatrician, and the School

As the health care provider for the student, the pediatrician has a responsibility to know what activities schools are involved with in the substance abuse prevention area. While clearly no physician can know the details of every school his patients might attend, the pediatrician must have a concept of what is being done, in order to offer support, counsel, and advice when indicated.

There are countless approaches to drug education and prevention, and it is clearly beyond the scope of this chapter to review these in detail. The reader is referred to one of the listed references for further information. Yet there are a number of pressing principles with which the pediatric consultant must be familiar. Goodstadt referred to them as the eight "dichotomies of drug education."[10]

1. Legal vs illegal drugs: that is, which should be the focus? Both must be addressed, as gateway substances may lead to the use of illicit drugs, and many adolescents are poly-drug abusers. Furthermore, many substances may be legal in some situations yet illegal in others. The principles of drug abuse apply to both licit and illicit substances.

2. Abstinence vs responsible use: that is, which policy should be promoted? Clearly there can be no "responsible" use of an illegal drug. Young people may lack the knowledge, judgment, and experience to measure "responsible use." Therefore, schools must espouse a policy of "NO DRUGS OR ALCOHOL" at school and any school-sponsored functions. Furthermore, all involved should promote the concept of "drug nonuse," that is, the conscious and deliberate decision not to use drugs.

3. Supply reduction vs demand reduction: that is, which part of the cycle should be addressed? Clearly neither method alone is effective, and all comprehensive programs must deal with both supply reduction and demand reduction.

4. Youth vs adults: that is, which age group should be targeted for prevention activities? Both groups are equally important. The earlier substance abuse is addressed, the better the results; theoretically, some of the most effective prevention activities would be directed initially at chil-

dren in the early grades. Nonetheless, adults serve as role models for children, and the problem of alcoholism and drug abuse in that group must be addressed as well.

5. Peers vs parents: that is, who is the stronger influence on a teenager? Certainly many students begin drinking to fit into the peer group they wish to join. Nonetheless, the importance of parental behavior as a societal norm cannot be ignored. Programs must direct students toward positive nonusing peer groups and provide support for parents with drug and alcohol problems.

6. Individual vs environment: that is, where does one direct energies—to the individual or to the group as a whole? Attention must be directed at the student as an individual, but studies show the importance of group involvement both in school and in the community.

7. Education vs legislation: that is, which is most effective? Education can be directed in different ways to all the components of drug use—the individual, the school, and the community. Laws about possession and use may be of no value, as nonusers do not need them, users ignore them, and we do not know the effect on those "on the fence" trying to decide what to do.

8. Education—help vs harm: that is, does drug and alcohol education promote (by glorifying) or discourage (by frightening) drug use? This is a very hard outcome to measure, since effects of education may vary by region of the country, type of school (public vs private), and content of the program.

Barriers to Intervention and the Student Assistance Program

Schools have a number of problems in dealing with student alcohol and drug abuse. These include the following: difficulty in identifying the user, as supervisors and teachers are not trained in diagnosing the problem; lack of expertise by school personnel in the area of intervention and referral; and the inherent conflict of interest that develops between safeguarding the student's confidentiality and protecting the teachers' and school's interests. Many schools have established programs modeled on employee assistance programs, commonly called student assistance programs (SAPs).[11]

SAPs characteristically are partnerships involving school personnel as well as outsiders—commonly chemical dependency experts, pediatricians, mental health personnel, business leaders, and law enforcement figures. The SAP must function somewhat independently as a "safe place," for if students are to seek counsel while in school, they must feel confident that their interests are being protected. Careful guidelines for confidentiality must be established.

The role of the SAP is to provide education, prevention, treatment, and support. It serves as a linkage between school and community and may offer counseling, intervention, group therapy, reentry groups (for those returning to school after a drug-related absence), referral, education, evaluation, parent support groups, and parent education meetings. Medical input is a major need of such groups.

Drug Testing

The issue of drug testing is an extremely controversial area, with implications in the medical, scientific, educational, and legal areas. While there is general agreement that drug use in schools must be eliminated, and those using and bringing drugs to school must be identified, there is great disagreement in the area of how these students are to be identified.

There are a number of conditions under which most authorities would consider drug testing to be appropriate. All adolescents with significant psychiatric symptoms or alteration of mental status should be tested, for these are youngsters at high risk, and therapy for the drug or alcohol problems must be included if a problem exists. Other high-risk adolescents, such as those with a history of chemical dependency, may be screened in order to initiate follow-up. Adolescents who have completed a chemical dependency program may be required to submit to periodic random screening as part of aftercare. Finally, at the physician's discretion, drug testing may be appropriate in the evaluation of recurrent symptoms such as cough, rhinitis, abdominal pain, dizziness, headaches, or other vague somatic complaints. Testing should be considered in those adolescents who appear to be especially accident-prone.

The American Academy of Pediatrics in 1989 made a number of recommendations in its statement on "Screening for Drugs of Abuse in Children and Adolescents."[12] The conclusions and recommendations are as follows:

1. The Academy condemns the nontherapeutic use of psychoactive drugs by children and adolescents.

2. Voluntary screening for the purposes of treatment is within the ethical tradition of health maintenance, but the psychosocial risks of such screening in the area of drug abuse warrant particularly careful attention to the requirements for informed consent and the maintenance of confidentiality.

3. "Voluntary" screening may be a deceptive term, in that there are often consequences for those who decline to volunteer.

4. Parental consent may be sufficient for the involuntary screening of the younger child who lacks the capacity to make informed judgments. Parental permission is not sufficient for involuntary screening of the older, competent adolescent, and the Academy opposes such involuntary screening. Consent from the older adolescent may be waived when there is reason to doubt competency or in those circumstances in which information gained by history or physical examination is strongly suggestive of a young person at high risk from substance abuse.

5. Referral of a child or adolescent to a health professional for evaluation, counseling, and treatment would be the appropriate response to suspicion of drug use within an educational or vocational environment.

6. The pediatrician's major role in this area should be counseling and treatment, not police work. They should, therefore, not perform drug screening for the primary purpose of detecting illegal use.

7. Student athletes should not be singled out for involuntary screening for drugs of abuse. Except for health-related purposes, such testing should not be a condition for participation in sports or any school function.

Specific Areas of Concern for the Pediatrician and the School

The pediatrician must be knowledgeable in a variety of areas in which consultation may be sought. Ideally, each pediatrician should make a commitment to drug-free children in drug-free schools, should be known to local school authorities, and should offer consultation and expertise in this area.

Common areas in which the pediatrician might interact with the school include the following possible requests:

1. To help set standards of tolerance for a school system.

   Macdonald suggests the following dictum: "Schools should treat drug abuse as a contagious disease."[7] That is to say, if the drug user is allowed to use in school, the message will be spread to others and the impression will be that the school does not care. Schools must monitor incidence, prevalence, and location of drug use in school. A strict policy must be announced and enforced, with appropriate penalties for violation. The pediatrician must cooperate with and insist upon careful control of the use of prescribed medications in school. Every effort should be made to avoid prescribing medications that must be taken during school, but if the need arises the physician must cooperate with the school's policy (see chapter 23). Controlled drugs, such as those used for attention deficit disorders, must be carefully monitored so that parents do not send excessive amounts to school.

2. To help define "excessive amounts" to school.

   Again, the message here must be strictly a "NO DRUGS AT SCHOOL" policy. Local pediatric societies and medical groups may be excellent resources to aid in support of drug-free extracurricular activities. The physician may serve by supporting community substance abuse awareness groups.

   It is especially important to keep in mind that prevention activities must be age-appropriate. The pediatrician must recognize that drug use begins at an earlier and earlier age, with many third to fifth graders reporting "peer pressure" to drink and use drugs. Ideally, the issue should be raised within the context of anticipatory guidance offered during routine pediatric health maintenance visits, beginning no later than fifth grade. Parents should be included in these discussions at the outset. They should be encouraged to participate in prevention activities, and the pediatrician should be a source of information and, if needed, an intervenor and counselor. By introducing the subject at a relatively early age, not only does one help head off possible involvement, but the subject can be raised in a nonthreatening manner long before the likelihood has arisen that a child is in trouble. Thus, the pediatrician assumes the role of concerned educator rather than inquisitor.

3. To consult about selection of a drug abuse prevention curriculum for a school system.

Drug and alcohol prevention and awareness should be part of the curriculum in every grade from kindergarten through high school. The theme should be sounded not only in health class. Literature classes can read materials that discuss alcoholism and chemical dependency. Mathematics and science classes can address the biological and chemical aspects. History and social studies classes can address the political and historical attempts to deal with the issue. The subject and its safety implications should be discussed in driver education, industrial arts, and home economics courses. Extracurricular activities, such as school newspapers and future professional clubs, provide excellent mechanisms for promoting further discussion of the issue. Clearly the tone and content must evolve through the years, but certain themes must be emphasized. These include the ongoing assertion of the harmfulness of drugs and alcohol, knowledge of what drugs do to the body, the social consequences of drug and alcohol use, the laws relating to childhood usage, promotion of the drug-free life-style and cultivation of resistance techniques, the need for community support in the form of drug-free activities, and the availability of intervention and treatment programs.[9]

4. To participate in faculty in-service education programs about substance abuse.

Pediatricians and educators are role models in any community. Thus, behavior in public should be closely monitored, and the argument can be made that both pediatricians and educators should avoid any public behavior that could be considered counterproductive to the "no drugs" message. The pediatrician, as well as the classroom teacher, should be prepared to deal with students' questions about the physician's personal drinking or drug use.

5. To speak about drugs to a health class.

This provides an outstanding forum for pediatrician-school interaction, and allows a community role model who may be well-known by many of the students to participate in the substance abuse curriculum. It furthermore identifies the pediatrician as a concerned expert in the field and a person to consult if the student or school has a problem in this area.

6. To consult with the school teacher, nurse, psychologist, or counselor about a child having problems that might be drug or alcohol related.

Many behavioral problems in adolescents, including those related to drugs and alcohol, will surface first in school. Just as the pediatrician should be a partner with the classroom teacher in the assessment and management of learning and attention problems, so must the pediatrician and school psychologist cooperate in the assessment and management of drug-related problems. Most adolescents who use alcohol or drugs on any regular basis will have increased incidence of school absenteeism and truancy. Somatic complaints may manifest, and the pediatrician must play an active role in ferreting out the nature of the problem. The key to getting school personnel to act on their suspicions of alcohol or drug use is to encourage them to consider such use and its manifestations to be a *medical* problem requiring medical attention, and to refer accordingly. Children who are intoxicated in class cannot function or learn. Teachers who identify suspicious behavior, such as lethargy, excessive moodiness, change in appearance or grades, etc, must be reminded to refer the young person for evaluation. The health care provider must make an appointment available at once, and take to heart the opinions of the school personnel.

7. To order drug testing on a student who appears intoxicated in class or is caught with drugs.

The pediatrician is neither a police officer nor a judge, but should cooperate with parents and school personnel in conducting appropriate evaluations. The pediatrician must respect confidentiality and, when consulted, use the information elicited within the context of the doctor-patient relationship. To avoid being seen by the student as an adversary, the physician must assume a helping stance and protect the rights of the student.

8. To evaluate physical findings suggestive of anabolic steroid abuse and render an opinion as to whether to allow a youngster to play competitive sports.

The pediatrician must insist on a "no use" philosophy and educate about the hazards of anabolic steroids. These drugs also are particularly toxic because abusers frequently will use up to 20 times the recommended dose. Coaches must remind players that these performance enhancers not only are dangerous but unethical, and be prepared to cut offenders at once. Team captains should be recruited as peer leaders and insist that their teammates avoid jeopardizing their health over personal and team achievement by abuse. Athletic teams and coaches can take a leadership role in espousing the "no drugs" message and supporting drug-free activities.

9. To participate in selecting a rehabilitation program for a student identified as a user.

It is the pediatrician's responsibility to be knowledgeable about drug intervention and rehabilitation programs within the community. Increasingly, in the age of health maintenance organizations and dwindling insurance coverage, it is the primary care provider (in some cases serving as case manager or gatekeeper) who must initiate and authorize treatment. Frequently, the most appropriate early intervention may be to refer the student back to the school, especially if there is a student assistance program in place.

Conclusions

The pediatrician and school authorities must see themselves as partners in the area of substance abuse treatment and prevention. Improved education of physicians in the area of adolescent chemical dependency will make this partnership function at an improved level. The pediatrician of the 1990s must be knowledgeable in all five areas of chemical dependency: (1) prevention, (2) education, (3) intervention, (4) treatment, and (5) recovery. Schools and health care providers, by working together, can facilitate each other's effectiveness in this challenging arena.

References

1. Johnston LD, O'Malley PM, Bachman JG. *Smoking, Drinking, and Illicit Drug Use Among American Secondary School Students, College Students, and Young Adults, 1975-1991, Volume 1: Secondary School Students.* Washington, DC: Government Printing Office; 1992. US Dept of Health and Human Services Publication No (ADM) 92-1920 (in press)

2. US Public Health Service. *Healthy People 2000: National Health Promotion and Disease Prevention Objectives.* Washington, DC: US Public Health Service; 1991. US Department of Health and Human Services Publication No (PHS) 91-50212

3. Schuckit MA. *Drug and Alcohol Abuse: A Clinical Guide to Diagnosis and Treatment.* 3rd ed. New York, NY: Plenum Publishing Corp; 1989

4. Kandel DB, Logan JA. Patterns of drug use from adolescence to young adulthood: Part I. Periods of risk for initiation, continued use, and discontinuation. *Am J Public Health.* 1984;74:660-666

5. Yamaguchi K, Kandel DB. Patterns of drug use from adolescence to young adulthood: Part II. Sequences of progression. *Am J Public Health.* 1984;74:668-672

6. Yamaguchi K, Kandel DB. Patterns of drug use from adolescence to young adulthood: Part III. Predictors of progression. *Am J Public Health.* 1984;74:673-681

7. Macdonald D. *Drugs, Drinking and Adolescents.* 2nd ed. Chicago, IL: Yearbook Medical Publishers; 1989

8. Jessor R, Jessor SL. *Problem Behavior and Psychosocial Development: A Longitudinal Study of Youth.* New York, NY: Academic Press; 1977

9. US Department of Education. *Drug Prevention Curricula—A Guide to Selection and Implementation.* Washington, DC: US Department of Education; 1988

10. Goodstadt MS. Drug education: the prevention issues. *J Drug Educ.* 1989;19:197-208

11. McGovern JP, DuPont RL. Student assistance programs: an important approach to drug abuse prevention. *J Sch Health.* 1991;61:260-264

12. American Academy of Pediatrics, Committee on Adolescence, Committee on Bioethics, and Provisional Committee on Substance Abuse. Screening for drugs of abuse in children and adolescents. *Pediatrics.* 1989;84:396-398

Suggested Readings

Adger H, Jr. Problems of alcohol and other drug use and abuse in adolescents. *J Adolesc Health.* 1991;12:606-613

American Academy of Pediatrics, Committee on Substance Abuse. In: Schonberg SK, ed. *Substance Abuse: A Guide for Health Professionals.* Elk Grove Village, IL: American Academy of Pediatrics; 1988

Anderson GL. *When Chemicals Come to School: The Student Assistance Program Model.* Greenfield, WI: Community Recovery Press; 1987

Bell C, Battjes R. *Prevention Research: Deterring Drug Abuse Among Children and Adolescents.* NIDA research monograph 63. 1985. Department of Health and Human Services Publication No (ADM) 85-1334

Chen TT, Winder AE. When is the critical moment to provide smoking education at schools? *J Drug Educ.* 1986;16:121-133

Davis S. Preventing adolescent pregnancy. In: Strasburger VC, Greydanus DE, eds. *Adolescent Med: State of the Art Rev.* 1990;1:113-126

Goldstein AP. Refusal skills: learning to be positively negative. *J Drug Educ.* 1989;19:271-283

Institute for Behavior and Health, Committee on the Future of Alcohol and Other Drug Use Prevention. In: DuPont RL, ed. *Stopping Alcohol and Other Drug Use Before It Starts: The Future of Prevention.* Rockville, MD: Office for Substance Abuse Prevention. Department of Health and Human Services Publication No (ADM) 89-1645; 1989

Jones R. Identification and management of the toxic adolescent. *Semin Adolesc Med.* 1985;1:239-245

Macdonald DI. Patterns of alcohol and drug use among adolescents. *Pediatr Clin North Am.* 1987;34:275-288

MacKenzie RG, Cheng M, Haftel AJ. The clinical utility and evaluation of drug screening techniques. *Pediatr Clin North Am.* 1987;34:423-436

Miller SK, Slap GB. Adolescent smoking: a review of prevalence and prevention. *J Adolesc Health Care*. 1989;10:129-135

National Commission on Drug-Free Schools. *Toward a Drug-Free Generation: A Nation's Responsibility*. Washington, DC; 1990

Rhodes JE, Jason LA. *Preventing Substance Abuse Among Children and Adolescents*. New York, NY: Pergamon Press; 1988

Rogers P, ed. Chemical dependency. *Pediatr Clin North Am*. 1987; 34:275-544

Tims F, Ludford J. *Drug Abuse Treatment Evaluation: Strategies, Progress and Prospects*. NIDA research monograph 51. 1984. Department of Health and Human Services Publication No (ADM) 84-1329

US Department of Education. *Growing Up Drug Free: A Parent's Guide to Prevention*. Washington, DC: US Department of Education; 1989

US Department of Education. *What Works—Schools Without Drugs*. Washington, DC: US Department of Education; 1989

CHAPTER 23

MEDICATION ADMINISTRATION IN SCHOOL

Many children and adolescents are able to attend school because of the effectiveness of their medication. The health circumstances requiring medication are diverse. Medications may be essential for continued functioning, either as a component of an elaborate treatment plan for the student with a complex disability or as the only treatment necessary for a student to maintain or regain control of his/her chronic illness. In rare instances medications may be necessary for life-threatening emergencies. For most students, the use of medication will be a convenient benefit to control acute minor or major illnesses, allowing a timely return to the classroom with minimal interference to others. Students may symptomatically benefit with nonprescription medications. Administration of these medications during the school day may be unnecessary. The overall purpose of medication is to benefit the child and school policies can be developed with this goal in mind.[1]

School Policy

The goal for the use of medications in school is to assist all students to participate at their fullest independent capacity. Handling, monitoring, and administering the variety of medications used to implement this goal sometimes challenges the school's efforts to ensure a safe, secure, and orderly environment. Differing characteristics, such as the size of the school and available health personnel, are additional factors that preclude the development of a medication treatment policy or protocol that would apply to all school settings. However, regardless of size and resources, each school is encouraged to establish a district policy regarding administration of medications. Furthermore, the presence of a school-based health service will significantly affect the scope of a treatment policy, and policy components essential for most schools may be irrelevant when licensed medical personnel are on-site.

The school board and the school superintendent in conjunction with other school personnel, most notably the school nurse, and in collaboration with the physician or medical advisory committee for each school (district), should develop a policy for the administration of medication in the school setting. The guidelines should indicate what age and/or class levels are included, such as kindergarten through grade 12 or, alternatively, separate guidelines for elementary school. Individual school districts also should seek the advice of counsel as they assume the responsibility for giving medication during school hours. Liability coverage should be provided for the staff, including nurses, teachers, athletic staff, principals, superintendents, and members of the school board. Any student who must take medication during regular school hours should do so in compliance with the school's regulations.

The AAP Committee on School Health recommends that each school include or consider the following sections in its medication policy.

Physician-Prescribed Medications

1. The school should require a written statement from the physician that provides the name of the drug, the dose, the times when the medication is to be taken, and the diagnosis or reason the medicine is needed, unless the reason should remain confidential.
2. The physician should alert the school when students may/will experience serious reactions while receiving prescribed medication. The school may facilitate this communication by having a check-off space on its medication form to highlight this possibility.
3. The physician also should alert the school when the medication prescribed may cause severe reaction even when administered properly. Any necessary emergency response should be outlined by the physician, either directly on the form or as an attachment describing the appropriate treatment.
4. The physician should state whether the child is qualified and/or able to self-administer the medication.
5. The parent or guardian should provide a written request that the school district comply with the physician's order. This may be a preprinted statement as a separate form, or the parent/guardian may indicate approval by signing on the same medication form used by the physician.

Parent- or Self-Prescribed Medications

The school must consider the symptomatic benefits of self-prescribed medications versus the issues of school safety and security of drug use. Medications are "prescribed" by parents who desire to facilitate their children's medical recovery and return to the school setting. Some schools may consider that any child who is ill enough to require medication should either stay at home or see a physician who can decide if it is safe for him/her to return to the school setting. The school realities include safeguarding other children and staff from contagious disease, preventing disruption to the classroom environment by symptomatic students, and concern about the sharing of medication at school between classmates. The social realities of working parents, often in jobs that do not allow for "sick day" benefits to attend to their children's illnesses, may require that parents send the child to school. Because of these realities, it may become necessary to consider the possibility of self- or parent-recommended medications for children.

Therefore, the AAP Committee on School Health recommends that schools consider developing guidelines for allowing children with minor illnesses into the classroom, with appropriate attention to recognized contagious disease policies and to pertinent state codes. It also recommends that students (especially older youth) be allowed to self-medicate at school with over-the-counter medications when the parent has provided an appropriate note to the school specifying the medication, the amount of medication to be given, the time it may be taken, and the reason for its administration. The parent's note should include a statement relieving the school of any responsibility for the benefits or consequences of the medication when it is parent-prescribed and self-administered and acknowledging that the school bears no responsibility for assuring that the medication is taken. The school should retain the note for at least the duration of time the medication is used at school. It is preferable that the note remain a permanent part of the student's school health record. The school should reserve the right to limit the duration of parent-prescribed medications and/or to require a physician statement for continued use of any medication beyond a specified time period. The school also should restrict the availability of the medication from other students, with immediate confiscation of the medication and loss of privileges if medication policies are abused or ignored.

Special consideration may need to be given to adolescents for self-prescribing medications without parental request. Depending on the school's size and need for security regarding drug use, the school may require the same policy as is required for younger children.

Security and Storage of Medication

All prescription medications brought to school should be in a container appropriately labeled by the pharmacist or the physician. All over-the-counter medications should be in their original container.

The school should make secure storage available for all medications, especially when school personnel administer the medication. The storage of self-administered medications is important when the school determines that the nature of the medication or the school environment requires greater security or when the student is too young or untrustworthy to personally maintain safe use. The parent or physician should request that medications be secured by the school when this is appropriate. Some medications will require refrigeration. All parenteral medications and all drugs controlled by the Drug Enforcement Agency must be appropriately secured by the school.

Students may be allowed to carry their own medication when it does not require either refrigeration or security as determined by the school, and when the school has granted permission for the students to take their own medication. The school may require that students demonstrate their capability for self-administration and for responsible behavior, and the school should develop standards that qualify students to carry and self-administer medication. The school may need to develop a "medication pass" that the student can show to any inquiring school personnel to verify the student has school permission for carrying and taking medication.

For selected medications or circumstances, the school should consider the convenience of retrieving and administering a medication when the treatment may have an impact on the medical outcome. Prepared syringes of epinephrine for treating serious allergic reactions are one example. Answers to questions, such as where the medication will be stored, who is responsible for the medication, and who will carry the medication for field trips, should be defined in advance in order to maintain medication security and safety while assuring timely treatment.

Supervision of Medication Administration

Designated personnel must be available to administer medication at agreed upon times and location. The person supervising the administration of medication must keep a written record.

Schools with full-time school nurse(s) should formally designate these professionals as the appropriate supervising personnel. The school's medication policy should specifically exclude teachers and other school staff from being responsible for independent requests from parents to administer medication.

Arrangements should be made for alternate personnel to supervise the administration of medication in schools in which full-time school nurses are not available. Even when a school nurse is only available part-time, the responsibility for coordinating and supervising the school's medication policy should be vested in this more qualified professional. Alternate personnel must know that they have been designated as responsible for supervising the administration of medication and must receive appropriate preparation and determination of capability. These alternate personnel should be certified in Basic Life Support.

The school should consider the frequency of administration and the degree of risk associated with medications in order to require a school nurse on location to supervise the administration of the medication. The Committee on School Health recommends that the administration of parenteral medications given on a scheduled basis should always be supervised by appropriately trained health professionals. Exception should be made in cases of potential emergencies, such as an epinephrine injection to abort a life-threatening allergic reaction. These injections should be given with prepared dosage kits and by personnel trained by a health professional in the administration of the dose. A school plan for requesting emergency professional support should be developed and communicated to all school staff. Guidance for the required competence of personnel to administer medication for specialized health needs is specifically outlined in a special interdisciplinary report issued in 1989 (Table 50).[2]

Field Trips

Out-of-school learning experiences represent special circumstances that may not be accommodated by an in-school medication policy. The issues are similar but need to be addressed as part of the preparatory arrangements for any student outing: Who will transport and/or secure the medication? Who will administer the medication? And, if the need is anticipated, who is trained to manage any adverse outcome from either the medication or from failure to administer the medication for those students who are dependent on regular medication doses? Well-planned field trips are valuable experiences for students, and sufficient staff supervision appropriate for the size and needs of the group is an important contributor to the trip's success. The additional staff time and attention necessary for the number of doses of medication to be administered must be considered when scheduling staff supervision for the trip.

When developing its medication policy, the school should consider whether transporting an epinephrine kit for all warm weather outings is a requirement.

Self-Administered Medications, Supervised

When the student is usually responsible for taking medication, the student should do so in school with parental consent. Physician consent also is needed if it is a prescription medication. The school personnel supervising the student should keep a record of medication to be taken by the student, including the dosage and frequency together with permission from the family and physician to allow the child to take this medication during school hours.

Medical Procedures for Disease Self-Monitoring

Students who are accustomed to self-administering medical testing procedures before taking medication, such as glucometer measurement of blood glucose for a diabetic student, should

Table 50. — Types of Medications Administered in Schools by Indicated School Personnel

MEDICATIONS: Medications may be given by LPNs and health aides only when the Nurse Practice Act of the individual state allows such practice, and under the specific guidelines of that Nurse Practice Act.

Medication	Physician Order Required	Registered Nurse	Licensed Practical Nurse	Certified Teaching Personnel	Related Services Personnel[1]	Paraprofessionals[2]	Others[3]
Oral	*	(A)	(S)	X	X	S/HA	X
Injection	*	(A)	(S)	X	X	X	X
Epi-Pen Allergy Kit	*	(A)	(S)	EM	EM	EM	EM
Inhalation	*	(A)	(S)	EM	EM	EM/HA	X
Rectal	*	(A)	(S)	X	X	EM/HA	X
Bladder Installation	*	(A)	(S)	X	X	X	X
Eye/Ear Drops	*	(A)	(S)	X	X	S/HA	X
Topical	*	(A)	(S)	X	X	S/HA	X
Per Nasogastric Tube	*	(A)	(S)	X	X	S/HA	X
Per Gastrostomy Tube	*	(A)	(S)	X	X	S/HA	X
Intravenous	*	(A)	(S)	X	X	X	X
Spirometer	*	(A)	(S)	X	X	S/HA	X

DEFINITION OF SYMBOLS

A — Qualified to perform task, not in conflict with professional standards
S — Qualified to perform task with RN supervision and inservice education
EM — In emergencies, if properly trained, and if designated professional is not available

X — Should not perform under any circumstances
O — Person who should be designated to perform task
HA — Health Aide only

[1] Related services include OT, PT, nutritionist, Speech/language pathologist
[2] Paraprofessionals include teacher aides, health aides, uncertified teaching personnel
[3] Others include secretaries, bus drivers, cafeteria workers, custodians

From The Joint Task Force for the Management of Children With Special Health Needs. *Report on the Delineation of Roles and Responsibilities for the Safe Delivery of Specialized Health Care in the Educational Setting.* Reston, VA: Council for Exceptional Children; 1989 be allowed this responsibility in the school setting after appropriate authorization and instructions from the family and the physician. The school must document the date, time, and results of the procedure. Any treatment is to be specifically defined by the physician. Complicated treatment regimens should be fully described by the physician in a letter.

Medication Form

A "medication form" used exclusively for recording and transmitting of information about the administration of medications for students should be uniform for the school system. A standardized form to be used by all school systems would be desirable for physicians who deal with multiple school systems but is unlikely to be immediately acceptable by all schools.

The AAP Committee on School Health recommends that medication forms include the following:

- The name and address of the school (at the top of the form)
- Name, birthday, and address of the student
- Relevant diagnosis(es)
- Name of medication
- Dosage, which should specify the amount to be given and the timing of administration
- Possible adverse reactions that should be reported to the physician
- Any special instructions for handling
- Dates for administration
- Date when form is completed
- Physician's signature, address, and how he/she can be reached
- Signature of parent/guardian authorizing the school to administer the medication
- A check-off square box allowing the physician to alert the school that a serious reaction could occur if the medication is not given exactly as prescribed.
- A check-off square box allowing the physician to indicate that a serious reaction can occur from the medication even when administered properly. Space should be available for the physician to describe what action or treatment should be rendered when an adverse reaction occurs.

The committee also recommends that the form be on paper of standard letter size (8 1/2 in x 11 in). This size corresponds to most filing systems and helps avoid the inadvertent loss of forms of smaller size, which can be misplaced between other pages of standard size. This size also facilitates photocopying and fax transmittal. Information can be formatted on letter-sized forms to accommodate folding if forms of smaller size are preferred. Printing on a distinct paper color can make the form readily identifiable and may facilitate its retrieval.

References

1. American Academy of Pediatrics, Committee on School Health. Guidelines for the Administration of Medication in School. *Pediatrics.* In press

2. The Joint Task Force for the Management of Children With Special Health Needs, American Federation of Teachers, Council for Exceptional Children, National Association of School Nurses, National Education Association. *Report on the Delineation of Roles and Responsibilities for the Safe Delivery of Specialized Health Care in the Educational Setting.* 1989

CHAPTER 24

PREGNANCY AND PREVENTION

A million American teenagers get pregnant every year—almost 1 out of every 10 women between the ages of 15 and 19. Almost half of these teen pregnancies occur to young women who are school age, ie, 17 and younger. Teenage mothers are significantly more likely to drop out of school and to fail to achieve their full potential in life. Many teen mothers require public assistance. It is estimated that 53% of households receiving Aid to Families With Dependent Children (AFDC) were started by women who had their first child when they were teens. Many pregnancies to teenagers are unplanned, and almost half of the pregnancies of school-age adolescents end in abortion.

Besides pregnancy, sexually active teens have high rates of sexually transmitted diseases and are at significant risk of infection with the human immunodeficiency virus. As of January 1991, almost 20% of AIDS cases had occurred in young people in their 20s. Many of these young adults became infected as adolescents.

Prevention

Schools can be important sites for primary prevention of pregnancy by providing appropriate sex education to include the virtues of delaying initiation of, or abstaining from, sexual intercourse. School personnel are often the first adults to recognize a teenager's pregnancy. Early pregnancy recognition (secondary prevention) affords the adolescent the fullest range of pregnancy options and ensures the best pregnancy outcomes. Tertiary prevention, or support of school staff during and after the pregnancy, can be crucial in preventing the potentially deleterious consequences: school dropout, underemployment and unemployment, rapid repeat pregnancy, and an unstable home life. This chapter will attempt to summarize the current state of our understanding of adolescent pregnancy, parenthood, and programs to prevent pregnancy and its potential adverse effects on youth. Throughout the chapter the role that school staff can play in alleviating the problems attendant with each stage of pregnancy and parenthood will be stressed.

Risk Factors for Early Sexual Activity and Parenthood

The most important determinant of an adolescent's risk of an early pregnancy is the age of initiation of sexual intercourse. The percentage of young people who are sexually experienced (ie, have had sexual intercourse at least once) increases rapidly between puberty and age 20. A series of adolescent health surveys between 1973 and 1988 have documented unprecedented increases in adolescent sexual activity. The proportion of sexually active adolescents aged 15 to 19 has increased from 30.4% in 1973 to 53% in 1988 (Table 51). Much of this increase has been among whites and more economically advantaged teens. Consequently, the traditional differences between blacks and whites and rich and poor have narrowed considerably.

The second most important influence on an adolescent's risk of early pregnancy is failure to use contraception. Adolescents are often poor users of contraception; many fail to use protection or fail to use it consistently. This is the result of a variety of developmental immaturities, fears, and concerns about using contraception. Young teens and teens who have recently initiated sexual activity are likely to be the worst users of contraception. Table 52 lists barriers to contraception utilization, and Table 53 lists reasons for delaying a first visit to a family planning clinic. Between 1973 and 1988, there were dramatic changes in adult and adolescent use of birth control. Data from 1988 suggests significantly increased use of condoms but a persistent "contraceptive gap" exists for many teens.

Given this increase in adolescent sexual activity, increased use of contraception, and some increase in use of abortion services, teen pregnancy and birth rates have not changed dramatically in the past 20 years. However, there have been dramatic increases in the numbers of teen mothers giving birth out of wedlock. Pregnancy is no longer a prelude to marriage for most teenagers.

An understanding of risk factors for early initiation of adolescent sexual activity and inconsistent use of contraception is as useful in preventing pregnancy as an understanding of cardiovascular risk factors would be in preventing heart disease and stroke. Risk factors are helpful in early *identification* of adolescents and in *design of school-based prevention*. A wealth of

Table 51. — Sexual Activity, Contraceptive Usage, and Pregnancy and Birth Rates Among American Women (Ages 15 to 19 Yr)*

	1971	1976	1979	1982	1988
Women in age group who are sexually active (%)[1,2]					
Total	30.4	43.4	49.8	47.1	53.2
White	26.4	38.3	46.6	44.5	52.4
Black	53.7	66.3	66.2	59.0	60.8
Hispanic	...	...	...	50.6	48.5
Women in age group using contraception at first intercourse (%)[2,3]					
Condoms	...	...	17.9	22.6	47.3
Oral contraceptives	...	...	8.7	8.3	8.2
Any method	...	...	48.9	47.9	65.0
Most recent method among those currently using contraception (%)[4]					
Oral contraceptives	...	...	...	64.0	59.0
Condoms	...	...	...	21.0	31.0
Diaphragm	...	...	...	6.0	1.0
Pregnancy rate (per 1,000)[5]					
Total	94	101	109	110	...
Birth rate (per 1,000)[5,6]					
Total	65	53	52	53	54
White	54	44	44	45	...
Black	135	105	102	97	...
Percentage of teen births out-of-wedlock[5,6]					
Total	31	40	46	51	66
White	17	25	30	37	...
Black	67	80	85	87	...

* Based on data from Zelnik and Kantner,[1] Forrest and Singh,[2] Zelnik and Shah,[3] Mosher,[4] Hofferth,[5] and National Center for Health Statistics.[6]

Table 52. — Percentage Distribution of Women, Age 15–19 Years, Who Did Not Use Contraception at First Intercourse by Reason Reported for Not Using a Method and According to Whether First Intercourse Was Planned*

Reason for Nonuse of Contraceptive	Planned	Unplanned
Wanted pregnancy or did not care if pregnancy resulted	3.5	4.6
Did not want to use contraceptives[†]	31.2	8.0
Did not know about contraception	19.8	12.4
Did not think about using contraceptives	13.5	24.3
Intercourse was not planned	0.0	31.8
Contraception was not available	14.4	12.9
Thought pregnancy was impossible	16.2	5.0
Other	1.4	1.0
Total	100.0	100.0

* From Zelnik M, Shah FK. First intercourse among young Americans. *Fam Plann Perspect.* 1983;15:64-70. Reprinted with permission.
† Includes partner's objection to the use of contraceptives.

research has suggested a number of clear risks for early initiation of sexual activity and inconsistent use of contraception. These are not certain predictors of behavior for any particular adolescent. They must be supplemented with a thorough individual assessment.

Poverty and its attendant problems have been classic determinants for teen parenthood. Recent studies suggest that poverty has become much less important as a determinant for early sexual experience but remains a strong risk factor for nonuse of contraception and, hence, teen pregnancy. Combined with less access to abortion services, poor teens still are the most likely to become teen parents.

Puberty and the physical and hormonal changes that attend it are clear risk factors for sexual interest and activity. Sexual activity is correlated with pubertal development as measured by Tanner stage. Early maturers are at greatest risk. Pubertal development proceeds independently of cognitive development so that early physical maturers may be "out of

Table 53. — Percentage Distribution of Reasons Cited by Teenage Women as Most Important for Delaying First Visit to a Family Planning Clinic and as Contributing to Their Delay of First Visit*

Reason	% Distribution by Most Important Reason	% Citing as Contributing Reason
Just didn't get around to it	15.6	38.1
Afraid my family would find out if I came	12.1	31.0
Waiting for a closer relationship with partner	12.0	31.0
Afraid to be examined	8.5	24.8
Thought birth control dangerous	7.9	26.5
Never thought of it	6.9	16.4
Did not think had sex often enough to get pregnant	3.6	16.5
Did not know where to get birth control help	3.3	15.3
Did not expect to have sex	3.3	12.8
Thought birth control I was using was good enough	3.1	7.8
Thought I was too young to get pregnant	2.8	11.5
Thought it cost too much	2.6	18.5
Partner opposed	2.5	8.4
Thought I had to be older to get birth control	2.1	13.1
Thought birth control wrong	1.1	9.2
Thought I wanted pregnancy	1.1	8.4
Forced to have sex	0.7	1.4
Sex with relative	0.1	0.7
Other	10.7	9.7
Total	100.0	. . .

*From Zabin LS, Clark SD. Why they delay: a study of teenage family planning clinic patients. *Fam Plann Perspect.* 1981;13:205-217. Reprinted with permission.

synch" developmentally and at increased risk. The outward signs of physical maturity are readily apparent. Because of adolescents' intrinsic concerns with body image, puberty can clearly be a "teachable moment."

Developmentally, adolescence is a time when peers begin to replace family in dictating the norms for behavior. Not surprisingly, therefore, having friends who are sexually active is a clear risk for early sexual experience. Best friends' behavior and the behavior of one's group of peers are both important influences on the likelihood that an adolescent will engage in sex.

Teens who engage in one kind of problem behavior often engage in others. The teen who is doing poorly in school, who is truant, who has had problems with the police, or who is using drugs tends to be more likely to be sexually active and less likely to use contraception. Often these troubled teens are well known to the school and unfortunately often drop out before help can be given. Conversely, teens who are engaged in prosocial activities (ie, clubs, athletics, volunteer service, and church-related activities) are "protected" to a degree, either because they delay sexual activity or because they are better users of contraception.

Families have important influences on many adolescent behaviors. Having a mother or a sister who was or is a teen mother puts a young woman at increased risk of parenthood. Mothers and daughters tend to reach menarche at similar ages and to initiate sexual activity about the same age. Parental supervision of dating seems to have a positive influence against early sexual experimentation. Despite parents being encouraged to provide good sex education, few parents are equipped for this role, and many parents are not talking at all to their adolescent sons and daughters. It is difficult to document the effects of family communication on initiation of sexual activity. There is some evidence that family communication may play a role in increasing contraceptive use. Families may be most important in teaching basic values to their children. This is best accomplished before the turmoil of adolescence begins.

International comparisons of adolescent fertility have been helpful in understanding the problems of teenage pregnancy in the United States. Compared to teens in other western countries, American teens are *not* more likely to be sexually active; however, they are twice as likely to become pregnant! Researchers point to lower rates of contraceptive use to call attention to a society that is less open about discussing sexuality than other western societies. Americans are more likely to be ambivalent about teenagers' use of contraception and more likely to stress abstinence as a solution. Efforts to reduce the incidence of teen pregnancy in this country are hindered by this lack of a national consensus on the role of contraception for sexually active adolescents.

Prevention Programs (School Based and Other)

Schools are potentially excellent sites for primary prevention programs for pregnancy and other health problems of adolescents. Unfortunately, schools often give health a low priority. Likewise, it is difficult to say what works in primary prevention. Teen pregnancy is the result of multiple influences, and single modality approaches are not likely to be effective. Comprehensive programs addressing a broad range of adolescent needs and concerns are needed.

Various health interventions have been attempted or suggested for schools. These include sex education, comprehensive health education, peer education, social skills training, values clarification, abstinence promotion, mentoring, peer counseling, community service, reproductive health services through school-based or school-linked clinics, condom distribution, community-school collaboration, and self-esteem enhancement. Evaluation of model programs would suggest that none of these is a panacea for the problem of teen pregnancy. For example, traditional approaches to sex education that stress reproductive biology increase knowledge but have little impact on adolescent sexual behavior. Comprehensive approaches to health education that stress social skills and values are needed. Programs which stress abstinence as the only option have shown little success, with the exception of programs using peer educators. Promotion of contraception to sexually active teens remains an essential component of comprehensive health education.

Recognition of Pregnancy by Nurses and Teachers (Secondary Prevention)

An understanding of these risk factors can be very helpful to school nurses and educators in identifying an "at-risk" adolescent. Some of these factors such as physical maturity, are readily apparent; some become apparent only after one gets to know the students in the school. Other risk factors may be discovered only after a careful and sensitive interview with a student. If pregnancy or possible pregnancy is suspected, the teenager should be referred to a school nurse or counselor who can conduct a careful and confidential assessment. If conducted by a medical professional, such an assessment should include a basic medical history; gynecological history, including the signs and symptoms of pregnancy; sexual history, including use of contraception; a social and family assessment; an exploration of the adolescent's feelings about any potential pregnancy; and a review of pregnancy options. The signs and symptoms of pregnancy may include amenorrhea, nausea, weight gain, tender breasts, frequent urination, and mood swings. If pregnancy is suspected, the adolescent should be referred for diagnosis and treatment and assisted in getting to the referral site.

Most state laws protect the privacy of an adolescent regarding the diagnosis and treatment of a pregnancy and the confidentiality of the interactions with a medical professional. School nurses and physicians should not disclose such facts to anyone, including parents and school administrators, without the permission of the teenager. Similar protection may not be available to educational staff. Anyone who counsels young people about pregnancy or other sensitive issues should be frank from the onset about any constraints on confidentiality that may apply.

Pregnancy Options

Diagnosis of pregnancy should occur in a clinic that can counsel a young person about medical options. These include parenthood, adoption, and abortion. A young person needs to receive unbiased and accurate information about the nature and consequences of each option. This should be provided in a supportive, nonjudgmental fashion. In most states, underage adolescents legally can receive treatment for pregnancy as if they were adults. The exception is often abortion, for which many states mandate parental notification. Usually a judicial waiver is possible if harm may come to the teenager whose parents are notified.

Counseling and referral by school health staff should begin when the pregnancy is suspected. This should include initial information about pregnancy options and about contraception. Young women whose pregnancy tests turn out to be negative are at high risk for pregnancy in the ensuing months and deserve close follow-up. School staff should be cognizant of their own feelings about teen pregnancy and avoid any attempt to pressure the student.

It is often very helpful to involve family, *with the teenager's consent*, in discussions of pregnancy options. This is especially true with very young adolescents. Many young teenagers do not know how to broach the issue of sexuality and pregnancy with parents. School staff can be helpful in initiating this dialogue. They must always be alert to potential adverse consequences from a dysfunctional parent.

Care of Pregnant Teens in School

A pregnant student can attend school without restriction unless her physician asks for a change in her educational program. Likewise, a teenager should not be restricted from returning to school postpartum unless so directed by her physician. The obstetrician is most likely to request restricted activity in the last trimester and particularly in the last month of the pregnancy. Home teaching can be very helpful for a student who has been put on bed rest.

Pregnant teens have a guaranteed right to attend school. Special schools for pregnant girls can be helpful in addressing the educational needs of the pregnant student; however, a student cannot legally be forced to leave her regular school. Parenting education, nutrition education, child development classes, and child care are several potential benefits of special schooling. Allowances should be made for the increased absenteeism created by the demands of prenatal care, delivery, postpartum recovery, and the continuing demands of child care. With proper support the tragedy of school dropout can be avoided.

Consequences of Adolescent Childbearing

It is now clear that the consequences of school-age parenthood are not as devastating as once thought. While it is true that teen parents are less likely to graduate and to succeed in life, many were clearly at risk of failing prior to getting pregnant. Much research currently is focused on understanding the relative importance of teen parenthood versus preexisting social circumstances in shaping a young mother's life course.

Among the known outcomes associated with teen childbearing are school dropout, underemployment and unemployment, reduced income, more rapid pace of childbearing and larger completed family size, and reduced family stability (single parenthood, divorce, etc). In the long run, many teen mothers overcome these initial adverse consequences. However, the long-term effects on the children of teen mothers may remain considerable.

The impact of elective termination of pregnancy in adolescents remains controversial. In the short-term, abortion has been associated with emotional distress and repeat pregnancy. In the long run, however, termination of pregnancy has been shown to improve social outcomes and overall life satisfaction. All cases in which the adolescent girl opts for abortion should have appropriate follow-up and professional counseling.

Summary

Public schools can be effective sites for prevention and care of adolescent pregnancy. School health education can provide adolescents with the knowledge, skills, and motivation to avoid pregnancy. School health services can aid in early diagnosis of pregnancy, in counseling, and in facilitating entry into the health care system. The school medical consultant can help to assure that school policy facilitates a young person's continued education. Schools, by combining comprehensive health education and health services, can become sites for effective prevention of "children having children."

References

1. Zelnik M, Kantner JF. Sexual activity, contraceptive use, and pregnancy among metropolitan-area teenagers: 1971-1979. *Fam Plann Perspect.* 1980;12:230-237

2. Forrest JD, Singh S. The sexual and reproductive behavior of American women, 1982-1988. *Fam Plann Perspect.* 1990;22: 206-214

3. Zelnik M, Shah FK. First intercourse among young Americans. *Fam Plann Perspect.* 1983;15:64-70

4. Mosher WD. Contraceptive practice in the United States, 1982-1988. *Fam Plann Perspect.* 1990;22:198-205

5. Hofferth SL, Kahn JR, Baldwin W. Premarital sexual activity among US teenage women over the past three decades. *Fam Plann Perspect.* 1987;19:46-53

6. National Center for Health Statistics. *Monthly Vital Statistics Report.* June 29, 1989;38(3)(suppl)

Suggested Readings

Armstrong E, Waszak C. *Teenage Pregnancy and Too-Early Childbearing: Public Costs, Personal Consequences.* 5th ed. Washington, DC: Center for Population Options; 1990

Donovan JE, Jessor R. Structure of problem behavior in adolescence and young adulthood. *J Consult Clin Psychol.* 1985;53:890-904

Furstenburg FF, Levine JA, Brooks-Gunn J. The children of teenage mothers: patterns of early childbearing in two generations. *Fam Plann Perspect.* 1990;22(2):54-61

Hansen H, Stroh G, Whitaker K. School achievement: risk factors in teenage pregnancies. *Am J Public Health.* 1978;68:753-759

Hayes CD, ed. *Risking the Future: Adolescent Sexuality, Pregnancy, and Childbearing.* Washington, DC: National Academy Press; 1987:414,454,457,460

Hofferth SL. Factors affecting initiation of sexual intercourse. In: Hayes CD, ed. *Risking the Future: Adolescent Sexuality, Pregnancy, and Childbearing.* Washington, DC: National Academy Press; 1987;2:7-35

Hogan DP, Kitagawa EM. The impact of social status, family structure, and neighborhood on the fertility of black adolescents. *Am J Sociology.* 1985;90:825-855

Holder AR. Minor's rights to consent to medical care. *JAMA.* 1987;257:3400-3402

Jones EF, Forrest JD, Goldman N, et al. Teenage pregnancy in developed countries: determinants and policy implications. *Fam Plann Perspect.* 1985;17:53-63

Mott FL, Haurin RJ. Linkages between sexual activity and alcohol and drug use among American adolescents. *Fam Plann Perspect.* 1988;20(3):128-136

Newcomer SF, Udry JR. Parent-child communication and adolescent sexual behavior. *Fam Plann Perspect.* 1985;17:169-174

Santelli JS, Beilenson P. Risk factors for adolescent sexual behavior, fertility, and sexually transmitted diseases. *J Sch Health.* 1992;62:271-279

CHAPTER 25

EATING DISORDERS: ANOREXIA AND BULIMIA NERVOSA

Definition and History

Anorexia nervosa is a condition in which a person, usually a young adolescent female, severely restricts food intake resulting in a relatively rapid and significant weight loss and the cessation of menstruation. Bulimia nervosa is characterized by recurrent episodes of eating extremely large amounts of food in a short period of time, and often associated with self-induced vomiting and the use of laxatives in order to avoid weight gain. In each condition, the individual has excessive concern with body weight and shape, intense fear of gaining weight, and an obsessional preoccupation with thoughts of food and eating. The major difference between the two groups of patients with eating disorders is whether the people involved persistently and rigidly restrict their caloric intake or whether they regularly consume extremely large amounts of food. A person may have symptoms of anorexia alone, bulimia alone, both conditions simultaneously, or may move back and forth between the two diagnoses at different times.

Anorexia and bulimia nervosa, contrary to popular opinion, are not new diseases unique to our modern postindustrial society. Anorexia first was described in the medical literature as long ago as 300 years, while bulimia was described by the Greek physician, Galen, as early as the 2nd Century AD. Sociocultural forces change with the times. Although the external or environmental stressor may vary, the psychophysiologic manifestation in the individual may be the same regardless of time. For example, a 13th Century adolescent may have fasted and denied herself comfort and pleasure in order to be more acceptable to God; the Victorian maiden may have refused food as a way of rebelling against a rigidly controlling patriarchal family, whereas a modern young woman may be experiencing the stress of societal demands for high achievement in all areas (ie, "superwoman") while she struggles with autonomy issues and separation from her overly intrusive and enmeshed parents.

Typology and Epidemiology

Feeling fat, wishing to lose weight, counting calories, worrying and feeling guilty after eating, and exercising to lose weight are becoming normative for US girls as young as age 7.[1] Although only 25% of American high school girls in one study were overweight, about half considered themselves fat, and more than two thirds wanted to lose weight.[2] College women are preoccupied with body appearance, and, on testing, many indicate anorexic-like symptoms. While not meeting the criteria for bulimia nervosa, a large majority of college women engage in binging and purging behaviors. These prevalent attitudes and behaviors are of concern because they constitute risk factors for the development of an eating disorder. However, they also raise the question as to whether eating disorders may merely be the extreme position on a continuum of normative behaviors and attitudes present in most women. For anorectic patients, current data do not support the above contention; while for bulimics there is insufficient data to distinguish pathologic behaviors from those that might be considered an expected response to a cultural focus on body weight and shape as equivalents of success, beauty, and control.

Anorexia occurs in about 1 in 100 adolescent girls in the upper middle class and upper class. The prevalence of bulimia in young women is much higher, estimated to be about 4% in female college populations. The highest social classes are at greater risk, as are those who look to their environment for validation and rely on others for their sense of self-worth. It follows that these would be the same women most vulnerable to family, peer, and societal pressures to achieve. Conversely, working class and minority women are less likely to develop an eating disorder.

Males constitute approximately 5% of patients with eating disorders, although up to one third of college male students report abnormal eating behaviors. Male patients with eating disorders are more likely to have unconventional psychosexual development and gender identity, and more male patients with eating disorders report homosexual or bisexual preference.

Eating disorders were once thought to occur with unusually higher frequency in Jewish, Italian, and Catholic adolescents; this impression no longer holds true and probably resulted from a reporting bias. Increasingly, patients are being diagnosed from all racial, ethnic, socioeconomic, and age groups. The following characteristics frequently are present: displacement from a culture that has no preference for a thin female physique to one that does; the existence of an upwardly mobile family orientation; and individual tendencies toward compulsivity, perfectionism, and high achievement.

Etiology and Risk Factors

The etiology of eating disorders is multifactorial. No single biological, psychological, or sociocultural determinant provides an explanation for their occurrence. These disorders almost certainly are the result of interactions between the family and cultural milieu. Within a developmental framework, the physical environment, the personality, and biological predisposing factors all contribute to the disorder. When a susceptible individual under cultural pressure to be thin begins to diet and lose weight, she or he may become trapped in a self-perpetuating cycle of psychological reinforcers and physiological changes that lead to the escalation of the symptoms to the level of a true eating disorder. Teachers and others who are important adults in the lives of children and adolescents can do much to counteract negative sociocultural influences. By gaining a knowledge and understanding of the determinants and risk factors for eating disorders, teachers and other school professionals will be able to recognize students at risk and intervene when appropriate.

The Role of the School Professional

The School Physician

In the role of health educator, the physician can make a major contribution to prevention programs for school personnel, students, parents, and the community. The physician can attempt to influence attitudes about what constitutes a desirable body size and shape, can try to offset media influences by pointing out incongruities in advertising, and can dispel myths regarding special diets, foods and supplements, exercise, and other "health promoting" practices such as prolonged fasting, colonic irrigations, and the use of laxatives.

The school physician should take action against any erroneous information or blatant distortion of data being presented in the classroom as scientific fact. The school physician should be aware of dietary and weight reduction advice given by uninformed peers and adults. When recommendations to lose weight to reach a particular weight for sports or dance participation are inappropriate, the physician should take steps to correct such advice.

The physician should be available to consult on patients suspected of having an eating disorder referred by the school nurse. A knowledge of the diagnostic criteria as well as the physical changes of anorexia and bulimia is required. Such detailed information is available in standard textbooks. If convinced that a student has an eating disorder, the school physician should assist in a referral to the student's primary care physician or other appropriate facility. The physician should assume responsibility, along with the school nurse, to see that follow-up care takes place.

The school physician can play an important role in the management of the patient with an eating disorder while the student is attending school and following return to school after hospitalization. Working with the primary care physician or specialist, the school physician can help monitor vital signs, weight, physical activity, and eating behaviors while at school. In consultation with the student's personal physician, the school physician also can help to determine what the student's activity level and degree of involvement in physical education should be after returning to school.

The physician may wish to serve as a resource to classroom teachers, providing lectures to large groups of students or meeting in small groups with students known to be engaging in food restriction or purging. Although it is unlikely that lectures or small group meetings of this kind can prevent or arrest a process already underway, it may help the student who is vulnerable but not yet fully affected.

The Child's Personal Physician

The personal physician for the patient with an eating disorder should serve as a bridge between the child, the family, the specialist or team treating the eating disorder, and the school. It is a vital role, in that education must continue during long absences from school due to hospitalization. Communication is essential during reentry into school, and the personal physician must be kept informed of any changes at school that may indicate poor compliance or relapse.

The School Nurse

The school nurse or nurse practitioner is a key person in a variety of areas: (1) as health educator; (2) as case finder; (3) as a resource to teachers and other personnel; (4) as a link between the student's physician and the school physician, teachers, and administration; (5) as a day-to-day provider and monitor of care, including monitoring of medication compliance; and (6) as a role model to students with regard to appropriate attitudes and behaviors regarding food, eating, and a commonsense perspective on physical appearance and attributes.

The educational activities described for the school physician apply to the school nurse as well. The nurse can become involved more directly in counseling individual students at high risk for, or already afflicted with, an eating disorder. The nurse can help plan the health instruction curriculum and ensure that the wide range of problems associated with eating disorders are addressed. She or he can monitor and promote a school environment and programs designed to counter existing school and community pressures for extreme thinness. By discouraging inappropriate dieting and minimizing anxiety regarding fitness, nutrition, and body size and shape, the nurse can bring balance to programs that encourage physical fitness through strenuous exercise and severe caloric restriction.

An alert nurse can "spot" students who appear unusually thin or emaciated. Moreover, the nurse can respond to teachers' reports of individual (or groups of) students involved in prolonged or intense dieting or self-induced vomiting or laxative abuse.

The nurse should be actively involved in the care of the ambulatory student with an eating disorder or the student returning from a long absence following hospitalization. Instructions should be obtained from the student's personal physician regarding frequency of weighing, vital signs, signs of relapse, and appropriate response to such frequent occurrences as syncope or episodes of weakness or muscle cramping.

Probably one of the most difficult tasks of the school nurse is educating other school professionals regarding the science of nutrition and physical fitness. Administrators, teachers, teacher's aides, coaches, health aides, and other school personnel are subject to the same misconceptions and biases as others in the community. Attitudes perpetuated by the media, misinformation disseminated through advertising by the health food industry, and misconceptions promoted by nonorthodox sources contribute to the well-intentioned, but misleading, lessons being taught. Nurses and physicians must first examine themselves for gaps in their knowledge and for biases, and then work with others to dispel myths and to correct erroneous beliefs. There are anecdotal reports of teachers instructing students to fast for 2, 3, or more days in order to "cleanse their systems." Recommendations have been given for health foods that will "lubricate your joints." Offhand comments such as, "you can never be too thin," may give the wrong messages. Wrestlers may attempt to "make weight" by eating only grapefruit for 2 or 3 days prior to a meet. Dance students may be encouraged through praise of performance to maintain below normal weights in spite of untoward effects such as decreased calcium deposition in bones and loss of menstrual periods. Many students are reinforced in their almost magical beliefs regarding "good" and "bad" foods and will eliminate essential components of their diet, often on the advice of a well-intentioned, but misinformed, adult. Students are very accepting of such information. Nurses should work to ensure that accurate information is provided to all school personnel and that unhealthful student and staff practices are discouraged.

The Classroom Teacher

The classroom teacher will usually not go beyond the scope of his or her expertise. The teacher can be helped to distinguish between what is accepted current nutrition knowledge and what constitutes a personal bias or belief. The teacher also must try to identify attitudes and prejudices within himself or herself that may influence students. Along with women physicians and other female professionals, female teachers are among a group likely to have had an eating disorder or to have dealt with similar stressors and feelings as those with an eating disorder.[3,4] One fourth of college women have extremely high levels of body preoccupation and anorexic-like symptoms;[5] 15% of female medical students give a history of lifetime struggles with an eating disorder;[4] 79% of college women report eating episodes beyond their control;[6] and self-induced vomiting is very common among college women.[3] It would appear that many classroom teachers bring with them into the classroom a past experience and orientation not different from that of many of their students. This allows positive identification with students, but it is important that teachers acknowledge these feelings when they are present and take steps to avoid overidentification to the point of accepting or excusing their students' attitudes and behaviors. It is equally important that teachers work actively to counteract such attitudes in their students.

Classroom teachers can be aware of particular students that are at high risk for developing an eating disorder. Those teaching in private schools and those with a large number of affluent students should anticipate encountering students with an eating disorder on a regular basis. For those teaching lower socioeconomic students in public schools, they should be alert for the minority student from a family that puts a high priority on academic achievement and economic success. The student who is perfectionistic, compulsive about her work, and who seems to achieve beyond her capabilities fits the description of many anorectic patients. Bulimic patients are more likely to have problems with impulse control, to be sensitive about rejection, to have a history of childhood maladjustment, and to be from a dysfunctional family.

Students who have a history of irregular menstrual periods may be more likely to develop anorexia. Those at high risk of developing an eating disorder include girls and young women who serve as role models for other females. These include ballet dancers, models, gymnasts, and cheerleaders. The teacher may wish to observe these students for excessive weight loss or to be watchful for signs of severe caloric restriction or alert to student conversations that might indicate group involvement in binging and vomiting.

When the classroom teacher becomes aware that a student has lost a large amount of weight, observes that the student is increasingly distractable and excessively physically active even while in class, learns that she or he is refusing to eat lunch, and sees that previously perfect school work has begun to deteriorate, a consultation with the school nurse is in order. It is preferable to consult first with the nurse, rather than to immediately talk with the parent.

It is difficult not to reinforce the student's striving for perfection and compulsive attitude about homework and classroom work. However, for individual students whose need to be perfect creates major anxiety, consultation with the nurse or school psychologist should be undertaken.

The Physical Education Teacher and Coach

Ideally, regular planning conferences should take place with the school physician, nurse, coaches, and physical education (PE) teachers. It is the responsibility of the school administration, school health program director, and the school physician to be sure that misinformation and/or unorthodox practices are not occurring in the classroom or on the playing field. A major problem is the imposition of personal feelings by a coach or teacher regarding what constitutes a healthful diet, a desired weight for a particular sport or dance, and the intensity of training or physical exercise required. Often these add to the stress of the individual vulnerable to developing an eating disorder or seriously jeopardize the health or recovery of the student already involved in one.

The coach and PE teacher are very valuable in identifying those students in need of help. Coaches and instructors who work with athletes for whom body appearance and size are vital to the sport or dance can function as case finders and also as members of the team handling eating disorders. Health professionals rely on coaches, instructors, and PE teachers to set limits on the timing of return to a particular activity and the intensity of that activity. Without their cooperation, the eating disorder recovery program can be seriously undermined.

Diagnosis, Initial Intervention, and Long-term Management

The diagnostic criteria for anorexia nervosa and bulimia nervosa have been standardized by the American Psychiatric Association. The approach to the diagnosis of eating disorders may be found in standard textbooks of pediatrics, adolescent medicine, and internal medicine as well as in many review articles. It is generally agreed that early diagnosis and intervention improve outcome, particularly for patients with anorexia. School personnel are in an excellent position to identify students with anorexia and, to a lesser extent, bulimia. Often parents are unaware of even major losses of weight in their adolescent children. This may be because they rarely see them undressed and because there may be an element of denial of the seriousness of the problem. Moreover, a majority of parents are pleased with the weight loss and dietary restrictions they observe in their children, becoming aware of the extent of weight loss or the binging and purging only very late in the process. School nurses monitor student weights and may have to deal with symptoms associated with an eating disorder such as syncopal episodes. Physical education teachers and coaches are among a limited number of people who can observe patients with eating disorders without the bulky clothing usually worn by anorectics and some bulimics. Teachers are often privy to conversations among students discussing a classmate's extreme dieting or about communal binging and purging. If school staff members act on their suspicions or information, they have done the student a great service.

Eating disorders are chronic and recurrent conditions, often necessitating repeated and extended absences from school. Administrators and teachers can be of great help by doing everything possible to allow the student to maintain good academic standing.

Anorectics and many bulimics are usually serious students who have much anxiety about falling behind. Teachers can be of great help in supporting the student undergoing treatment. By working with the hospital-based teacher, school personnel can ensure that examinations can be administered in hospital under the proctorship of the hospital-certified teacher. School administrators and counselors can assist by arranging for special tutors if it becomes necessary.

For a few students with eating disorders, it may become necessary to provide skilled career counseling. Particularly for anorectic students, helping the students realize their capabilities and limitations can be of major import, but it must be accomplished with much sensitivity and tact. Many anorectics achieve far beyond their capabilities, but at great emotional expense. Most patients with eating disorders, with the exception of many bulimics, feel a pressure to achieve. Both anorectics and bulimics rely excessively on the environment, particularly their parents, for their sense of self-worth, also making them very vulnerable to cultural pressures to achieve. They are more likely to experience anxiety, depression, and to be very sensitive to criticism by others. Suicidal behavior is not uncommon. Many are socially isolated. It is understandable that the professional who elects to counsel the young person regarding changes in career goals must do so with attention to these personality characteristics in the student. On the other hand, it is more humane to help the patient deal realistically with career goals prior to embarking on what may be too difficult a task, than to suffer devastating failures later.

Prevention

Until more is known about the etiology of eating disorders, approaches to prevention will continue to be empiric. Attempts to reduce societal pressures that equate thinness with beauty, success, and control should be encouraged. In this area, schools can do much to counter media messages and existing attitudes. Parenting is another area in which schools can exert influence. Parenting classes not only can stress more appropriate attitudes about body size and appearance, but also can address normal development and the emotional needs of children and adolescents. Measures can be taken to reduce enmeshment between children and parents in order to encourage the timely development of autonomy. A reasonable and balanced approach to exercise and diet can be stressed in school health curricula. Early education of students with regard to the fallacy of using weight and appetite control as a way of coping and gaining control over their emotions is another area of education that deserves emphasis.

Prognosis and Outcome

The prognosis for most young people with an eating disorder is relatively good if intervention occurs early and the treatment is multidimensional and of high quality. The outcome for both anorexia and bulimia depends on the severity and the number of risk factors present in the individual. The risk factors have to do with: (1) the patient's psychological makeup, including personality, body image, self-image, and sexuality; (2) the patient's family; (3) the patient's early development, particularly the process of separation; and (4) genetic and biological influences, including genetic influences on temperament, hunger, appetite, and neuroendocrine function. Outcome depends on the intensity of therapy directed at the above factors, including a response to medication, and the level of family, community, and school support available. Of course, much depends on the individual patient's capacity for insight, willingness to work at changing, and ability to change in the face of often severe emotional deficits.

References

1. Maloney MJ, McGuire J, Daniels SR, Specker B. Dieting behavior and eating attitudes in children. *Pediatrics*. 1989;84:482-489

2. Huenemann RL, Shapiro LR, Hampton MC, Mitchell BW. A longitudinal study of gross body composition and body conformation and their association with food and activity in a teen-age population: views of teen-age subjects on body conformation, food, and activity. *Am J Clin Nutr*. 1966;18:325-338

3. Halmi KA, Falk JR, Schwartz E. Binge-eating and vomiting: a survey of a college population. *Psychol Med*. 1981;11:697-706

4. Herzog DB, Pepose M, Norman DK, Rigotti NA. Eating disorders and social maladjustment in female medical students. *J Nerv Ment Dis*. 1985;173:734-737

5. Schwartz DM, Thompson MG. Do anorectics get well? Current research and future needs. *Am J Psychiatry*. 1981;138:319-323

6. Hawkins RC, Clement PF. Development and construct validation of a self-report measure of binge eating tendencies. *Addict Behav*. 1980;5:219-226

CHAPTER 26

SCHOOLS AND SEXUALITY EDUCATION

Sexuality Education

Today's children and youth are growing up in an increasingly complex world, bombarded by sexual messages and conflicting and confusing cultural messages about sexual values and morality. The need for sexual literacy is acute. High percentages of teenagers are involved in intimate sexual relationships before they leave high school, or even junior high school. The family structure in the United States has continued to change as a result of rising out-of-wedlock births, high divorce rates, emerging reproductive technologies, and changing gender roles. The HIV/AIDS epidemic has made even more imperative the need to help young people make responsible sexual choices.

Sexuality education is the lifelong process of acquiring information and forming attitudes, beliefs, and values about identity, relationships, and intimacy. School-based sexuality education is more than teaching young people about anatomy and the physiology of reproduction. It includes an understanding of sexuality in its broadest context—sexual development, reproductive health, interpersonal relationships, affection and intimacy, body image, and gender roles. Parents, peers, schools, religion, the media, friends, and partners all influence learning about sexuality for people at every stage of life.[1]

Sexuality Education in the United States

Only a few US communities offer comprehensive sexuality education programs at all grade levels. Although between two thirds and three fourths of students say they have received some sexuality education by the time they graduate from high school, few have participated in programs from kindergarten through the 12th grade.[2] Most school systems wait until junior high school or high school to teach human sexuality. Sexuality education topics are most likely first introduced in the 9th and 10th grade as part of a discussion of another subject, often health or physical education. The average amount of time spent on these topics is under 12 hours in seventh grade and only 18 hours by 12th grade.[3] Most teachers think that materials dealing with sexually transmitted diseases (STDs) and teenage pregnancy should be taught by the end of the seventh grade; but, in reality, they frequently are not taught until high school.[4]

Most professional educators believe it is important for school systems to implement comprehensive kindergarten through 12th grade (K-12) programs, with the subject matter and content of the course appropriate to each age and grade/developmental level. In the earlier grades, sexuality education topics can be integrated into comprehensive health education programs and can help children learn about family relationships, growth and development, self-esteem, and good health habits. They can help children begin to identify peer pressure and develop decision-making skills. These programs will become more specific about human sexuality as the children approach puberty.

Children need comprehensive health education from preschool through college. Comprehensive health education should include broad-based sexuality related issues, not just anatomy and abstinence. Ideally, schools would offer independent sexuality courses as part of an overall health education initiative. Sexuality courses are able to address the broadest range of sexual issues in the context of health education and health promotion. In many communities, however, sexuality education will be integrated into existing health courses. Some communities gradually phase in sexuality education, first offering a special elective taught by community professionals, then moving to integrate it into the health program.

Goals and Content of Sexuality Education

Sexuality Education Programs: Four Important Goals

Information: Young people will have accurate information about human sexuality including: growth and development, human reproduction, anatomy, physiology, masturbation, family life, pregnancy, childbirth, parenthood, sexual response, sexual orientation, contraception, abortion, sexual abuse, HIV/AIDS, and other sexually transmitted diseases.

Attitudes, Values, and Insights: Young people will question, explore, and assess sexual attitudes and feelings in order to develop their own values, increase their self-esteem, develop their insights concerning relationships with members of both genders, and understand their obligations and responsibilities to others.

Relationships and Interpersonal Skills: Young people will develop interpersonal skills, including communication, decision making, assertiveness, peer refusal skills, and the ability to create satisfying relationships. Sexuality education programs should prepare students to understand their sexuality effectively and creatively in adult roles, for example, as spouse, partner, parent, community member, and citizen. This includes helping them develop capacities for caring, supportive, noncoercive, and mutually pleasurable intimate and sexual relationships.

Responsibility: Young people will exercise responsibility in their sexual relationships by understanding abstinence and how to resist pressures to become prematurely involved in sexual intercourse, as well as by encouraging the use of contraception and other sexual health measures. Sexuality education should be a central component of programs designed to reduce the prevalence of sexually related health problems, including teenage pregnancies, sexually transmitted diseases (including HIV infection), and sexual abuse.

Education regarding HIV and AIDS should take place within the context of comprehensive health and sexuality education. It should not be taught as an isolated program but should rather be integrated into an approach that includes the objectives listed above. The HIV/AIDS unit should address five primary objectives:

1. *Reducing Misinformation:* Eliminate misinformation about HIV infection and transmission and reduce the panic associated with the disease.
2. *Delaying Premature Sexual Intercourse:* Help young people delay premature sexual intercourse; this includes teaching young people to recognize the implications of their actions and to gain the communication skills with which to confront peer pressure and negotiate resistance.
3. *Supporting Safer Sex:* Help teenagers who are sexually active to use condoms each and every time they have any

kind of intercourse or only practice those sexual behaviors that do not place one at risk of pregnancy, sexually transmitted diseases, or HIV infection.

4. *Preventing Drug Abuse:* Warn children about the dangers of drug use and teach young people the skills with which to confront peer pressure and negotiate resistance.

5. *Developing Compassion for People With AIDS:* Encourage compassion for people with AIDS and for people who are infected with HIV.

In 1991 the Sex Information and Education Council of the United States (SIECUS) convened a national task force of health, education, and sexuality professionals to develop national guidelines for sexuality education. Task force members included representatives from the US Centers for Disease Control, the American Medical Association, the National School Boards Association, the National Education Association, the March of Dimes Birth Defects Foundation, and the Planned Parenthood Federation of America, as well as experienced school-based sexuality education teachers.

The task force developed national guidelines for a comprehensive K-12 approach to sexuality education. Six key concepts representing the highest level of generality of knowledge of human sexuality and family living were generated. These key concepts form the basis of a comprehensive sexuality education program to be taught at an age-appropriate level in all grades. Table 54 lists these key concepts and important topics to be covered. A complete copy of the guidelines is available from SIECUS, 130 W 42nd St, Suite 2500, New York, NY 10036.

Values in Sexuality Education Programs

The question of values is one of the most difficult ones facing HIV/AIDS and sexuality education programs. Each community, school board, and school has to decide which values will be part of its program. School-based education programs must be carefully developed to respect the diversity of values and beliefs represented in each community.

Some people believe that sexuality and HIV/AIDS education should be "value-free." Yet, because sexuality represents the most intimate part of people's lives, sexuality and HIV/AIDS education cannot be taught without a discussion of values and

Table 54. — Key Concepts and Topics to be Covered in a K–12 Curriculum

KEY CONCEPT 1: Human development is characterized by the interrelationship between physical, emotional, social, intellectual, and spiritual growth.

TOPICS
Reproductive anatomy and physiology
Reproduction
Puberty
Body image
Sexual orientation

KEY CONCEPT 2: Relationships play a central role throughout our lives.

TOPICS
Families
Friendships
Love
Dating
Marriage and divorce
Parenthood

KEY CONCEPT 3: Healthy sexuality requires the development and use of specific personal and interpersonal skills.

TOPICS
Values
Decision making
Communication
Assertiveness
Negotiation
Finding help

KEY CONCEPT 4: Sexuality is central to being human and individuals express their sexuality in a variety of different ways.

TOPICS
Sexuality through the life cycle
Masturbation
Shared sexual behaviors
Abstinence
Human sexual response
Fantasy
Sexual dysfunction

Table 54. — Key Concepts and Topics to be Covered in a K–12 Curriculum (continued)

KEY CONCEPT 5: Promotion of sexual health requires that individuals have information, knowledge, and attitudes necessary to avoid unwanted consequences of their sexual behavior.

TOPICS
Contraception
Abortion
HIV and STDs
Sexual abuse
Reproductive health

KEY CONCEPT 6: Social and cultural environments shape the way individuals learn about, experience, and express their sexuality.

TOPICS
Gender roles
Sexuality and the law
Sexuality and religion
Sexuality in the arts
Diversity
Sexuality and the media

attitudes. Indeed, one of the hallmarks of a comprehensive sexuality education program is that it gives young people the opportunity to develop their own values about sexual issues.

Some communities in the United States have taken a lesson from Sweden, where a practical approach to sexuality education has been developed. The curriculum is divided into "fundamental values" and "controversial values" – those values that are to be treated without taking sides by the school.

If the program is to be accepted and supported, it is wise to base the core values of the program on the shared values of the community. Also it is important to state the values of the program specifically and share them with parents, teachers, school administrators, and the community.

It is, of course, essential that sexuality and HIV/AIDS education programs respect and recognize the diversity of values about such issues as contraception, abortion, and premarital intercourse. In the words of New York State Governor Mario Cuomo, "It seems to me clear that responsible sex education

that recognizes and respects the different moral values in our society . . . is an appropriate part of the public school curriculum."[5] The following statements are likely to be accepted as "core values" in most American schools:
- Sexuality is a natural and healthy part of living.
- Sexuality is more than sex.
- Abstaining from sexual intercourse is the best method of pregnancy and HIV prevention for many teenagers.
- Young people who are involved in sexual activity and relationships need access to information about health care services.
- People should respect the diversity of values and beliefs about sexuality that exist in a community.
- Sexual relationships should never be coercive or exploitative.
- All children should be loved and cared for.
- It is wrong to spread disease knowingly.
- Knowledge about sexuality is helpful; ignorance is harmful.
- Every person has dignity and self-worth; enhanced self-esteem helps in making healthy and responsible decisions.
- All sexual decisions have effects or consequences; each person has the right to make responsible sexual choices.
- Everyone benefits when children are able to discuss sexuality with their parents and/or other trusted adults.

In many communities, teaching about controversial issues represents one of the most difficult aspects of sexuality and HIV/AIDS education.[6] It *is* possible to teach about sexuality and HIV/AIDS without discussing controversial issues, but it is not likely to be very effective if controversial issues are ignored. Basic information about anatomy and reproduction can be integrated into a biology class without much discomfort, as well as information about HIV infection, epidemiology, and disease symptoms. However, it is very unlikely that such discussions will encourage or assist young people in adopting safer sexual behaviors or the ability to have meaningful interpersonal relationships.

Four issues – abortion, contraception, masturbation, and homosexuality – often dominate the controversy over what is to be taught in sexuality education. According to the Alan Guttmacher Institute, more than 40% of the teachers at the high school level who are providing sexuality education do *not* teach about condom use, sexual orientation, abortion, and safe sex practices.[7] Even fewer discuss the pleasures of sexuality.

Many parents feel that a crucial objective of sexuality education is lost if the course is less than comprehensive. Young people's sexual decision-making skills cannot be enhanced unless they are made aware that they do have options and choices – especially in the "controversial areas." These parents stress that a range of varying and/or conflicting views, attitudes, and judgments exist and that students should be exposed to the whole range. Following such discussions in classes, young people can be urged to discuss these subjects with their parents, religious advisors, and other trusted adults.

In Connecticut, there is a State Board of Education policy on teaching controversial issues that may be appropriate for adaptation by other states and communities:

> Learning to deal with controversial issues is one of the basic competencies all students should acquire. . . . Controversy is inherent in the democratic way of life. The study and discussion of controversial issues is essential to the education for citizenship in free society. Students can become informed individuals only through the process of examining evidence, facts and differing viewpoints, by exercising freedom of thought and moral choice, and by making responsible decisions. . . . Teachers should also endeavor to develop a flexibility of viewpoint in students so that they are able to recognize the need for continuous and objective re-examination of issues in the light of changing conditions in society and as new and significant evidence becomes available to support a change of view. . . . Teachers do not have the right to indoctrinate students with their personal view.[8]

Teachers and school boards need to decide how to approach controversial issues. Teachers often need special training or preparation to deal with these issues. Many teachers advocate presenting both sides (or all the sides, if there are more than two). For example, schools can invite representatives of "pro-choice" organizations to send speakers to their programs; this can be balanced the next day with a speaker from a group that is "pro-life." It is generally not wise to set up debates between outside organizations; these usually become confrontations with more heat generated than clarification of issues for students.

Debates among students, however, can be used as an effective learning activity. For example, students can be randomly assigned to research the following debate question: "Teenagers need parental permission to obtain birth control." One group of students could develop arguments for the "pro" side; the other could develop arguments for minors' rights; and a debate could ensue.

At times, school policies have stated that certain topics cannot be part of the curriculum. One way for programs to handle these issues is to have a written policy that those who teach sexuality education can answer students' questions on subjects not covered in the approved curriculum. This will protect the teachers, provide a way to be responsive to the students' needs, and allow for group discussion.

Some communities decide that certain issues need not be presented as controversial. They clearly state the values of the program and, although respectful and tolerant of other points of view if expressed by students, they do not actively present those. For example, most sexologists believe that masturbation is a natural and nonharmful behavior and that no one should be made to feel guilty for masturbating. Thus, most communities do not present the view that masturbation is sinful or dangerous. Other programs underscore the value that sexually active teenagers need information about sources of contraception and present the view that it is proper to tell teens about family planning.

Support for Sexuality Education

It is a tribute to the common sense of the American people that despite all the attempts to make sexuality and HIV/AIDS education appear "controversial," most adults support school-based programs. More revealing is the fact that those parents most concerned – the parents of children who are in school – are found to favor this education even more strongly than the general public. More than 8 in 10 parents want sexuality education taught in high schools; three fourths of adults in a national sample (which includes both parents and nonparents) agree.[9] A majority of parents say these courses should teach about premarital sex, sexual intercourse, abortion, and homosexuality.[9]

Support for AIDS education in schools is even higher; 94% of parents think public schools should have an HIV/AIDS education program, and only 4% think they should not. More than 8 out of 10 parents want their children to be taught about safe sex as a way of preventing AIDS.[10]

Parents of students provide their support for sexuality education in another way. When parents are given the option of excusing their children from sexuality education classes, less than 1% to 5% do so.[9]

National health and education organizations support sexuality education. More than 35 national organizations have passed policies in support of sexuality education, and more than 60 national organizations have joined together as the National Coalition to Support Sexuality Education, a coalition of organizations that support the goal that all children and youth will receive sexuality education by the year 2000. Coalition members include such national organizations as the American Medical Association, the National Education Association, the YWCA of the United States, the American Nurses Association, the Children's Defense Fund, the American School Health Association, and the National Urban League.[11] A list of coalition members current as of 1992 is Table 55.

School Health Services and Sexuality Education

Classroom-based sexuality education programs should be coordinated with the school health services. In the primary grades, the school nurse and school social worker can play an important role in supplementing classroom teachers' presentations of this subject matter. In junior and senior high schools, the programs should be taught by especially prepared teachers. School health personnel can offer their expertise to teachers and provide lectures on specific medical topics such as growth and development and contraception. Further, these personnel should examine how the health service can support the programs in the classroom. Medical and nursing personnel can provide information to the teachers on students' sexual health concerns, as well as provide confidential counseling and support to young people with questions. Special efforts can be made to reach those young people at highest risk for the morbidity of sexual behaviors –

Table 55. — The National Coalition to Support Sexuality Education

The following organizations have joined together to assure that all children and youth receive comprehensive sexuality education.

The Alan Guttmacher Institute
American Association for Marriage and Family Therapy
American Association on Mental Retardation
American Association of School Administrators
American Association of Sex Educators, Counselors, and Therapists
American College of Obstetricians and Gynecologists
American Counseling Association
American Home Economics Association
American Library Association
American Medical Association
American Nurses Association
The American Orthopsychiatric Association, Inc
American Psychological Association
American Public Health Association
American School Health Association
American Social Health Association
Association for the Advancement of Health Education
Association of Reproductive Health Professionals
Association of State and Territorial Directors of Public Health Education
Astraea National Lesbian Action Foundation
B'nai B'rith Women
Catholics for a Free Choice
Center for Population Options
Child Welfare League of America
Children's Defense Fund
Coalition on Sexuality and Disability, Inc
Commission on Family Ministries and Human Sexuality, National
    Council of the Churches
ETR Associates
Girls, Inc
Hetrick-Martin Institute for Gay and Lesbian Youth
The Institute for Advanced Study of Human Sexuality Alumni Association
Midwest School Social Work Council
National Abortion Rights Action League
National Association of Counties
National Association of School Psychologists
National Coalition of Advocates for Students

Table 55. — The National Coalition to Support Sexuality Education (continued)

National Council on Family Relations
National Council of State Consultants for School Social Work Services
National Education Association Health Information Network
National Family Planning & Reproductive Health Association
National Gay and Lesbian Task Force
National Information Center for Children & Youth With Disabilities
National League for Nursing
National Lesbian and Gay Health Foundation
National Mental Health Association
National Network of Runaway & Youth Services
National Organization on Adolescent Pregnancy & Parenting
National Resource Center for Youth Services
National School Boards Association
National Urban League
Planned Parenthood Federation of America, Inc
Sex Information and Education Council of the United States
Society for Adolescent Medicine
Society for Behavioral Pediatrics
Society for Public Health Education, Inc
Society for the Scientific Study of Sex
Unitarian Universalist Association
United Church Board for Homeland Ministries
United States Conference of Local Health Officers
United States Conference of Mayors
University of Pennsylvania
YWCA of the United States

teenagers engaging in unprotected sexual intercourse as well as those involved in substance abuse and those at risk for dropping out of school. The school medical and nursing personnel should be comfortable providing such services to heterosexual and gay and lesbian youth. Further, the health service can provide pamphlets and booklets on such health concerns as birth control, STDs, decision making about sexuality, and sexual orientation issues. School health services should develop a referral list of community services, such as clinics dealing with family planning and STDs, prenatal clinics, hot lines, mental health centers, and gay and lesbian community centers.

The community-based pediatrician has an important role to play in supporting school-based sexuality education programs. Pediatricians are important members of community advisory boards, which are mandated in many areas. These community advisory boards often assist in curriculum design and selection as well as community education. Pediatricians may be able to assist with the presentation of medical information and they can be persuasive advocates for the program at community and school board meetings. They can also help train teachers in child and adolescent growth and development. The local medical society can pass resolutions in support of the program.

Resources for More Information

Numerous resources exist for helping school systems develop and implement sexuality and HIV/AIDS education programs. Some states have developed curricula guidelines for school programs and have resource people in the State Department of Education to assist local communities. The Sex Information and Education Council of the United States (SIECUS), has developed national guidelines for sexuality education programs and a step-by-step guide for implementing programs in a community. There are numerous curricula and teaching materials available from many publishers. Several organizations such as the American Association of Sex Educators, Counselors, and Therapists; the National Council of Family Relations, and the Society for the Scientific Study of Sex offer continuing education programs for teachers. Local colleges and universities may also offer training courses. While a complete list of resources is beyond the scope of this chapter, the addresses and phone numbers of key national organizations that provide resources in sexuality education is provided in the Resource List.

Resource List

The Alan Guttmacher Institute
111 Fifth Ave
New York, NY 10010
212/254-5656

American Association of Sex Educators,
Counselors and Therapists (AASECT)
Suite 1717
Chicago, IL 60611-4067
312/644-0828

American School Health Association
7263 State Route 43
PO Box 708
Kent, OH 44240
216/678-1601

Centers for Disease Control and Prevention,
Division of Adolescent and School Health
1600 Clifton Rd NE
Mail Stop K-31
Atlanta, GA 30333
404/488-5362

ETR Associates
PO Box 1830
Santa Cruz, CA 95061-1830
408/429-9822

National Council on Family
Relations (NCFR)
3989 Central Ave NE
Suite 550
Minneapolis, MN 55421
612/781-9331

Planned Parenthood Federation of America (PPFA)
810 Seventh Ave
New York, NY 10019
212/603-4632

Sex Information and Education Council of the United States (SIECUS)

130 W 42nd St
Suite 2500
New York, NY 10036
212/819-9770

Society for the Scientific Study of Sex (SSSS)

PO Box 208
Mt Vernon, IA 52314
319/895-8407

References

1. Position Statement. Sex Information and Education Council of the United States, January 1990

2. Sonenstein F, Pittman K. The availability of sex education in large city school districts. *Fam Plann Perspect*. 1986;16(1):19-25

3. Forrest J, Silverman J. What public school teachers teach about preventing pregnancy, AIDS, and sexually transmitted diseases. *Fam Plann Perspect*. 1989;21(2):65-71

4. Donovan P. *Risk and Responsibility: Teaching Sex Education in America's Schools Today*. New York, NY: Alan Guttmacher Institute; 1989

5. Cuomo M. *Speech to the Family Planning Advocates of New York Annual Meeting*. Albany, NY; 1990

6. Haffner D, DeMauro D. *Winning the Battle: Developing Support for Sexuality and HIV/AIDS Education*. New York, NY: SIECUS; 1991

7. Donovan P. *Risk and Responsibility: Teaching Sex Education in America's Schools Today*. New York, NY: Alan Guttmacher Institute; 1989;8-11

8. *Teaching About Controversial Issues*. Policy adopted by Connecticut State Board of Education; October 4, 1978

9. Gallup A, Clark D. *The 19th Annual Gallup Poll of the Public's Attitudes Towards the Public School*. Gallup Polls; 1987;69(1):13

10. Gallup A, Clark D. *The 19th Annual Gallup Poll of the Public's Attitudes Towards the Public School*. Gallup Polls; 1987;69(1):42

11. Haffner D. *Sex Education 2000: A Call To Action*. New York, NY: SIECUS; 1990

CHAPTER 27

THE STUDENT ATHLETE

Why Sports?

Intramural and interscholastic athletic programs can provide valuable educational experiences for all participants. School intramural athletic programs should strike a balance between maximizing participation and allowing for skilled and un-skilled athletes to participate at levels commensurate with their abilities. The school sports programs, both intramural and in-terscholastic, should safeguard athletes' health by stressing proper conditioning and providing good coaching, capable offici-ating, proper equipment and facilities, and adequate health supervision.

More than 5 million American high school boys and girls com-pete in interscholastic sports each year. Sports can foster a degree of self-confidence in youth, although this may not be the case if humiliation, sarcasm, and negative feedback are used as coaching techniques. Experiencing the "thrill of victory" as well as the "anguish of defeat" can help prepare the athlete to cope with the inevitable successes and failures of adult life. If the students participate in team sports, they learn how to cooperate while competing. Learning to make "self-sacrifices" for the good of the team can assist the person in later life when faced with choices involving personal gain versus that which would be good for the group (such as the company or the family). The young person who becomes interested in athletics might also be condi-tioned to follow as an adult a life-style that includes regular physical activity, with its benefits of longevity, weight control, and positive self-image.

The Risks

The major scholastic competitive sports are not free of risks. Football is by far the most dangerous high school sport, at least when measuring the frequency of injuries. More than 600,000 high school players are injured each year, defining injury as one severe enough to cause the athlete to suspend activities for at least a day.[1] Each high school football team will average one player hospitalized with an injury each season, and another player will require surgery at a later time. About five boys are rendered quadriplegic each year in the United States playing high school football, and a similar number sustain a fatal injury, generally an intracranial hemorrhage. Ice hockey has proportionally more catastrophic neck injuries than does football.[2] Wrestling and girls gymnastics are generally the next two sports, after football and ice hockey, in which a significant risk for injury exists. All parents and student athletes should be aware of these risks, and the school should maintain a valid consent form for each participant. The benefits accruing from the athletic experience would seem to outweigh the possible risks, with the sole exception of boxing, a "sport" that both the Academy and the American Medical Association condemn.

Girls in Sports

As there are no significant differences in the average physical size or ability between prepubescent boys or girls, there is no medical reason to separate them for interscholastic or intramural sports, or for that matter, any recreational activity. However, by the time a girl has completed puberty, most boys of similar chronological age are well into their own pubertal growth and are bigger, faster, and stronger. Gender-specific sports participation after puberty begins is therefore reasonable and gives girls an opportunity to excel when competing against each other.

Some high school girls have attempted to compete for a place on the "boys'" team when there were no girls' teams in the same sport, such as wrestling and ice hockey. Most school districts have had rules preventing this, presumably in the belief that girls, being on the average smaller and less strong, would be more likely to be hurt when competing against boys, particularly in collision sports such as football or ice hockey. However well-meaning the original reason for the rule was, it does not stand up to either logical or judicial scrutiny. In every high school, there will be a number of boys who are not as big and strong as many of the girls, yet there are no rules preventing those smaller and lighter boys from competing for the boys' team. Many girls who were prevented from competing have taken their cases to court, and they have *invariably* won the right to compete on the boys' team. The AAP legal counsel reviewed the judicial experiences regarding this question in 1986 and concluded that there was no legal justification for a school rule that would prevent a girl from competing for a place on a boys' athletic team *in a sport in which there was no girls' team in that school*. In fact, to do so would be a violation of the 14th Amendment.[3] Girls should therefore be allowed to compete for positions on teams in sports in which there are no teams specifically for girls, even wrestling.

However, the courts are split as to whether "reverse discrimination" (ie, keeping boys off girls' teams) is unconstitutional. The AAP legal counsel review indicated that while some court cases sustained the boys' position, others upheld the school rule.

Team Physicians

A school should obtain the services of qualified, sports-trained, and sports-oriented physicians to act as team physicians, at least for the sports associated with a high frequency of injury (football, ice hockey, and wrestling). This kind of task is usually a voluntary one, as very few public schools have the resources to pay for physician services. The team physician should report administratively to the principal or school superintendent rather than to the team coach or director of athletics. This gives the physician more authority when making recommendations to the coaches regarding incorrect conditioning techniques, unsound coaching practices, or student athlete exclusions. There are many opportunities for pediatricians to become educated about sports medicine by attending the many continuing medical education courses offered each year by the American College of Sports Medicine, the Academy, and other organizations.

Primary Responsibilities of the Team Physician

1. To approve medical eligibility of athletes for participation in the sport.
2. To approve medical eligibility of athletes to resume activity after illness or injury.

3. To know the availability of medical services at athletic events (eg, first aid procedures, arrangement for transportation to hospitals).
4. To provide immediate care to all injuries and arrange for follow-up care if that is necessary.
5. To supervise the certified athletic trainer, if one is available, during an athletic event attended by the team physician.
6. To contribute to the selection of training practices with health implications such as diets and conditioning, encourage the use of protective equipment, and participate in programs to counter drug and steroid use.

The team physician must have the final authority to determine whether any particular athlete competes. This policy should be obtained in writing from the school administration before the season, and the physician's authority should be understood by trainers, athletic directors, coaches, students, and their parents. In some states, it is written in the education code. Although an athlete's personal physician or orthopedic surgeon treating a serious injury or illness should approve the resumption of physical activity, the team or school physician should review each situation before making the final decision about a student returning to competition.

The team physician should evaluate the interim health history form (Fig 5), which should be completed by the family and/or athlete at least annually, and then decide whether a physical examination is necessary. If preparticipation physical examinations cannot be done by the athletes' personal primary care physicians, the team physician may decide to do a mass physical examination with volunteer assistants (see section on Sports Preparticipation Examination). Legal requirements also may dictate practices within each state.

When attending an athletic event the team physician should sit on the bench with the players so that injuries can be observed firsthand and minor ones can be managed at the side of the playing field. The team physician should arrive at least 30 minutes before the event to see if any of the athletes have been injured since the last game or have any current medical problems; to find out where the closest available telephone is located; to know how to summon emergency transportation to that site;

Interim Health History

This form should be used during the interval between preparticipation evaluations. Positive responses should prompt a medical evaluation.

1. Over the next 12 months, I wish to participate in the following sports:
   a. _____
   b. _____
   c. _____
   d. _____

2. Have you missed more than 3 consecutive days of participation in usual activities because of an injury this past year?
   Yes _____ No _____
   If yes, please indicate:
   a. Site of injury _____
   b. Type of injury _____

3. Have you missed more than 5 consecutive days of participation in usual activities because of an illness, or have you had a medical illness diagnosed that has not been resolved in this past year?
   Yes _____ No _____
   If yes, please indicate type of illness:
   _____

4. Have you had a seizure, concussion, or been unconscious for any reason in the last year?
   Yes _____ No _____

5. Have you had surgery or been hospitalized in this past year?
   Yes _____ No _____
   If yes, please indicate:
   a. Reason for hospitalization _____
   b. Type of surgery _____

6. List all medications you are presently taking and what condition the medication is for.
   a. _____
   b. _____
   c. _____

7. Are you worried about any problem or condition at this time?
   Yes _____ No _____
   If yes, please explain: _____
   _____
   _____

I hereby state that, to the best of my knowledge, my answers to the above question are correct.

Date _____

Signature of athlete _____

Signature of parent _____

Fig 5. Sample of interim health history form.

to inform the other team's coach of the presence of a physician; and to inspect the playing area for potentially dangerous conditions. The physician should then observe the contest closely in order to personally see any injuries that may occur.

Prior to the athletic season the team physician should meet with the players and their parents to discuss the health risks of that particular sport, ie, "making weight" in wrestling by using unwise crash weight-loss programs, taking anabolic steroids to "bulk-up" for playing football and ice hockey, and using outdated nutritional practices such as eating a meal that includes a large steak a few hours prior to an athletic event in the belief this will make the athlete stronger.

Legal Liability

Team physicians have the same responsibilities as physicians in private practice, plus an additional obligation to have professional knowledge about the medical and traumatic problems inherent in the sports they cover. To avoid or minimize legal liability, team physicians should insist on written contracts that clearly state their authority and obligations; and they should maintain complete records of medical findings and recommendations. Many states have the language of their "Good Samaritan" statutes such that acting as a volunteer physician at a school athletic event would be covered by the statute, and the physician would be immune from medical liability lawsuits. Individuals interested in such activities are strongly urged to investigate local liability issues.

Certified Athletic Trainers

Ideally, each high school should have an athletic trainer on the staff who is available to care for acute injuries during practices as well as during athletic events. Certification by the National Athletic Trainers Association should ensure a high degree of professional competence. High schools should also have a training room with weight training equipment and the equipment that would allow the trainer to apply physical therapeutic techniques to minor soft-tissue injuries.

Coaches

As most schools will have neither trainers nor physicians available at athletic practices, all school coaches should be trained in basic cardiopulmonary resuscitation. In all cases, the coaches should be knowledgeable about safe conditioning practices and be cognizant of the current philosophy of adolescent development that emphasizes positive rewards rather than negative feedback in coaching techniques.

Sports Preparticipation Examination

The two most common kinds of "sports physicals" are the health maintenance examination in a physician's office and the mass examination. *As usually performed, that is without a musculoskeletal assessment, both are notoriously ineffective in detecting abnormalities* that would either affect the athlete's performance or pose an undue risk during athletic participation. If the examination takes place in the physician's office, there is at least an opportunity to offer anticipatory guidance and assess the need for more formal counseling completely unrelated to athletics. One study indicated that about 80% of high school athletes undergoing a sports preparticipation examination had *no other annual health assessment* by a physician during the school year, so physicians should try to convert the office "sports physical" into a health maintenance examination whenever possible.[4]

A third kind of preparticipation examination—that done by a group of physicians and other personnel in "stations"—has been shown to be very effective in finding physical abnormalities. An advantage of this kind of examination is that it has volunteer physicians who frequently self-select for this task because of an interest in sports medicine and who therefore have a greater knowledge about performing the musculoskeletal component of the examination. A disadvantage is that the physician is not able to administer anticipatory guidance or perform the other components of a health maintenance examination.

After the history, the musculoskeletal component of the examination is the most productive part in revealing abnormalities that usually are residual of previous injuries and could lead to other injuries unless rehabilitative exercises are performed. Unfortunately, most physicians still concentrate on detecting medical abnormalities such as a heart murmur or inguinal hernia during preparticipation sports examinations. One large study of high school football players indicated that musculoskeletal abnormalities were detected in 10% of the players when the examination included a component quite similar to the "two-minute orthopedic examination" described in Table 56.[5]

Frequency

Health maintenance examinations should be performed at least every 2 years throughout adolescence. An interim medical history should be obtained at least annually, and the school can use it to determine whether a physical examination is necessary. Because of state laws, most school districts only require an annual physical examination. This means that an athlete could sustain an ankle sprain playing football but it would not be known when he tried out for the basketball team since he was still "covered" by the examination performed before the football season began. This is why the Academy advocates an interim medical history be completed at least annually.

Laboratory Examinations

Although a urinalysis and hemoglobin/hematocrit determination have been traditional components of sports examinations, they are not necessary for sports-related purposes. They may well be included if the examination is part of a health maintenance examination.

The Medical History

Figure 6 consists of the history component of the AAP sports participation health record.

The Examination

The preparticipation health evaluation should be conducted at least 4 to 6 weeks before the beginning of the athletic season so that previous injuries can be identified in time to be treated with rehabilitative exercises in an attempt to prevent reinjury. When the examination cannot be performed on an individual basis in a physician's office, it frequently will be conducted at the school,

Health History

To be completed by athlete and parent

		YES	NO
1. Have you ever had an illness that:			
	a. required you to stay in the hospital?	___	___
	b. lasted longer than a week?	___	___
	c. caused you to miss 3 days of practice or a competition?	___	___
	d. is related to allergies? (ie, hay fever, hives, asthma, insect stings)	___	___
	e. required an operation?	___	___
	f. is chronic? (ie, asthma, diabetes, etc)	___	___
2. Have you ever had an injury that:			
	a. required you to go to an emergency room or see a doctor?	___	___
	b. required you to stay in the hospital?	___	___
	c. required x-rays?	___	___
	d. caused you to miss 3 days of practice or a competition?	___	___
	e. required an operation?	___	___
3. Do you take any medication or pills?		___	___
4. Have any members of your family under age 50 had a heart attack, heart problem, or died unexpectedly?		___	___
5. Have you ever:			
	a. been dizzy or passed out during or after exercise?	___	___
	b. been unconscious or had a concussion?	___	___
6. Are you unable to run a half mile (2 times around the track) without stopping?		___	___
7. Do you:		___	___
	a. wear glasses or contacts?	___	___
	b. wear dental bridges, plates, or braces?	___	___

8. Have you ever had a heart murmur, high blood
pressure, or a heart abnormality?   _____ _____

9. Do you have any allergies to any medicine?   _____ _____

10. Are you missing a kidney?   _____ _____

11. When was your last tetanus booster? _____

12. For Women
    a. At what age did you experience your first
      menstrual period? _____
    b. In the last year, what is the longest time you
      have gone between periods? _____

EXPLAIN ANY "YES" ANSWERS _____

_____

_____

_____

I hereby state that, to the best of my knowledge, my answers to the
above questions are correct.

Date _____

Signature of athlete _____
Signature of parent _____

Fig 6. History component of AAP sports participation health record.

in which case a "stations" format is most efficient. Regardless of
the location of the examination, a complete musculoskeletal
examination (Table 56) should be performed carefully.

Stations Examination

The only requirements are a room large enough to accommodate
all the waiting examinees simultaneously and quiet office areas
adjacent to the larger room. This arrangement allows all exam-

Table 56. — The 2-Minute Orthopedic Examination

Instructions	Observation
Stand facing examiner	Acromioclavicular joints, general habitus
Look at ceiling, floor, over both shoulders; touch ears to shoulders	Cervical spine motion
Shrug shoulders (examiner resists)	Trapezius strength
Abduct shoulders 90° (examiner resists at 90°)	Deltoid strength
Full external rotation of arms	Shoulder motion
Flex and extend elbows	Elbow motion
Arms at sides, elbows 90° flexed; pronate and supinate wrists	Elbow and wrist motion
Spread fingers; make fist	Hand or finger motion and deformities
Tighten (contract) quadriceps; relax quadriceps	Symmetry and knee effusion; ankle effusion
"Duck walk" four steps (away from examiner with buttocks on heels)	Hip, knee, and ankle motion
Back to examiner	Shoulder symmetry, scoliosis
Knees straight, touch toes	Scoliosis, hip motion, hamstring tightness
Raise up on toes, raise heels	Calf symmetry, leg strength

inees to be given instructions at one time, yet it provides privacy for the portions of the examination requiring the athlete to disrobe.

The area should be divided into examination stations, which should be marked clearly with large printed numbers. Each station should have a chair/desk or a chair and a clipboard. An examination table will be needed at the station where the abdominal examination is done.

Efficient examination of 30 or more athletes within 2 hours requires a team of six: two physicians and four nonphysician medical personnel (nurses or certified athletic trainers). In addition, the coach of the sport involved should be present to ensure order and good attendance.

The athletes must be present at least 10 minutes before the examination is scheduled to begin. Boys should wear gym shorts; girls should wear gym outfits.

The history is the most important aspect of the preparticipation health evaluation. Because medical histories of minors require parental signatures, these forms should be completed prior to their arrival. Young adult athletes could complete this history at the time of the examination while waiting.

The athlete moves from one examination station to the next in the order given here. Only three stations—4, 5, and 7—require a physician; if only two physicians are present, 4 and 5 can be combined in one station. A description of the stations follows.

Station 1: Blood pressure, taken by health care professional. Right arm, with person sitting. Values demanding repeat determinations or referral for further evaluation are: 6 to 11 years: >125/80 mmHg (boys), >120/75 mmHg (girls); 12 years and older: >135/90 mmHg (boys), >130/85 mmHg (girls).

Station 2: Visual acuity, evaluated by health care professional. Uncorrected vision less than 20/40 requires referral for further evaluation.

Station 3: Skin-mouth-eyes, tested by physician, nurse, or athletic trainer. Examination for pustular acne, herpes, dental prosthesis, severe caries, pupil inequality, rashes, tinea pedis, and other infections.

Station 4: Chest examination, performed by physician. Cardiac-related history is reviewed and examination performed.

Station 5: Lymphatics, abdomen, and genitalia, examined by physician looking for cervical adenopathy, abdominal organomegaly, testicular abnormalities, inguinal hernia (in males), and Tanner pubic hair sexual maturity rating of both male and female adolescents competing in contact sports.

Station 6: Musculoskeletal examination by physician or athletic trainer. *This "two-minute orthopedic examination" is the most productive part of the examination after the history;* it is here that an abnormality affecting athletic performance and causing undue risk of injury is most likely to be detected. The AAP recommended examination form includes this musculoskeletal examination.

Table 57. — Classification of Sports

Contact/ Collision	Limited Contact/ Impact	Noncontact		
		Strenuous	Moderately Strenuous	Nonstrenuous
Boxing	Baseball	Aerobic	Badminton	Archery
Field	Basketball	dancing	Curling	Golf
hockey	Bicycling	Crew	Table	Riflery
Football	Diving	Fencing	tennis	
Ice hockey	Field	Field		
Lacrosse	High jump	Discus		
Martial arts	Pole vault	Javelin		
Rodeo	Gymnastics	Shot put		
Soccer	Horseback	Running		
Wrestling	riding	Swimming		
	Skating	Tennis		
	Ice	Track		
	Roller	Weight		
	Skiing	lifting		
	Cross-			
	country			
	Downhill			
	Water			
	Softball			
	Squash,			
	handball			
	Volleyball			

Station 7: Review, by a physician, of the results of the various components of the history and examination, as recorded on the examination forms. The physician may repeat those parts of the examination reported to be abnormal or equivocal and then make the final decision about the athlete's degree of participation.

Recommendations for Participation in Competitive Sports

To assist physicians in deciding whether athletes should be allowed to participate in particular sports, the American Academy of Pediatrics in 1988 compiled a list of recommendations for participation. Athletic events are divided into groups depending on degree of strenuousness and probability for collision (Table 57). These groups of sports are then considered in light of medical and surgical conditions to determine whether partici-

Table 58. — Recommendations for Participation in Competitive Sports[1]

	Contact Collision	Limited Contact Impact	Noncontact		
			Strenuous	Moderately Strenuous	Nonstrenuous
Acute illnesses	*	*	*	*	*
Needs individual assessment, eg, contagiousness to others, risk of worsening illness					
Atlantoaxial instability	No	No	Yes*	Yes	Yes
*Swimming: no butterfly, breast stroke, or diving starts					
Cardiovascular					
Carditis	No	No	No	No	No
Hypertension					
Mild	Yes	Yes	Yes	Yes	Yes
Moderate	*	*	*	*	*
Severe	*	*	*	*	*
Congenital heart disease	†	†	†	†	†
*Needs individual assessment.[2]					
†Patients with mild forms can be allowed a full range of physical activities: patients with moderate or severe forms, or who are postoperative, should be evaluated by a cardiologist before athletic participation.[2]					
Eyes					
Absence or loss of function of one eye	*	*	*	*	*
Detached retina	†	†	†	†	†
*Availability of American Society for Testing and Materials (ASTM)-approved eye guards may allow competitor to participate in most sports, but this must be judged on an individual basis.[3,4]					
†Consult ophthalmologist					
Inguinal hernia	Yes	Yes	Yes	Yes	Yes
Kidney: absence of one	No	Yes	Yes	Yes	Yes
Liver: enlarged	No	No	Yes	Yes	Yes
Musculoskeletal disorders	*	*	*	*	*
*Needs individual assessment					

Table 58. — Recommendations for Participation in Competitive Sports[1] (continued)

	Contact Collision	Limited Contact Impact	Noncontact		
			Strenuous	Moderately Strenuous	Nonstrenuous
Neurologic					
History of serious head or spine trauma, repeated concussions, or craniotomy	*	*	Yes	Yes	Yes
Convulsive disorder					
Well controlled	Yes	Yes	Yes	Yes	Yes
Poorly controlled	No	No	Yes†	Yes	Yes‡
*Needs individual assessment					
†No swimming or weight lifting					
‡No archery or riflery					
Ovary: Absence of one	Yes	Yes	Yes	Yes	Yes
Respiratory					
Pulmonary insufficiency	*	*	*	*	Yes
Asthma	Yes	Yes	Yes	Yes	Yes
*May be allowed to compete if oxygenation remains satisfactory during a graded stress test					
Sickle cell trait	Yes	Yes	Yes	Yes	Yes
Skin: boils, herpes, impetigo, scabies	*	*	Yes	Yes	Yes
*No gymnastics with mats, martial arts, wrestling, or contact sports until not contagious					
Spleen: enlarged	No	No	No	Yes	Yes
Testicle: absence or undescended	Yes	Yes*	Yes	Yes	Yes
*Certain sports may require protective cup.[3]					

[1]Adapted from American Academy of Pediatrics, Committee on Sports Medicine and Fitness. Recommendations for participation in competitive sports. Pediatrics. 1988;81:737-739

[2]Sixteenth Bethesda Conference. Cardiovascular abnormalities in the athlete: recommendations regarding eligibility for competition. J Am Coll Cardiol. 1985;6:1186-1232

[3]Dorsen PJ. Should athletes with one eye, kidney, or testicle play contact sports? Phys Sportsmed. 1986;14:130-138

[4]Vinger PF. The one-eyed athlete. Phys Sportsmed. 1987;15:48-52

pation would create a substantial risk of injury (Table 58). Certain activities such as skiing are not inherently "contact sports," yet when competitors hit a tree, they are as much at risk as participants in the more traditional collision/contact sports. Such sports are, therefore, included in the group called "limited contact/impact." These recommendations should only be used as a guideline; the physician's clinical judgment should remain the final arbiter in interpreting these recommendations for a specific patient.

References

1. Powell J. 636,000 injuries annually in high school football. *Athletic Training*. 1987;22:19-22

2. Tator CH, Edmonds VE. National survey of spinal injuries in hockey players. *Can Med Assoc J*. 1984;130:875-880

3. Brief on file at the American Academy of Pediatrics. Elk Grove Village, IL; 1986

4. Goldberg B, Saaniti A, Whitman P, et al. Preparticipation sports assessment: an objective evaluation. *Pediatrics*. 1980;66:736-745

5. Thompson TR, Andrish JT, Bergfeld JA. A prospective study of preparticipation sports examinations of 2670 young athletes: methods and results. *Cleve Clin J Med*. 1982;49:225-233

CHAPTER 28

DENTAL HEALTH

Three major dental health issues are most relevant to school programs. These are dental caries, periodontal disease, and oral trauma.

Dental caries occurs when acid, over time, demineralizes teeth. Oral microorganisms, residing in plaque, metabolize dietary carbohydrates to produce this acid. If the caries process continues unchecked, the microorganisms infect the dental pulp producing pain. This infection, known as pulpitis, may progress to periapical infection. Periapical infection, if untreated, may lead to facial cellulitis and hospitalization.

Periodontal disease may begin as early as age 3. Poor oral hygiene allows plaque to accumulate and inflame the gingiva. If oral hygiene remains poor over a 20- to 30-year period, tooth loss results. The process is insidious, similar to unrecognized chronic hypertension, and end-stage treatment is often not possible.

Oral trauma may be physical in nature, associated with accidents, altercations, and child abuse, or secondary to the irritation of smoked or smokeless tobacco products.

Magnitude of Oral Disease

The dental caries rate is decreasing but continues to affect the permanent teeth of 50% of school-age children.

Gingival infections are experienced by 60% of 15 year olds, and 36% of people over age 65 have lost all their natural teeth.

The incidence of oral physical trauma is increasing, while the oral cancer rate is stable at about 30,500 new cases per year and 8,350 deaths per year.

Risk Factors

The following indicators, either singularly or in combination, increase oral disease risk:
- Lower socioeconomic group
- Specific population group:
    Native Americans
    Migrant workers

Those who dwell in urban ghettos
Rural poor
- Developmentally disabled
- No or limited access to topical and systemic fluoride, dental sealants, and professional oral care
- Long-term nocturnal and on-demand nursing bottle or breast-feeding
- Sporadic oral hygiene practices
- Tobacco use, both smoked and smokeless
- Athletes and physical education students are at risk for oral trauma

What Can Be Done?

Oral disease can be prevented or controlled by daily toothbrushing with a fluoride dentifrice, daily consumption of fluoridated water, regular meals with minimal snacking, the timely use of dental sealants, periodic professional visits, timely mouth guard use, and abstinence from tobacco.

The school health professional should promote oral health by developing a program that takes advantage of local resources and encourages involvement of local oral care professionals. A menu of suggested program ideas and resources follows:

Programs

- A daily in-school brushing program using a fluoride dentifrice.
- Support community water fluoridation and, in nonmetropolitan areas with low fluoride concentrations in the school water supply, consider fluoridating the school water system or instituting a weekly supervised fluoride rinse program.
- Classroom oral health education including the importance of daily brushing with a fluoride dentifrice and a regular meal schedule.
- Promote the use of dental sealants for permanent teeth to prevent biting surface caries.
- Encourage low caries diets in school breakfast and lunch programs and remove high sugar snacks from school vending machines.
- Oral health screening in conjunction with Children's Dental Health Month each February.

- Include dental examinations as part of the physical examination for athletics or as a suggested requirement before entering school.
- Require use of a mouth guard in all school-sponsored athletic programs and physical education classes.
- Sponsor an inservice program on healthy life-styles and disease prevention for school faculty and staff.

Resources

- Recruit parents, especially those with dental care experience, and retired or semiretired dental professionals to organize and administer oral health programs.
- Work with local dental society leadership to identify offices willing to provide support for school oral health programs. Dentists are often interested in working with athletic programs to provide mouth guards and oral trauma care.
- Contact local or state health departments for educational materials or human resources. Contact members of Congress at the federal level.
- Dental schools, dental hygiene schools, and dental assisting programs often are interested in involving themselves in classroom activities.
- Contact national dental organizations such as the American Academy of Pediatric Dentistry or American Dental Association.

Implications

Distribution of information on oral disease prevention with encouragement to apply this information can be accomplished in schools with the following positive effects:

- Healthy children have a better opportunity to learn.
- Schools, working in concert with parents and local professionals to promote health for children, project a very positive public image.
- Increased awareness of disease and prevention may establish lifelong healthy habits and reduce the morbidity and mortality associated with dental caries, periodontal disease, oral trauma, and oral cancer.
- Pleasing dental appearance fosters a positive self-image.
- Preventing oral disease reduces health care costs.

School oral health programs have contributed to the steady reduction in oral disease accomplished during the last two decades. School health professionals should continue these programs and look for ways to improve and expand them in order to continue disease reduction into the next century.

Suggested Readings

Allensworth DD, Wolford CA. Schools as agents for achieving the 1990 health objectives for the nation. *Health Educ Q.* 1988;15(1):3-15

Equity and Access for Mothers and Children. Strategies From the Public Health Service Workshop on Oral Health of Mothers and Children. Washington, DC: US Department of Health and Human Services; 1990. DHHS Publication No. HRS-MCH-90-4

Giblin PT, Poland ML. Health needs of high school students in Detroit. *J Sch Health.* 1985;55(10):407-410

Horowitz AM, Frazier PJ. Effective oral health programs in school settings. In: Clark J, ed. *Clinical Dentistry.* New York, NY: Harper & Row; 1976;2(16)

Johnson K, Siegal M. Resources for improving the oral health of maternal and child populations. *J Public Health Dent.* 1990;50(6):418-426

National Goals for Education. US Dept of Education. Washington, DC; 1990

Oda DS, DeAngelis C, Berman B, Meeker R. The resolution of health problems in school children. *J Sch Health.* 1985;55(3):96-98

Public health service workshop on oral health of mothers and children. Background issue papers. *J Public Health Dent.* 1990;50(6)special issue

US Department of Health and Human Services. Healthy People 2000 Conference; September 1990; Washington, DC. National Health Promotion and Disease Prevention Objectives. *Oral Health.* Chapter 13

CHAPTER 29

SCHOOL TRANSPORTATION SAFETY

According to Special Report 222 of the Transportation Research Board of the National Research Council, approximately 400,000 school buses are used to transport 25 million children nearly 4 billion miles to and from school and school activities each year in the United States. Approximately 85% of these buses are the large, "Type I" school buses that carry more than 16 passengers. Children riding in small school buses built in accordance with federal safety standards, including lap belts, fared very well in 24 crashes investigated by the National Transportation Safety Board. Children in Type I school buses fared less well; however, the school bus safety record is considerably better than the safety record for private vehicles.

Given the high numbers of children transported and miles traveled annually, the levels of fatalities and injuries to children as a result of crashes related to school buses are relatively light. Of the approximately 150 people killed in such incidents each year, only 12% are passengers on the bus: 8% student passengers, 2% adult passengers, and 2% drivers. The remaining fatalities are occupants of other vehicles (55%), bicyclists (3%), and pedestrians (30%). Of the fatally injured pedestrians, 84% were school-aged, and 16% were adults. Of those, 70% were struck by school buses. The majority of pedestrians killed were young children who were struck by their own school bus. The number of injuries related to school bus incidents is estimated to be 19,000 per year, and most injuries are minor. One half of these injuries are sustained by school bus passengers. An estimated 4% of injuries are sustained by pedestrians and are typically more severe.[1]

Public outcry and demands for change predictably surface when tragic crashes occur, even though the frequency of on-board fatalities and injuries on school buses remain lower than outside-the-bus incidents. Expectations for school bus safety should be upheld not as a result of reactions to the loss of children's lives or the injury of children, but rather from an ongoing commitment from communities and states to assuring the safest ride possible for children on school buses every day.

Pediatricians can help by serving as resources, educators, consultants, and advocates for school bus safety, since travel in the school bus consumes such a consistent and long-term role in the daily lives of children from preschool through high school.

The National Traffic and Motor Vehicle Safety Act of 1966 authorizes the Department of Transportation to issue minimum standards for new school buses manufactured for sale in the United States.[2] This act was amended in 1974,[3] and the National Highway Traffic Safety Administration (NHTSA) developed the current minimum performance standards for school buses manufactured after April 1, 1977.[4] In recent years, school bus safety in the United States has again been closely scrutinized, and, although certain topics continue to be controversial, there is strong consensus regarding most issues. The AAP Committee on School Health is in the process of revising its 1985 statement on "School Bus Safety." The following recommendations, which are under consideration, are derived from several recent studies.[1-9] These recommendations can enhance community systems for addressing school bus safety education, awareness, and practices. Pediatricians can assist in this process through active sharing of these recommendations at both the community and state levels.

School Bus Safety

1. Many school systems provide for the transportation of preschool-age children. The use of child safety seats and other restraint systems on school buses for preschool-age children is recommended as a necessary practice to keep them secured on the school bus seat. All restraint systems used during school bus transport should meet the requirements of Federal Motor Vehicle Safety Standard (FMVSS) 213.[4] The Academy recommends that school districts provide appropriate and federally approved child restraint systems for children riding in school buses who are prekindergarten age. Cases of children with special needs who require restraint above prekindergarten age should be evaluated on an individual basis to determine the most appropriate restraint that meets their needs for positioning during travel. All children with special needs should be provided with the most appropriate restraint possible,

regardless of age, weight, and height. Further recommendations are outlined in the AAP policy statement on transportation of children with special needs.[8]

2. Compartmentalization, keeping child passengers confined to a padded compartment in a crash, is the major principle by which school bus passengers are currently protected. In general, the higher the seat back and the closer the spacing between rows, the better the "compartmentalization" of students in a crash. Current provisions are for a seat back height of 20 inches above a reference point (about 22 inches measured from the seat surface). A study committee of the National Transportation Safety Board has issued a recommendation that NHTSA revise FMVSS 222 (School Bus Safety and Interiors) to require that seat backs be 24 inches above the "reference point." Seat backs would be slightly over 26 inches from the seat surface.[1] The Academy supports this recommendation.

3. The issue of school bus safety has been linked frequently with concerns over whether school buses should be required to have safety belts for all passengers. It is estimated that the use of seat belts on large buses (Type I) may reduce deaths and injury by 20% but that usage rates are only 50%.[1] Belt usage rates can be significantly increased through education and monitoring, and, therefore, effectiveness estimates can be enhanced when all students wear the belts correctly all the time. An additional benefit of seat belt use is the behavioral reinforcement of the important habit developed through consistent use of seat belts in private vehicles. While cost-effectiveness of seat belt use on school buses may remain controversial, the American Academy of Pediatrics recommends the installation of seat belts on all newly purchased school buses. School districts that provide seat belts on school buses must ensure appropriate education of administrators, students, teachers, drivers, and parents to assure they are used consistently and correctly.

4. Radial tires improve driver control of the school bus and provide added safety.

5. All school buses should be equipped with the following in order to prevent pedestrian accidents: (a) eight warning

and loading lights (two flashing red and two flashing amber on both front and back); (b) stop signal arms; and (c) crossview mirror system. The bus should meet all current recommendations for mirrors, including two large round mirrors that allow the driver to view more fully the front of the bus. Additionally, districts should consider strobe lights for reduced visibility conditions, an external loud speaker system to enable the driver to communicate with children outside the bus, and loading and backing alarms or pulsating back-up horns.[9] Electronic sensor systems are available but have not been adequately evaluated.[1]

6. Brake retarder systems may be effective in reducing serious injuries and death due to sudden stops.

7. Mandatory state school bus inspections are recommended.

8. It is recommended that, in addition to regular annual school bus inspections, the state highway patrol (or other independent agency) make detailed, unexpected, random school bus inspections.

9. All school buses, including private, "for hire," and parochial school buses, should be in compliance with all federal regulations. Buses manufactured prior to 1977 should be retired from use by any transportation provider.

10. The use of wheelchairs for school bus transportation of children with disabilities is a common practice. The Academy recommends that states adopt the requirements for use of wheelchairs on school buses outlined in the 1990 National Standards for School Buses.[9]

School Bus Driver Selection and Training

School bus drivers should annually meet the following requirements:

1. Maintain a valid commercial driver's license.

2. Be a minimum of 21 years of age.

3. Show proof of a yearly health examination, including vision and hearing, that documents the absence of problems that might compromise driving and child supervision.

4. Maintain a satisfactory driving record as determined by the school district and successfully pass a check for a criminal record.
5. Attend a minimum of 6 to 12 hours of instruction covering: (a) driver duties; (b) bus operating procedures; (c) traffic and school bus laws and regulations; (d) record keeping; (e) emergency and accident-related procedures; (f) first aid; (g) very basic knowledge of the developmental stages and needs of school-age children; (h) child supervision responsibilities; and (i) transportation of special-needs pupils.
6. Successfully complete a written or oral test covering topics described in Recommendation 5, as well as a driving performance test, and demonstrate safe loading and unloading procedures.
7. Submit to mandatory drug testing, if not already required by the district.

School Bus Passenger Instruction

Passengers of all ages should be taught safe riding and pedestrian behavior, even if the passenger is an infrequent rider. Instruction should include: (1) safe pedestrian practices going to and from bus stops; (2) safe behavior while waiting at the bus stop; (3) safe practices for boarding and disembarking; (4) safe behavior on the bus; and (5) procedures for emergencies.

School Bus Passenger Supervision

Adult supervision on school buses should focus on: (1) ensuring that passengers stay seated, use seat belts, and keep arms and heads inside windows; (2) assisting in the handling of emergencies; (3) assisting with special-needs passengers; and (4) escorting children across busy roadways. These objectives can best be met by a second adult (other than the driver) serving as a monitor on the school bus.

School Bus Routes and Stops

Planning routes and stops should involve attention to: (1) avoiding the need for the bus to back up; (2) minimizing traffic disruptions; (3) providing a good field of view at all stops; and (4) minimizing the need for children to board or leave the bus on, or to cross, a busy roadway. It is recommended that children be supervised by an adult when they must cross a roadway after leaving a school bus.

The Pediatrician's Role

Community Level

1. Inquire about current policies relating to transportation. Find out mechanisms for proposing needed changes and serve as a resource to this decision-making body.
2. Inquire about types of training being offered at the local level for bus drivers. Provide direction in making test materials to evaluate driver competency in areas related to child development. Volunteer to participate in local training sessions for bus drivers in areas relating to child development, behavior, child safety seat use and positioning needs, and safety belt use.
3. Share the preceding recommendations at local school district meetings and advocate for their implementation, if not currently in place.
4. Encourage the development and distribution of educational materials on school bus safety through the local school systems.
5. Serve as consultants to local transportation directors, state directors of school transportation, or school boards on the physical and emotional development of preschool-age children and assist in developing training materials for transportation providers.

State Level

1. Contact state directors of school transportation and request a copy of current state specifications for school buses. Compare this information with recommendations posed by National School Bus Safety Standards and urge revisions of state specifications, if necessary, through appropriate decision-making channels at state level.
2. Volunteer to serve on writing committee for state specifications. Share information contained in this chapter and recommendations by National School Bus Safety Standards.

3. Contact state departments of education and recommend development of information materials on school bus safety for statewide distribution to elementary schools.

4. Serve as resource/consultant to state department of education regarding training of bus drivers in areas relating to child passenger safety and child development and behavior.

References

1. National Research Council, Transportation Research Board. *Special Report 222— Improving School Bus Safety*. Washington, DC: National Research Council; 1989

2. *National Traffic and Motor Vehicle Safety Act of 1966*. (Public Law 102-240). 1992

3. US Department of Transportation, National Highway Transportation Safety Administration. *School Bus Vehicle Safety Report. Report of the Secretary of Transportation to the United States Congress Pursuant to Section 103 of the 1976 Amendments to the National Traffic and Motor Vehicle Safety Act of 1966*. Report No. (DOT) HS-802 191. 1977

4. *Code of Federal Regulations: Transportation 49*. (Parts 400-999). Washington, DC: US Government Printing Office; 1992

5. National Transportation Safety Board, Bureau of Safety Programs. *Safety Study—Crash Worthiness of Large Poststandard School Buses*. Washington, DC: National Transportation Safety Board; 1987

6. National Safety Council. *Policy on Protecting Pupil Passengers in School Buses*. Chicago, IL: National Safety Council; 1984

7. Colorado School Bus Safety Committee, Governor's Traffic Safety Advisory Committee. *Colorado School Bus Safety Report*. 1989

8. American Academy of Pediatrics, Committee on Injury and Poison Prevention. Transporting children with special needs. *AAP Safe Ride News*. Winter 1993

9. Eleventh National Conference on School Transportation. *National Standards for School Buses and National Standards for School Bus Operations*. Revised ed. Chicago, IL: National Safety Council; 1990

CHAPTER 30

VIOLENCE IN SCHOOLS: CURRENT STATUS AND PREVENTION

Magnitude of the Problem

According to the Children's Defense Fund, 135,000 children bring guns to school daily.[1] In 1990, some 12,000 students in grades 9 through 12 in urban areas throughout the country were asked, "During the past 30 days, how many times have you carried a weapon, such as a gun, knife, or club, for self-protection or because you thought you might need it in a fight?" Nearly 20% reported that they had carried a weapon at least once during that period (and more than a third of those answering "yes" said they carried a weapon six or more times during the 30 days). Among the weapons carried, knives or razors were most common (more than half the time). Firearms, generally handguns, accounted for more than 20% of the weapons carried.[2]

The results have been tragic. Every 36 minutes, a child is killed or injured by a firearm (14,600 annually), usually by a handgun, and usually by another child either in school or in the neighborhood.[3] The fatal shooting of two students by another in 1992 at New York's Thomas Jefferson High School caught the nation's attention for an agonizing moment. But a scant few months before, in November 1991, another student had been gunned down, and a teacher wounded in Jefferson's halls. And, as the headline of the *Newsweek* story accompanying the account of Jefferson's double murder noted, "It's not just New York . . . Big cities, small towns: more and more guns in younger and younger hands."[4]

In the four academic years beginning 1986 there were at least 761 fatal shootings on school grounds. Six of the victims were school employees. Another 201 persons were severely wounded, and there were almost 250 incidents of hostage-taking at gunpoint. These incidents, compiled by the Center to Prevent Handgun Violence, occurred in 35 states and the District of Columbia. "Besides the most populated states having the most incidents," noted the authors, "there was no clear geographic pattern for gun violence in school. It seemed to strike every area of the country." And while two thirds of these incidents took place in high schools, another quarter took place in junior high schools. (Incidents also were recorded in elementary school and even in preschool; most often these involved violence by adults in which children were the victims.)[5]

Because of the information noted above, the National Education Association adopted a policy supporting control of guns and other deadly weapons through legislation.

How do students perceive the safety of their school environment? In 1989, as part of its ongoing National Crime Victimization Survey, the US Department of Justice asked more than 10,000 students age 12 to 19 years about their experience and perceptions regarding violence and crime at school. (The sample is representative of the estimated 21.6 million students ages 12 to 19 years enrolled in the nation's public and private schools between January and June 1989.)

An estimated 9% of the students reported having been the victim of a crime in or around their school during the previous 6 months. Most of these incidents involved property crimes, but 9% (432,000 if the sample is projected to the total population) were victims of violence. Younger students were more likely to be victimized than older ones, and crime rates were similar across racial and ethnic groups. Fifteen percent of the students reported the presence of gangs at their schools, and those students also reported the highest levels of victimization and fear of violence. Similarly, while only a minority of students reported that alcohol and drugs were available at school, these students also were most likely to report the fear of victimization. (The connection between alcohol and other drugs and violence has been widely noted.)[6,7] Finally, 16% of the respondents claimed that a teacher had been threatened or attacked by a student at their school in the preceding 6 months.[8]

In this chapter, we explore some of the interventions that have been developed to address the problem of youth and violence. Violence in schools is a problem for all school personnel, students, parents, and other members of the community. However, as we consider a variety of interventions that address school climate, education programs, and behavior change, we will note places in which school health personnel can make a special contribution. In large part, this unique vantage point from which they can address youth violence reflects the relatively recent understanding that violence is a public health problem.

Violence, Public Health, and Schools

The level and lethality of school violence has increased dramatically in recent years, as has the general level of violence in society. In response to the need to understand and prevent violence, for more than a decade public health researchers and practitioners have examined the patterns and risk factors that characterize violence, worked with colleagues in many disciplines to develop interventions, and served as advocates to raise the awareness of society that violence, like other forms of injury and disease, can be controlled or prevented.[9]

Public health provides an epidemiologic basis for understanding violence and for developing interventions. Injuries caused by violence, like all other forms of injury, result from the interaction of a host, an agent, and the environment. For example, a drunk driver (host), a car with faulty brakes (agent), and a slick, winding road (environment) each play a role in a resulting collision. Because it is the *interaction* of the three components that results in the collision, changing any one component can reduce the risk of injury. An alcohol-impaired person, a gun, and a dark, noisy bar (which together create an extremely high risk for serious violence) fit the same model. The second important contribution of public health to the understanding and potential prevention of violence is that frequently the perpetrators and victims of violence know each other, and injury results from an escalating argument. This is particularly important when dealing with violence in schools.

The third important contribution from public health is to enumerate three basic approaches to designing interventions against serious population-wide health problems, and to assert that the most powerful interventions try to combine elements of each. *Legislation and enforcement* interventions seek to protect large numbers of people simultaneously (eg, gun control laws). *Technological or engineering* interventions are directed at modifying the environment in which injuries can occur (eg, using metal detectors to keep guns out of schools). And *education or behavior change* interventions address the human component of the host-agent-environment equation (eg, violence prevention curricula).[10]

Successful interventions must be multidisciplinary as well. They require the expertise and commitment of teachers, school administrators, counselors, and others. School health personnel—nurses, physicians, and health aides—and pediatricians in the community have a unique role to play in school violence prevention.

Because establishing and maintaining school safety is essential to any preventive strategy, we will begin by considering interventions that directly address school climate. Then we will focus on interventions designed to reduce violence through education and behavior change. First, however, it is important to note that violence and violence prevention mean different things for children of different ages.

The most dramatic, most lethal violence has been among high-school-age students, and it is in this environment that the majority of violence prevention initiatives have been carried out. However, there is increasing evidence that younger adolescents (ages 10 to 15 years) are both victims and perpetrators of severe violence[11] but still are at a developmental stage at which patterns of thought and behavior regarding violence are changeable.[12] Thus, the need for intensive violence prevention efforts at the middle school level has received support from the federal Centers for Disease Control and Prevention (CDC).[13]

At the elementary and even preschool levels, teachers and students need assistance in identifying and moderating patterns of thought and behavior that express themselves in aggressive actions and that can lead to the kinds of violence witnessed among adolescents.[14] Even the youngest children in some urban areas often are placed at greater risk of psychological damage and potential later violent behavior by frequent exposure to community violence.[15] Despite these needs, and the development of some interventions for younger children,[16] the emphasis has been on programs for older children in urban areas. However, to successfully reduce violence throughout the country, interventions must be adapted to all student populations.

Interventions for a Safer School Environment

"School climate" includes everything from the safety of the physical plant to the degree of mutual respect accorded students, teachers, and other school personnel in their dealings with each other. In California, for example, the state constitution defines an "inalienable right to attend campuses which are safe, secure, and peaceful,"[17] and the state supreme court has interpreted this to mean that "safe and welcoming schools" must be free from criminal behavior.[18]

The general policies and practices that encourage the maintenance of a good school climate have been amply documented in publications of the National School Safety Center and will not be repeated here.[19] More specific information about the problem of gangs in schools is available as well.[20] The most recent reviews of substance abuse prevention interventions, including programs to reduce the availability of drugs in and around schools, are cited in the references at the end of this chapter.[21-23] However, in an increasing number of schools, disarmament is the essential precondition to establishing effective discipline and a reasonable school climate.

A wide variety of tactics have been employed by administrators to reduce the in-school "arms race." The use of metal detectors is perhaps best known, although they have been employed in a limited number of schools. Random locker searches and requirements that students carry only clear plastic or mesh book bags to preclude hidden weapons also have been tried successfully.[24]

The most detailed discussion of weapons-related interventions was prepared for the CDC Forum on Youth Violence in Minority Communities in 1990.[25] The authors describe educational, legal, and technological interventions and indicate what is known about their effectiveness. Among the educational interventions reviewed are firearm safety courses, public information campaigns, counseling programs, classroom education, peer education and mentoring, and crisis intervention. "Educational strategies are widely used because they are persuasive rather than coercive," they conclude. "Yet, we know little about the effectiveness of educational efforts concerning firearms and other weapons; education alone may not lead to changes in practice among large numbers of people. [It] is a gradual process. The effects of educational campaigns may not be seen for a year or more."

After reviewing the myriad of local, state, and federal firearms laws, the authors state that "Despite the proliferation of gun control laws in the United States, there still remains some uncertainty about the effectiveness of previous legislative attempts to restrict availability and use of firearms." (They do note, however, that a widely reported recent study comparing gun control laws and homicide rates in Vancouver, British Columbia, and Seattle, Washington, found that the Canadian city's significantly lower homicide rate may be a consequence of its restrictive gun ownership laws.)[26]

The technological and environmental interventions described in the paper prepared for the forum include modifying weapons to make them less easily fired, modifying ammunition to reduce the severity of injury, and the use of dress codes and metal detectors in schools. In assessing the use of metal detectors, the authors conducted interviews and compared the experiences of New York City, where 1,500 to 2,000 weapons are confiscated every school year, with Los Angeles.

In New York City, the 2-year-old metal detector program has met largely with success. School security staff, wielding handheld metal detectors, randomly search students in the lobbies of 16 high schools at the start of school days. Portal metal detectors, such as those used in airports, were judged to be more expensive and time-consuming (ushering thousands of students through one doorway can delay school start-up for several hours). Searches are conducted once a week, unannounced, in each of the schools. The program requires a mobile staff of 120 teachers. Sites chosen were the schools where the highest numbers of weapons were being found. (The shootings at Thomas Jefferson High School occurred the day after a once-weekly random check was made; metal detectors will now be used daily instead.) As a result of the confiscation of weapons, attendance has improved in several of the schools and students have reported an increased sense of security.

According to the director of security, a key to the program's success was the multilayered orientation program. The orientations among school administration, staff, students, and parents involved both meetings and demonstrations of the equipment. This groundwork, he believes, is what has allowed the program to proceed without legal suits, political controversy, or community distress. The detector program is conducted in the context of a broader violence prevention program in the schools that includes curricula, peer mediation programs, and crisis intervention teams. At the current level of effort, the program costs $300,000 per school per year.

The Los Angeles school system has decided that while weapons in schools are a growing problem, metal detectors are not a desirable or practical option. Because schools are in use—but not protected—well beyond traditional school hours (for afterschool activities, night meetings, etc), persons who want to get a weapon into the school can do so. Further, the district believes the greater threat of weapon-related violence is from nonstudents and that any new security measures will deal with intensifying a buffer there. Portal metal detectors also have been rejected as too time-consuming.

In many school systems, the authors suggest, a rejection of metal detectors is founded more on philosophy than practicality. Opponents see them as an image-creating attempt to demonstrate concern about students' safety. Other opponents question whether metal detectors violate or are an excessive infringement of civil liberties of students. Because of this debate, the authors note, few technological and environmental strategies have been tried or evaluated thus far.

The Role of School Health Personnel

Many of the interventions designed to improve school climate require more than administrative decisions or new regulations and procedures. Because maintaining and improving school climate is the responsibility of all school personnel, there is a role for school nurses, physicians, and other health workers. School health personnel also may play an important role as advocates for wider policies that affect school climate. For example, as health professionals, they can support the availability of substance abuse prevention and treatment services for adolescents. As other health professionals have, they can advocate for policies designed to reduce the number of firearms available in the community.[27] And they can work within their own professional organizations to develop a greater understanding of the problems of violence in schools. Some other unique and important roles that health professionals can play in schools are discussed in the next section.

Educational Interventions

In terms of the classic public health paradigm, the previous section focused primarily on interventions that exemplify the approaches of legislation and enforcement or technology and engineering. In this section we turn to those educational interventions for which schools are best suited.

In 1990 and 1991, with the support of the Carnegie Corporation and the CDC, the Education Development Center, Inc (EDC) carried out two surveys of violence prevention interventions for young adolescents and reported the results in a series of papers.[28-31] The survey found that a wide variety of educational interventions are being employed to prevent youth violence. Such programs fall into the following three categories: interventions to build male self-esteem, conflict resolution skills and mediation education, and public education interventions. The category of self-esteem development includes the following: (1) manhood development curricula; (2) mentors and role models; and (3) immersion schools. Subcategories within conflict resolution and mediation are (1) curricula, training, and technical assistance; (2) crime prevention/law-related education; (3) handgun violence education; and (4) life skills training. Public education interventions include (1) public service announcements; (2) educational videos; (3) video conferences; and (4) media education.[32]

After reviewing many examples of these educational interventions, the authors concluded, "No one program claims it has *the* solution to the problem of minority youth violence. For example, some programs have as a goal to help minority youth develop the skills that will enable them to resolve the conflicts in their lives without violence. Because the target population for these programs [all students] is not one that, for the most part, is currently engaged in violent behavior, it is extremely difficult to determine whether the program has been effective."[32]

There are a great many interventions designed to prevent youth violence, as the review indicated. At a time of crisis, when the need to *do something* is felt strongly, programs proliferate. And some grow and become widely disseminated. But which programs work? Determining which violence prevention programs have proved effective by rigorous evaluation was the goal of the Violence Prevention for Young Adolescents Project supported by the Carnegie Corporation in 1990.

A survey of 83 programs was conducted (to which 51 programs responded) to determine the basic features of location, funding sources, program goals, populations served, major activities, identifiable barriers to success, and whether any evaluation had been carried out. For 11 programs that had been the subject of some outcome evaluation, more detailed information was obtained through a second survey and case studies were developed.[33]

The programs identified below were selected because in each case the evaluation indicated that they hold promise as interventions and also because the evaluation raised issues about the nature of program evaluation. The programs are:

- Boston Conflict Resolution Program (Cambridge, MA)
- Conflict Management/Peer Mediation Program (Topeka, KS)
- Gang Prevention and Intervention Program (Garden Grove, CA)
- The Paramount Plan: Alternatives to Gang Membership (Paramount, CA)
- Project Stress Control: School-Based Curriculum (Atlanta, GA)
- Project Stress Control: Youth Development Centers (Atlanta, GA)
- Resolving Conflict Creatively Program (New York, NY)
- Second Step: A Violence Prevention Curriculum (Seattle, WA)
- Viewpoints Training Program (Santa Barbara, CA)
- Violence Prevention Curriculum Project (Newton, MA)
- Violence Prevention Project (Boston, MA)

For addresses and telephone numbers of these programs, see the Resource List at the end of this chapter.

Although these are the best-evaluated programs to date, those evaluations could not support judgments as to which among them were the most effective. In each case, and largely due to the limited resources that have been devoted to program evaluation, methodological and design flaws, inadequate data collection, or insufficiently rigorous analysis made it impossible to "prove" that a program met its goals and achieved its objectives. But if we do not know everything we would like to know, we already know a great deal: the results of these programs have been promising and we can learn a great deal from their continued implementation and evaluation.

Behavior Change Interventions and School Health Personnel: A Model

In the public health model, the distinction between education and behavior change is sometimes blurred, but for the purpose of this discussion it is useful to think of many of the interventions discussed in the previous sections as educational. They are designed to alter the knowledge or attitudes of a group of students (eg, an entire class) in the hope of influencing their health-related behavior. Behavior change interventions, on the other hand, can be seen as more intensive activities, often focused on the individual student and designed to address specific health risks or to effect specific behavior change. The distinction is useful only to a point, but it will help us to identify the special role for health professionals and health staff in addressing school violence.

This is not to say that school health personnel do not have an important role to play in educational interventions. On the contrary, when violence prevention activities are incorporated into a comprehensive school health education framework, school nurses, physicians, and other health personnel can support health educators by participating in curriculum design and by direct involvement in classroom instruction. Former Massachusetts Commissioner of Public Health, Dr. Deborah Prothrow-Stith, author of a widely disseminated violence prevention curriculum,[34] began as a concerned medical student to bring the realities of violence to inner-city high school classrooms. Certainly a presentation on the number of gunshot-injured youth who survive but are paralyzed for life can be a powerful moment in a violence prevention course. But it is in their interactions with individual students that health personnel can play a unique role.

Let us consider the pivotal developmental stage of young adolescents. As a setting, we will choose a middle school that includes a school-based clinic. These are not common, but the number of school-based or school-linked clinics is growing; the model has been successful in some sites, and it allows us to highlight activities that can be adapted to different models of school health delivery.

Early adolescence is a time of transition and important developmental tasks: gaining autonomy, independence, and mastery; pursuing intimacy; and separating from parents as new identities are formed.[35] Young adolescents begin to make decisions about self-worth, the value of education, health, work, and citizenship. Adolescents are more likely to adopt positive health behaviors if they believe they are susceptible to specific threats that have serious consequences. They must think it is within their control to take protective action and that such action is socially and culturally acceptable.[36,37] Further, they must recognize the pressures impelling them toward risk behaviors and gain the motivation (eg, self-esteem and a concern for personal well-being) and skills necessary to resist those pressures.[38]

School-based health clinics have been found to be partially successful in providing health care to medically unserved or underserved adolescents.[39] Generally, such clinics provide both preventive and primary health care services, diagnostic and treatment services for acute and chronic problems, health and dental screening, mental health counseling, updating immunizations, and referrals to a variety of backup services. The utilization rates are high, and children seek services for a variety of reasons: because of injuries or other acute conditions, for mental health counseling, and physical examinations or other preventive services.[40]

It also would be possible to initiate services by bringing each student (who has received parental consent to use the clinic) to the clinic for an interview and initial assessment. The assessment could focus on a variety of health risks, including violence, sex-related risks, alcohol and substance abuse, and other high-risk behaviors. Based on the assessment, other appointments could be scheduled and a variety of clinic-based or referral services provided.

Health care providers, in school clinics or in the community, can establish confidential, supportive relationships with their patients and take positive steps to influence their attitudes and behaviors around violence. However, to do so requires both special training and practical tools. Ideally, in collaboration with health educators and other school staff, school health personnel should be trained to jointly provide health messages addressing prevention of violence and other health risks (especially alcohol and substance abuse, given the high correlation between alcohol use and violence). Such training is essential both to increase the knowledge and skills of clinicians in recognizing and responding to the sensitive psychosocial issues related to the health risks that youth face and to allow youth to confront their own violence-related values and fears.

A violence prevention protocol can help school health and community providers make this serious risk for adolescents a standard part of routine health care. One such protocol has been developed and pilot tested by EDC and staff of Boston's Violence Prevention Project. The protocol (including training materials, slides, and posters) assists health care providers in assessing and discussing violence with their adolescent patients. It is designed to be used both with patients who present with a violence-related (or apparently violence-related) injury and with all patients who receive routine services.[41] "Although it is true that some youth are particularly at high risk for violence and the injury and death that can follow," the authors caution, "it should be remembered that adolescence *alone* is a significant risk factor for violence." Similarly, it is recommended that the protocol be used with both male and female patients.

The protocol covers four major topics: (1) violence history, (2) weapons, (3) anger management, and (4) strategies to avoid fights. The taking of a violence history is strongly recommended to ask questions about recent violent behavior and, moving backward, to past fights. Questions about the origin of a fight not only should include such prompts as, "How did it start?" but also, "How much had you been drinking?" The protocol's authors state, "Experience has shown that questions will be most effective if phrased to suggest that it is acceptable for teens to be candid with you about drinking, fighting, etc. In other words, 'How often do you fight?' is more effective than 'Do you ever fight?' " as a question to use in interviewing.

The protocol emphasizes that anger is a normal emotion for adolescents and that it may require different, safer outlets. The final section of the protocol includes a discussion with the patient about possible specific steps that can be taken to avoid potentially violent confrontations. At least one of the pilot test sites has added a "violence" section to its examination form as a prompt to all clinicians and to help ensure that the issue is addressed. A similar prompt could be added to school clinic records. A similar model has been described by Stringham and Weitzman.[42]

One of the most serious barriers to asking school health personnel or community providers to elicit information from their patients about violence is the availability of referral sources. "I was able to find kids that were either presently engaged in violent behavior or were at very high risk," reported a physician at one of the pilot test sites, "but without any real intervention resources available in the community, I didn't think I was able to intervene."[43] Thus, the protocol recommends the development of a directory of in-house and community referral resources, a model for which has been developed by Boston's Violence Prevention Project.

Although, as we noted, school-based clinics have been successful at providing services to underserved adolescents, evidence of their ability to alter high-risk behaviors such as violence and improve related health outcomes is not available.[44] However, recommendations have been made to strengthen clinics that bear on this critical need. Such recommendations include the following: (1) better identification and targeting of students engaged in high-risk behaviors; (2) conducting more outreach within the school; and (3) developing community-wide programs.[45] In each of these approaches, school health personnel and community providers can play an important role.

Violence in schools is a serious health and safety problem, but it cannot be addressed in isolation from general issues of school environment and climate or other problems of adolescent high-risk behavior. "A variety of indices indicate that we are suffering heavy casualties during the years of growth and development," wrote Carnegie Corporation president, David

Hamburg, recently, "and these casualties not only are tragic for the individuals but also bear heavy costs for American society."[46] Schools cannot "solve" the problem, but through comprehensive approaches to health education and through the provision of health services they can make a powerful contribution to finding that solution.

Resource List

Boston Area Educators for Social Responsibility
11 Garden St
Cambridge, MA 02138
617/492-8820

Kansas Child Abuse Prevention Council
715 SW 10th St
Topeka, KS 66612
913/354-7738

Turning Point Family Services, Inc
12912 Brookhurst St
Suite 150
Garden Grove, CA 92640
714/229-0689

The Paramount Plan
Human Services Department
City of Paramount
16400 Colorado Ave
Paramount, CA 90723
213/220-2140

Wholistic Stress Control Institute, Inc
3480 Greenbriar Pkwy
Suite 310B
Atlanta, GA 30311
404/344-2021

Resolving Conflict Creatively
New York City Public Schools
163 Third Ave #239
New York, NY 10003
212/260-6290

Committee for Children
172 20th Ave
Seattle, WA 98122
206/322-5050

Viewpoints Training Program
University of Illinois at Chicago
Center for Research on Aggression
Department of Psychology
PO Box 4348 M/C 285
Chicago, IL 60680
312/413-2624

Education Development Center, Inc
55 Chapel St
Newton, MA 02160
617/969-7100 (x328)

Health Promotion Program for Urban Youth
1010 Massachusetts Ave
Boston, MA 02118
617/534-5196

References

1. Children's Defense Fund. *The State of America's Children 1991.* Washington, DC: Children's Defense Fund; 1991

2. Centers for Disease Control. Weapon-carrying among high school students—United States, 1990. *MMWR.* 1991;40:681-684

3. Slavin S, Stiber J. Decade of the child. *Adm Radiol.* April 1990: 15-17

4. Kids and guns: a report from America's classroom killing grounds. *Newsweek.* March 9, 1992:22-30

5. Smith D, Lautman B, Scherzer V, Sternberg J. *Caught in the Crossfire: A Report on Gun Violence in Our Nation's Schools.* Washington, DC: Center to Prevent Handgun Violence; 1990

6. US Department of Health and Human Services. In: De La Rosa M, Lambert EY, Gropper B, eds. *Drugs and Violence: Causes, Correlates, and Consequences.* NIDA research monograph 103. Washington, DC: US Department of Health and Human Services; 1990

7. Cohen S. *Alcohol-Related Injuries: The State of the Art in Interventions.* Secretary's National Conference on Alcohol-Related Injuries. March 23-25, 1992; Washington, DC: Office of Substance Abuse Prevention

8. Bastian LD, Taylor BM. *School Crime: A National Crime Victimization Survey Report.* Washington, DC: Bureau of Justice Statistics, US Department of Justice; 1991

9. Rosenberg ML, Fenley MA, eds. *Violence in America: A Public Health Approach.* New York, NY: Oxford University Press; 1991

10. National Committee for Injury Prevention and Control. *Injury Prevention: Meeting the Challenge.* New York, NY: Oxford University Press; 1989

11. Treatser J. Teen-age murderers: plentiful guns, easy power. *The New York Times.* May 24, 1992:1

12. Jackson AW, Hornbeck DW. Educating young adolescents: why we must restructure middle grade schools. *Am Psychol.* 1989;44(5): 831-836

13. Education Development Center, Inc. *Aggressors, Victims, and Bystanders: An Assessment-Based Middle School Violence Prevention Curriculum.* Newton, MA: Education Development Center, Inc. In press

14. Parke RD, Slaby RG. The development of aggression. In: Mussen PH, ed. *Handbook of Child Psychology, IV.* 4th ed. New York, NY: Wiley; 1983;4:547-641

15. Pynoos RS, Nader K. Psychological first aid and treatment approach to children exposed to community violence: research implications. *J Traumatic Stress.* 1988;1:445-473

16. Hendrix K, Molloy PJ. Interventions in early childhood. Presented at the Forum on Youth Violence in Minority Communities: Setting the Agenda for Prevention. Dec 10-12, 1990; Atlanta, GA

17. Cal Const Article I, §28(c)

18. *Brosnahan v Brown.* 32 Cal. 3d 236, 651 P.2d 274, 186 Cal. Rptr. 30; 1982

19. National School Safety Center. *School Safety Check Book.* Malibu, CA. Pepperdine University Press; 1988

20. National School Safety Center. *Gangs in Schools: Breaking Up Is Hard To Do.* Malibu, CA: Pepperdine University Press; 1988

21. Dryfoos JG. *Adolescents at Risk: Prevalence and Prevention.* New York, NY: Oxford University Press; 1990

22. US Congress, Office of Technology Assessment. *Adolescent Health—Volume II: Background and the Effectiveness of Selected Prevention and Treatment Services.* Washington, DC: Office of Technology Assessment; 1991. OTA-H-466

23. US Department of Education. *What Works: Schools Without Drugs.* Washington, DC: US Department of Education; 1986

24. US Department of Justice, Office of Juvenile Justice and Delinquency Prevention. Weapons in schools. *Juvenile Justice Bulletin.* Washington, DC: US Department of Justice; 1989

25. Northrop D, Hamrick K. Weapons and Minority Youth Violence. Presented at the Forum on Youth Violence in Minority Communities: Setting the Agenda for Prevention. Dec 10-12, 1990; Atlanta, GA

26. Sloan JH, Kellerman AL, Reay DT, et al. Handgun regulations, crime, assaults, and homicide: a tale of two cities. *N Engl J Med.* 1988;319:1256-1262

27. Education Development Center, Inc and the Johns Hopkins Injury Prevention Center. *Educating Professionals in Injury Control (EPIC): Firearm Injuries.* Newton, MA: Education Development Center, Inc; 1990

28. Wilson-Brewer R, Cohen S, O'Donnell L, Goodman IF. *Violence Prevention for Young Adolescents: A Survey of the State of the Art.* Washington, DC: Carnegie Council on Adolescent Health; 1991

29. Cohen S, Wilson-Brewer R. *Violence Prevention for Young Adolescents: The State of the Art of Program Evaluation.* Washington, DC: Carnegie Council on Adolescent Development; 1991

30. Wilson-Brewer R, Jacklin B. Violence prevention strategies targeted at the general population of minority youth. Presented at the Forum on Youth Violence in Minority Communities: Setting the Agenda for Prevention. Dec 10-12, 1990; Atlanta, GA

31. Northrop D, Jacklin B, Cohen S, Wilson-Brewer R. Violence prevention strategies targeted towards high risk minority youth. Presented at the Forum on Youth Violence in Minority Communities: Setting the Agenda for Prevention. Dec 10-12, 1990; Atlanta, GA

32. Wilson-Brewer R, Jacklin B. Violence prevention strategies targeted at the general population of minority youth. Presented at the Forum on Youth Violence in Minority Communities: Setting the Agenda for Prevention. Dec 10-12, 1990; Atlanta, GA

33. Wilson-Brewer R, Cohen S, O'Donnell L, Goodman IF. *Violence Prevention for Young Adolescents: A Survey of the State of the Art.* Washington, DC: Carnegie Council on Adolescent Health; 1991

34. Prothrow-Stith D. *Violence Prevention: Curriculum for Adolescents.* Newton, MA: Education Development Center, Inc; 1987

35. Hechinger FM. *Fateful Choices: Healthy Youth for the 21st Century.* New York, NY: Carnegie Council on Adolescent Development; 1992

36. Rosenstock IM. The health belief model. In: Glanz K, Lewis FM, Rimer BK, eds. *Health Behavior and Health Education: Theory, Research, and Practice.* San Francisco, CA: Jossey-Bass; 1990:chap 3

37. Rosenstock IM, Strecher VJ, Becker MH. Social learning and the Health Belief Model. *Health Educ Q.* 1988;15:175-183

38. Miller BC, Card JJ, Paikoff RL, Peterson JL, eds. *Preventing Adolescent Pregnancy.* Newbury Park, CA: Sage; 1992

39. Kirby D, Waszak CS, Ziegler J; Donovan P, ed. *An Assessment of Six School-Based Clinics: Services, Impact and Potential.* Washington, DC: Center for Population Options; 1989

40. US Congress, Office of Technology Assessment. *Adolescent Health—Volume III: Crosscutting Issues in the Delivery of Health and Related Services.* Washington, DC: Office of Technology Assessment; 1991:11. OTA-H-467

41. Education Development Center, Inc. *Identification and Prevention of Youth Violence: A Protocol for Health Care Providers.* Boston, MA: Violence Prevention Project, Department of Health and Hospitals, City of Boston; 1991

42. Stringham P, Weitzman M. Violence counseling in the routine health care of adolescents. *J Adolesc Health Care.* 1988;9:389-393

43. Wright SM. *Report on the Pilot Test of the Protocol for Health Care Providers Addressing Adolescent Acquaintance Violence During Routine Health Care Visits.* Newton, MA: Education Development Center; 1989. Unpublished manuscript

44. US Congress, Office of Technology Assessment. *Adolescent Health—Volume III: Cross-Cutting Issues in the Delivery of Health and Related Services.* Washington, DC: Office of Technology Assessment; 1991:53. OTA-H-467

45. Kirby D, Waszak CS, Ziegler J; Donovan P, ed. *An Assessment of Six School-Based Clinics: Services, Impact, and Potential.* Washington, DC: Center for Population Options; 1989:12-13

46. Hamburg DA. *Today's Children.* New York, NY: Times Books; 1992

CHAPTER 31

ENVIRONMENTAL HAZARDS IN SCHOOLS

Environment hazards for a school can be described from a number of perspectives: physical, chemical, infectious, psychological, or natural. We will define environmental hazard as any risk factor that can cause acute or chronic illness or injury to a school's students, faculty, or staff.

Traditionally, schools have limited their focus on environmental hazards to preparation and drills for fires, natural disasters, climactic control, and generic accident prevention. More recently, additional environmental hazards have been recognized, including air pollution, radon gas, asbestos, and lead (see Table 59). Because a number of these environmental hazards are addressed under specific legislated laws developed during the 1980s, school districts increasingly have needed to define and address to what degree these hazards pose a risk to their schools.

One approach to sorting out school hazards is to categorize them as either safety or health hazards. Safety hazards usually result in acute injuries, are more obvious in nature, and often are the primary focus of a school district's accident prevention program. Areas commonly addressed include: fire, electrical, material handling (ie, chemicals, heavy lifting), ladders, tools, and slips or falls. Conversely, health hazards may not be as obvious, often result in chronic disease that may be asymptomatic, or have a prolonged latent period. The important step to addressing a school's health hazards is to be aware of existing risk factors in the district and to try and anticipate what hazards may be discovered in the future.

Clearly the most important action needed to reduce safety and health hazards is to have a regular process that screens and identifies the problems. The key to a successful program is for the process to be periodic and conscientious, not perfunctory. To achieve this, school districts often have health and safety committees to oversee the development of a policy and the operations process and to periodically review the program. A Hazard Survey Form (Fig 7) is included at the end of this chapter to assist schools or districts in identifying potential health or safety hazards in the school environment.

Resources

National Education Association, Affiliate Services. *Health and Safety Handbook for Education Employees*. Washington, DC: National Education Association; 1988

This handbook outlines and details the steps to be taken in developing a health and safety policy. Particularly helpful is their hazards survey, which could provide a start to identifying a district's environmental hazards.

National Institute for Occupational Safety and Health (NIOSH), Centers for Disease Control and Prevention (CDC). Atlanta, GA: US Public Health Service

US Environmental Protection Agency. *Environmental Hazards in Your School: A Resource Handbook*. Washington, DC: US Environmental Protection Agency; 1990. (TS-799), Pub No 2DT-2001, 1990

This handbook spells out in detail important information needed to develop approaches and policies on asbestos, radon, lead in drinking water, indoor air quality, and other hazardous problems. The handbook identifies school districts' legislated responsibilities and available resources (eg, technical assistance or additional information).

Table 59. — Environmental Hazards in School

Issues	Asbestos	Indoor Air Quality (IAQ)	Radon	Lead in Drinking Water
Risks	Malignancy Lung cancer Especially in employees	Allergic disease, chemical irritation/chronic absorption, airborne infectious disease	Lung cancer	If drinking water contains ≥ 20 ppb of lead, there may be a risk of brain injury and subsequent consequences
Legislation/ responsibility	AHERA,* 1986 (EPA)† Mandated activities	SARA,‡ Title IV, 1986	Same as Indoor Air Quality	Safe Drinking Water Act, 1976; Lead Ban Amendment, 1986, 1988; Lead Containment Control Act, 1988
Assessment/ management	Inspections Management plans Education of staff and parents Follow-up every 3 yr	"Diagnosis of Sick Building Syndrome," address 1) Indoor chemical sources 2) Inadequate ventilation 3) Contaminated outdoor air 4) Microbial contaminations	Standards by Radon Measurement Proficiency (RMP) of EPA and National Radon Contractor Proficiency Program (RCP) of EPA	EPA† recommends 1) Develop plumbing profile 2) Ongoing testing program 3) Correction of outlet (ie, ≥20 ppb of lead)
Available resources	ASHAA (EPA) Loans (100% cost) Grants (50% cost)	Information/guidance from Indoor Air Division, Office of Air/Radiation of EPA Fact Sheet: Sick Buildings Public Information Center (PM-211B) US, EPA Washington, DC 20460	Interim & final reports by EPA for Radon Measurement and Reduction Techniques in Schools. Discussion: *J Sch Health.* 1989;59(10):441-443	*Lead in School Drinking Water* Stock # OSS-000-C0281-9, Superintendent of Documents US Printing Office Washington, DC 20402
Contacts	TSCA Hotline (EPA) 202/554-1404 Asbestos Hotline 800/368-5888	IA Division (ANR-445) Office Air and Radiation, US, EPA Washington, DC 20460	Regional EPA or designated state office	Regional EPA or designated state office

* AHERA -Asbestos Hazard Emergency Response Act.
† EPA -Environmental Protection Agency.
‡ SARA -Super Fund Amendment and Reorganization Act

Hazard Survey Form

1. What chemicals are in use in your work area? Please list.

   _____

2. Is there a Material Safety Data Sheet (MSDS) for each chemical on file in the office?

   a. ☐ Yes   b. ☐ No

   If no, please identify the following:

   Trade name(s) (if applicable):

   _____

   Chemical name(s):

   _____

   Manufacturer(s):

   _____

3. How often are employees exposed to chemicals?

   a. ☐ Very Frequently   c. ☐ Seldom
   b. ☐ Frequently   d. ☐ Never

4. In what quantity are employees exposed to chemicals?

   _____

5. How are chemicals used? (Check all that apply)

   a. ☐ Dry   c. ☐ Mixed
   b. ☐ Wet   d. ☐ Dumped

6. Are there any radiation sources in the work area? (Check all that apply)

   a. ☐ X-rays   c. ☐ Ultraviolet
   b. ☐ Microwave   d. ☐ None

7. Is there excessive noise?

   a. ☐ Yes   b. ☐ No

8. Is there excessive heat?

   a. ☐ Yes   b. ☐ No

9. Have noise or environmental surveys (eg, air sampling) been conducted by the district?

   a. ☐ Yes   b. ☐ No

   If yes, specifically what kind(s) of survey(s) was(were) conducted?

   _____

   Who conducted the survey(s)?

   _____

10. Are there engineering controls (ie, ventilation, hoods, enclosures) to reduce exposure to:
   a. ☐ Chemicals   c. ☐ Noise
   b. ☐ Radiation   d. ☐ Heat

11. Is there adequate ventilation to reduce air contamination and heat?
   a. ☐ Yes   b. ☐ No

12. Are pollution and other contamination-reduction equipment maintained regularly?
   a. ☐ Yes   b. ☐ No

13. Are ventilation ducts and dust collection ducts cleaned out daily? (Check all that apply.)
   a. ☐ Yes, ventilation ducts
   b. ☐ Yes, dust collection ducts
   c. ☐ No (neither are cleaned daily)

14. Are cleaning and changing facilities provided?
   a. ☐ Yes   b. ☐ No

15. Are eye-wash stands available in areas where acids/caustics are used?
   a. ☐ Yes   b. ☐ No

16. Are work clothes provided by the employer?
   a. ☐ Yes   b. ☐ No

17. Are work clothes laundered by the employer?
   a. ☐ Yes   b. ☐ No

18. Do certain jobs have high absence or quit rate?
   a. ☐ Yes   b. ☐ No

19. Are there medically related disabilities or retirements among employees for such reasons as cancer, heart, or respiratory disease? (Check all that apply.)
   a. ☐ Yes, medically related disabilities
   b. ☐ Yes, medically related retirements
   c. ☐ No (medically related disabilities or retirements)

20. Are the following conditions or symptoms present in work areas? (Check all that apply.)
   a. ☐ Visible airborne dust, smoke, or mist
   b. ☐ Accumulations of dust, liquids, or oil on floors or window sills
   c. ☐ The odor of solvents or cleaning vapors or gases
   d. ☐ Employees develop a "bad taste" when in certain areas
   e. ☐ Employees' eyes burn or their noses and throat get irritated
   f. ☐ Employees feel extreme heat or cold
   g. ☐ Employees hear noise

Hazard Survey Form (continued)

21. Do employees suffer from the following problems or exhibit the following symptoms? (Check all that apply.)
    a. ☐ Dermatitis or skin rash
    b. ☐ Nagging coughs or persistent colds
    c. ☐ Dizziness or headaches
    d. ☐ Irritability
    e. ☐ Nausea
    f. ☐ Fatigue
    g. ☐ Loss of appetite
    h. ☐ Backaches
    i. ☐ Loss of hearing or ringing in the ears
    j. ☐ Recurring infections
    k. ☐ Respiratory ailments such as tight chest or heavy breathing

22. What personal protective equipment is available? (Check all that apply.)
    a. ☐ Respirators   d. ☐ Boots
    b. ☐ Goggles   e. ☐ None
    c. ☐ Gloves

23. Are there frequent injuries in the work area?
    a. ☐ Yes   b. ☐ No
    If yes, please explain:

    _____

24. Are there frequent illnesses in the work area?
    a. ☐ Yes   b. ☐ No
    If yes, please explain:

    _____

25. What are the conditions of floors and stairways? (Check one for each.)

	Excellent	Good	Fair	Poor
Floors	_____	_____	_____	_____
Stairways	_____	_____	_____	_____

26. Are there enough exits?
    a. ☐ Yes   b. ☐ No

27. Are the exits well marked?
    a. ☐ Yes   b. ☐ No
28. How much lifting is required?
    a. ☐ Very frequent   c. ☐ Little
    b. ☐ Frequent   d. ☐ None

29. Are there provisions for assistance with lifting?
    a. ☐ Yes   b. ☐ No

30. Do you think workers are feeling "stressed out"?
    a. ☐ Yes   b. ☐ No
    If yes, please explain:

Fig 7. Hazard survey form from National Education Association. *Health and Safety Handbook for Education Employees.* Washington, DC: National Education Association. Reprinted with permission.

CHAPTER 32

PHYSICIAN EDUCATION IN SCHOOL HEALTH

Physicians' roles and activities in school health have evolved with the changing health needs of children in America. Rapid social change and biomedical advances have created new sets of developmental, behavioral, and social problems. Pediatricians in primary care who have become involved with schools often have responded to parents' requests for service[1] and recognized the value of physician-school collaboration.[2] Many of the problems caused by the new morbidity are best handled by focusing on disease prevention and health promotion.[3] To this end, physicians serving as school consultants have participated in health education programs and have recommended educational strategies for children with disabilities.

Pediatric education generally has not kept pace with the needs of children or the demands of practice. Although a large proportion of pediatricians engage in some form of school health activities, many have received limited relevant training during medical school and residency.[4,5] One study of practicing pediatricians found 50% received no useful knowledge in developmental pediatrics during medical school, and 20% indicated that residency was of no value in this area.[6] Despite the strong recommendations of the Task Force on Pediatric Education (1978), many recent graduates still lack sufficient exposure to the biosocial and developmental aspects of pediatrics.[7,8]

While pediatric department chairpersons and residency training program directors have usually acknowledged a need to follow the Task Force recommendations, they cite inadequate funding, lack of appropriately trained faculty, and an already full curriculum as barriers to full compliance. Clearly those who seek to implement curricula in school health and related developmental areas must provide sound educational reasons and benefits.

The discrepancy between physician education and later patient care needs is the best justification for the inclusion of school health content in medical school, residency, and continuing education curricula. A structured curriculum has proven more effective than an unstructured approach with loosely specified goals, methods, and plans for evaluation.[9] It also has been well documented that resident participation in a structured curriculum in developmental-behavioral pediatrics does not reduce knowledge of the more traditional organic aspects of pediatrics.[10] The growing biosocial and developmental morbidity of pediatric practice, the placement of technology-dependent children in schools, the support for school health education to prevent drug abuse and other life-style diseases, and the use of school-based health services to overcome barriers of access to medical care highlight the importance of education in school health to the pediatrician of the future.

Level of Training

Training in school health should begin during medical school, continue during residency, and be updated by postgraduate educational experiences. A basic level of knowledge is important to pediatric subspecialists, as well as generalists, whose patients will be identified and served by school screening and intervention programs. A small number of pediatricians will choose to make school health a major aspect of their careers and will need further training to be specialists in school health.

Medical Student Education

The school health curriculum for medical students aims to provide a base on which to build later learning experiences and a minimum level of competence for any physician. Medical students should become aware of the range of normal development, factors that cause developmental deviations and impair school performance, and school programs for screening and intervention. They should be able to communicate effectively with schools concerning the cognitive, behavioral, and social effects of medical conditions and treatments. Interviewing skills should be learned that allow them to elicit the concerns and feelings of parents about their child's development and school achievement, appraise the home learning environment, and gather accurate and complete information about the child's past and current behavior.

Objective 1: To demonstrate introductory knowledge of the normal growth and development of school-age children and adolescents: cognitive, neuromuscular and physical, emotional, and social.

Objective 2: To develop basic knowledge of the evaluation and treatment of developmental dysfunction and common behavior problems of the school-age population: learning disabilities, communication disorders, attention deficits, motor problems, sensory impairments, mental retardation, school refusal, depression, psychosomatic disorders, enuresis, encopresis, and problems due to child abuse and neglect.

Objective 3: To become aware of the psychosocial and developmental aspects of chronic illness and how children with chronic medical conditions are managed in the schools and served by community resources.

Objective 4: To describe the key state and federal laws for special education: identification and review process, types of disabilities that receive assistance, services provided, parental rights, and role of the physician.

Objective 5: To discuss the most common health screening procedures used in schools and criteria for evaluating their efficacy.

Objective 6: To acquire introductory knowledge of the environmental influences on development and academic achievement: family, cultural, social, school, and early intervention programs.

Objective 7: To develop sufficient understanding of the operation of school systems to know how to communicate effectively with schools concerning student health and illness.

Objective 8: To develop interviewing skills necessary to acquire basic information about child development and behavior, social adjustment and school achievement, and parental concerns and expectations.

Methods in Medical School Curriculum

Medical student education in school health should consist of a combination of readings; didactic and audiovisual presentations; and small group discussions of core topics, cases, and school experiences. An essential component of the curriculum should expose medical students to the school setting and allow them to observe school-age children in the school environment. They should observe regular and special education classes and watch how a school nurse manages student illness and health information. A multidisciplinary team (physician, nurse, guidance counselor, educational diagnostic staff, and classroom teacher) should be observed planning an educational program for a pupil with a medical or developmental problem. Medical students should interview healthy and disabled pupils about their perceptions and attitudes about school, peers, family, and health-related topics. Families of healthy and disabled pupils should be interviewed concerning their observations, feelings, and expectations of their child's early development and school achievement, behavior, and social-emotional adjustment.

The years of the medical school curriculum during which school health is taught and the department that coordinates instruction may vary depending on the resources and interests of each institution. Some of the educational objectives may be achieved in a basic science course in preventive medicine or psychiatry and others in a clinical clerkship directed by pediatrics, family medicine, community medicine, or psychiatry.

Pediatric Residents

All physicians specializing in the care of children and adolescents must have knowledge and skill to identify and manage school-related problems. The content of the pediatric resident curriculum in school health should, therefore, include the core elements necessary for the competent functioning of a pediatrician in general practice or in a subspecialty such as cardiology. There should be elective opportunities for residents with a special interest in school health to develop more advanced management and consultative expertise. The elective curriculum will overlap with the content of clinical training at the fellowship level. It should not be assumed that competency sufficient for later practice will occur automatically in the course of residency training.[11] Satisfactory training in school health requires the development of a specific curriculum and clinical experiences that are integrated into the framework of the general training program.

A feature that distinguishes training at the residency level from medical student training is a greater emphasis on the application of knowledge through clinical experiences. Residents need experiences beyond the medical role of physical examination and the direct provision of health care to prepare them for future activities as consultants to school health services and health education programs.[12] In addition to the objectives listed for medical student education, residents in pediatrics should accomplish the following objectives.

Objective 1: Describe the incidence, clinical manifestations, diagnostic criteria, natural history, and approaches to prevention and prognosis of common developmental and behavioral disorders: mental retardation, cerebral palsy, learning and communication disorders, hearing and visual disabilities, and major psychopathological conditions.

Objective 2: Understand the role of school-based professionals, school programs, and community resources in the evaluation and management of children with developmental-behavioral variation and chronic illnesses.

Objective 3: Describe and assess the general organization of school systems and typical schools: governance structure and role descriptions at state, local district, and school building levels.

Objective 4: Demonstrate a basic understanding of common psycho-educational tests and school testing programs: developmental screening and readiness tests, group and individual achievement tests, intelligence and aptitude tests, tests of speech and language, and tests of visual and fine motor and gross motor skills.

Objective 5: Perform preliminary assessments of children with the common developmental and behavioral disorders noted above: perform developmental screening and observe performance in basic academic areas, review school records and results of previous evaluations, obtain observations from school and community personnel, coordinate referrals for diagnostic evaluation and intervention, advise parents and provide an explanation for the child, and integrate findings into a written report for use in educational and medical management.

Objective 6: Describe the health education programs in schools and basic considerations in planning, conducting, and evaluating a health education program.

Objective 7: Participate as a member of a school multidisciplinary diagnostic and planning team: understand barriers to physician-school communication and apply basic knowledge of group process.

Objective 8: Serve as medical consultant to a school or community program for children: describe steps in the consultation process, discuss common obstacles of consultation and how to overcome them, and compare and contrast the physician's activities as primary care provider with activities as consultant for common school-related clinical issues and problems.

Methods in Residency Curriculum

Because of the variability in faculty resources and program structures in different pediatric training sites, objectives of the residency curriculum will be met in different ways. Some of the curriculum can be incorporated into existing lectures and case conferences in general or developmental pediatrics. Traditional clinical experiences in continuity clinics and developmental evaluating centers also can be utilized. Factual knowledge in school health should be provided during the first year of residency and will be particularly valuable for those who had limited instruction in medical school. Regardless of the method of learning and the program's resources, the resident's knowledge should be applied in clinical and school settings with close supervision provided by faculty who have expertise in the area of school health. Participation in multidisciplinary evaluation and/or planning meetings and school consultation experiences should occur during the second and/or third year of residency, after sufficient knowledge and clinical skill have been acquired.

Adequate training necessitates maintaining a continuing relationship with parents and school professionals participating in the long-term management of children with some of the most common developmental-behavioral variations and chronic medical conditions. Learning the basic principles of consultation (Objective 8) requires that the resident spend a minimum of a half day per week for three consecutive months functioning as a school physician. A more complete understanding of the social system of schools, how schools work, and how to work with schools would be achieved by providing consultative services over a full school year. There is no substitute for direct school involvement that allows the resident to observe various pupil activities, functions of school personnel, and regular and special education classrooms and programs.

Fellowship/Advanced Training in School and Community Health

The physician interested in school or community health as a career will need further training to broaden and deepen the knowledge and skills learned at the resident level. This will require clinical experience with a wide spectrum of children with longer follow-up as well as long-term consultative experience with exposure to a large variety of school health programs for students throughout the pediatric age range. Fellowship or specialist training also is differentiated from training at the resident level by emphasis on the development of teaching, research, and leadership skills.

Objective 1: To attain in-depth knowledge of assessment and management of developmental and behavioral disorders.

Objective 2: To develop clinical knowledge necessary to function effectively as medical consultant to each component of a comprehensive school health program: health services, health education, physical education and athletic programs, environment and safety, school-site health promotion, food service, and school counseling.[13]

Objective 3: To develop knowledge and skills in consultation: system entry and needs assessment, rationale for and components of a written contract, methods of evaluating consultation activities, and reasons and ways to terminate a consultation agreement.

Objective 4: To develop teaching skills: basic education principles and methods in clinical and didactic settings, manuscript and slide preparation, and methods of evaluating trainees and curriculum.

Objective 5: To develop ability to plan, execute, and evaluate research: introductory statistics, research methodology, scientific writing and presentation, and grant writing.

Objective 6: To develop leadership and administrative skills: basic principles of group process, planning and conducting meetings and conferences, time management and job stress control, and basic concepts of personnel management.

Methods of Advanced Education

Advanced training for physicians in school health most often will be available at medical schools in departments of pediatrics

Postgraduate fellowships are typically 2 to 3 years in duration, with longer programs providing more training in teaching and research. Other sources of training include schools of public health and colleges of education, the latter offering course work in health education, child development, and special education/learning disabilities. It generally would take a minimum of 2 years to adequately cover all of the objectives at the fellow level. Individuals not interested in a full-time academic career could achieve clinical competency in less time if they had extensive school health training during residency. Some physicians may effectively pursue advanced training by devising an individual course of study, utilizing multiple courses and sources of instruction.

While much can be learned about assessment and management of developmental-behavioral disorders at a hospital or evaluation center, the central component of fellowship training should be longitudinal consultation with schools. In school- and community-based sites, clinical and consultation knowledge and skills are applied and refined with faculty-preceptor supervision. The fellow should participate as both member and leader of multidisciplinary assessment teams. Problems in areas of health services, health education, and school environment would be addressed by working through the stages of consultation from system entry to final evaluation and termination. Medical students, residents, and school staff would be taught under supervision after sessions with faculty on education processes. After course instruction in statistics and research design, fellows would be expected to develop and implement a research project for presentation and/or publication. Administrative and leadership skills would be learned by course work on management and group process, and developed by assuming supervised organizational responsibilities.

Evaluation

Successful training at any level includes an evaluation component that measures the learning of each trainee and the overall effectiveness of the curriculum. An essential step in evaluation is specifying goals and objectives for attitudes, knowledge, and skills according to measurable parameters. Attitudes and skills can be assessed by ratings completed by the student, instructor, and community and school professionals. A survey of perceived competence or self-efficacy is a reliable method of following trainee growth in several areas over a period of time. Knowledge and skills may be directly observed in teaching, clinical, and administrative situations; assessed from tape recordings; and tested during simulated case examinations. Clinical knowledge and skills also can be determined by chart and diagnostic report reviews. Knowledge can be measured more objectively by written tests. Ratings by students and residents are needed to evaluate a fellow's teaching skills. Review of abstracts, manuscripts, and scientific presentations can be used to evaluate skills necessary for research.

Evaluation of the overall curriculum in school health is particularly important in establishing and maintaining the support of pediatric department chairpersons and residency training program directors. Most pediatric departments administer the American Board of Pediatrics in-training examination. The results from this test can be analyzed to develop an aggregate estimation of the cognitive ability of each Pediatric Resident Level (PL 1,2,3) group in content areas related to school health, providing an indication of the teaching effectiveness of the training program.[14] In addition, students, residents, and program graduates should offer feedback on what aspects of the curriculum they like or dislike and what they find valuable.[15] If a comparable control group is available, a scientifically sound evaluation can be designed that can attribute learning to participation in a specific component of the curriculum.

Continuing Medical Education in School Health

Residency training would ideally provide the physician an opportunity to achieve basic competency in dealing with school-related problems that may present in his/her practice. Through elective rotations during residency and fellowships, those with special interests could develop advanced clinical and consultation skills. As noted, the inadequacy of training in this area is well documented. Fortunately, there are numerous ways for the practicing pediatrician to acquire and improve competency in school health.

Self Education: By far the most common approach involves listening to videotapes and reading texts and journals with chapters and articles devoted to school health topics. In addition to pediatric publications, the literature of related disciplines, such as special education, psychology, psychiatry, neurology, sports medicine, infectious disease, public health, health education, and school nursing, contains useful information. Much can be learned by developing liaisons with a local school or school district that allow the physician to become involved with school nursing, pupil evaluation teams, athletics, and health education. The physician should be reimbursed for these activities.

Lectures on School Health: Pediatric grand rounds at hospitals and medical schools and periodic AAP chapter scientific meetings are logical forums for school health presentations. The state chapters' school health committees can play an organizing role to ensure that this area of pediatrics is given adequate coverage. Lecture topics may include:

- The Role of the Pediatrician in Schools
- School Refusal and Phobia
- Attention Deficits and Hyperactivity
- The Child With HIV in School
- Care of the Chronically Ill Child in Schools
- Models for Teaching Sex and Drug Education in Schools
- Early Intervention Programs
- School-Based Health Services
- Schools: How They Work and How to Work With Them
- Planning for and Managing Medical Emergencies in School
- Normal Development During Middle Childhood
- School Underachievement: Evaluation and Intervention
- Fitness and Physical Education in Schools
- Communicable Disease Control in Schools
- Special Education: Laws and Services
- The Pediatrician's Role in Comprehensive Health Education
- Psychoeducational Testing
- Managing the Emotionally Disturbed Child in the Classroom
- Screening for School Readiness
- School Screening Programs
- School Sports Medicine

- School Absenteeism
- Teenage Pregnancy
- Child Abuse and Neglect

Seminars and Workshops: Round tables, seminars, and section scientific sessions at the AAP Annual and Spring Meetings and AAP-sponsored 2- to 3-day continuing medical education courses usually provide more intensive instruction in school health. Half-day or full-day symposia also are offered by medical schools, scientific meetings of related disciplines, and state departments of health and education. Seminars and workshops may vary from a review of the major aspects of school health to in-depth "state-of-the-art" review of a single area.

Mini-Fellowships: These could be 1- to 3-month full-time experiences or involve longitudinal participation (eg, half a day per week for 6 months) in the clinical areas of school health programs. This type of experience is not widely available but may be provided by recognized programs in academic centers on request. Such courses should be individually designed with clearly defined learning objectives and expectations, faculty supervision, and structured evaluations.

References

1. Burnett RD, Bell LS. Projecting pediatric practice patterns. *Pediatrics.* 1978;62(suppl):625-680

2. Marshall RM, Wuori DF, Hudler M, Cranston CS. Physician/school teacher collaboration. Some practical considerations. *Clin Pediatr.* 1987;26:524-527

3. Nader, PR. A pediatrician's primer for school health activities. *Pediatr Rev.* 1982;4:82-92

4. Chilton LA. School health experience before and after completion of pediatric training. *Pediatrics.* 1979;63:565-568

5. Black JL, Nader PR, Broyles SL, Nelson JA. A national survey on pediatric training and activities in school health. *J Sch Health.* 1991;61:245-248

6. Dworkin PH, Shonkoff JP, Leviton A, Levine, MD. Training in developmental pediatrics. How practitioners perceive the gap. *Am J Dis Child.* 1979;133:709-712

7. Weinberger HL, Oski FA. A survey of pediatric resident training programs 5 years after the Task Force report. *Pediatrics.* 1984;74:523-526

8. Zebal BH, Friedman SB. A nationwide survey of behavioral pediatric residency training. *J Dev Behav Pediatr.* 1984;5:331-335

9. Phillips S, Friedman SB, Zebal BH. The impact of training in behavioral pediatrics: a study of 24 residency programs. *J Dev Behav Pediatr*. 1985;6:15-21

10. Philips S, Friedman SB, Zebal BH, Parrish JM. Residents' knowledge of behavioral pediatrics. *J Dev Behav Pediatr*. 1985;6:268-272

11. Yancy WS, Coury DL, Drotar D, Gottlieb MI, Kohen DP, Sarles RM. A curriculum guide for developmental-behavioral pediatrics. *J Dev Behav Pediatr*. 1988;9(suppl):1S-8S

12. Sklaire, MW. The role of the pediatrician in school health. *Pediatr Rev*. 1990;12:69-70

13. Allensworth DD, Kolbe LJ. The comprehensive school health program: exploring an expanded concept. *J Sch Health*. 1987;57:409-412

14. Kappelman MM, Lewis JM. Utilization of in-training examination results. *Am J Dis Child*. 1986;140:188-189 (Letter)

15. Niebuhr VN, McCormick DP, Barnett SE. School health training during pediatric residency. *Am J Dis Child*. 1991;5:79-84

PART IV

APPENDIX

AAP Policy Statements Related to School Health Issues

Following is a list of AAP policy statements relating to school health issues. These statements represent a consensus of the Academy and leading pediatric experts.

To order the complete text of individual policy statements listed below, call the AAP Publications Department at 708/228-5005, or mail your order to: AAP Publications Department, 141 Northwest Point Blvd, PO Box 927, Elk Grove Village, IL 60009-0927. All reprints are $.95 each—prepaid orders only. No shipping or handling charge on reprint orders less than $10.

Committee on Adolescence

Adolescent Pregnancy

Alcohol Use and Abuse

Contraception and Adolescents

Counseling the Adolescent About Pregnancy Options

Education to Strengthen the Family

Homosexuality and Adolescence

Marijuana: A Continuing Concern for Pediatricians

On the Terminology of Adolescent/Adolescence

Role of the Pediatrician in Management of Sexually Transmitted Diseases in Children and Adolescents

Sexuality, Contraception, and the Media

Suicide and Suicide Attempts in Adolescents and Young Adults

Tobacco Use by Children and Adolescents

Committee on Bioethics

Principles of Treatment of Disabled Infants

Religious Exemptions From Child Abuse Statutes

Screening for Drugs of Abuse in Children and Adolescents

Committee on Careers & Opportunities

Supervision of Pediatric Nurse Practitioners

Committee on Child Abuse and Neglect

Guidelines for the Evaluation of Sexually Abused Children

Council on Child and Adolescent Health

Age Limits of Pediatrics

Committee on Children With Disabilities

Children With Health Impairments in School

Doman-Delacato Treatment of Neurologically Handicapped Children

Learning Disabilities, Dyslexia, and Vision

Medication for Children With an Attention Deficit Disorder

Pediatrician's Role in Development and Implementation of an Individual Education Plan (IEP) and/or an Individual Family Service Plan (IFSP)

Prevocational and Vocational Education of Children and Adolescents With Developmental Disabilities

Provision of Related Services for Children With Chronic Disabilities

School-Aged Children With Motor Disabilities

Committee on Communications

Impact of Rock Lyrics and Music Videos on Children and Youth

Committee on Community Health Services

Health Care for Children of Migrant Families

Health Needs of Homeless Children

Committee on Drugs

Medication for Children With an Attention Deficit Disorder

Committee on Environmental Health

Smokeless Tobacco

Committee on Infectious Diseases

Chemotherapy for Tuberculosis in Infants and Children

Universal Hepatitis B Immunization

Committee on Injury and Poison Prevention

Bicycle Helmets

Children and Fireworks

School Bus Safety

Committee on Nutrition

Megavitamins and Mental Retardation

Megavitamin Therapy for Childhood Psychoses and Learning Disabilities

Statement on Cholesterol

Committee on Practice and Ambulatory Medicine
Vision Screening and Eye Examination in Children

Committee on Psychosocial Aspects of Child and Family Health
Pediatrician and Childhood Bereavement

Committee on School Health
Administration of Medication in School

AIDS Education in Schools

Alcohol Abuse Education in School

Children With Health Impairments in School

Concepts of School Health Programs

Corporal Punishment in Schools

CPR Training in the School

Education to Strengthen the Family

Guidelines for Urgent Care in School

Health Education and Schools

Impedance Bridge (Tympanometer) As a Screening Device in Schools

Medical Guidelines for Day Camps and Residential Camps

Medically Indicated Home, Hospital, and Other Non-School Based Instruction

Organized Athletics for Preadolescent Children

Nursing Personnel Delivering Health Services in Schools

Physical Fitness and the Schools

The Potentially Suicidal Student in the School Setting

The Role of the Physician in School

School-Based Health Clinics

School Bus Safety

School Health Assessments

Committee on Sports Medicine and Fitness
Amenorrhea in Adolescent Athletes

Anabolic Steroids and the Adolescent Athlete

Atlantoaxial Instability in Down Syndrome

Exercise for Children Who Are Mentally Retarded

Human Immunodeficiency Virus (AIDS) in the Athletic Setting

Physical Fitness and the Schools

Risks in Distance Running for Children

Sports and the Child With Epilepsy

Strength Training, Weight and Power Lifting, and Body Building
by Children and Adolescents

**Task Force on the Future Role of the Pediatrician in the Delivery
of Health Care**

Report on the Future Role of the Pediatrician in the Delivery
of Health Care

Provisional Committee on Pediatric Aids

Education of Children With HIV Infection

Guidelines for HIV-Infected Children and Their Foster Families

Ad Hoc Task Force on Definition of the Medical Home

The Medical Home

Section on Allergy and Immunology

Exercise and the Asthmatic Child

INDEX

Page numbers followed by *f* indicate figures. Page numbers followed by *t* indicate tables.